Cardiovascular Hemodynamics for the Clinician

Cardiovascular Hemodynamics for the Clinician

SECOND EDITION

EDITED BY

George A. Stouffer MD

Henry A. Foscue Distinguished Professor of Medicine
Chief of Cardiology
University of North Carolina School of Medicine
Chapel Hill, NC
USA

ASSOCIATE EDITORS

J. Larry Klein MD

Division of Cardiology
University of North Carolina School of Medicine
Chapel Hill, NC
USA

David P. McLaughlin MD

Harrisonburg Medical Associates
Harrisonburg, VA
USA

WILEY Blackwell

This edition first published 2017 © 2008, 2017 by John Wiley & Sons Ltd

Registered Office
John Wiley & Sons Ltd, The Atrium, Southern Gate, Chichester, West Sussex, PO19 8SQ, UK

Editorial Offices
9600 Garsington Road, Oxford, OX4 2DQ, UK
The Atrium, Southern Gate, Chichester, West Sussex, PO19 8SQ, UK
111 River Street, Hoboken, NJ 07030-5774, USA

For details of our global editorial offices, for customer services and for information about how
to apply for permission to reuse the copyright material in this book please see our website at
www.wiley.com/wiley-blackwell

Library of Congress Cataloging-in-Publication data applied for

9781119066477 [paperback]

A catalogue record for this book is available from the British Library.

Wiley also publishes its books in a variety of electronic formats. Some content that appears in print may
not be available in electronic books.

Cover image: ©SCIEPRO/gettyimages

Set in 9/12pt Meridien by SPi Global, Pondicherry, India

Printed in the UK

Contents

List of contributors, viii

Part I: Basics of hemodynamics

1 Introduction to basic hemodynamic principles, 3
James E. Faber and George A. Stouffer

2 The nuts and bolts of right heart catheterization and PA
catheter placement, 17
Vickie Strang and George A. Stouffer

3 Normal hemodynamics, 37
Alison Keenon, Eron D. Crouch, James E. Faber and George A. Stouffer

4 Arterial pressure, 56
George A. Stouffer

5 The atrial waveform, 69
David P. McLaughlin and George A. Stouffer

6 Cardiac output, 82
Frederick M. Costello and George A. Stouffer

7 Detection, localization, and quantification of intracardiac shunts, 91
Frederick M. Costello and George A. Stouffer

Part II: Valvular heart disease

8 Aortic stenosis, 103
David P. McLaughlin and George A. Stouffer

9 Hemodynamics of transcatheter and surgical aortic valve replacement, 119
*John P. Vavalle, Michael Yeung, Thomas G. Caranasos
and Cassandra J. Ramm*

10 Mitral stenosis, 129
Robert V. Kelly, Chadwick Huggins and George A. Stouffer

11 Aortic regurgitation, 143
George A. Stouffer

12 Mitral regurgitation, 154
Robert V. Kelly, Mauricio G. Cohen and George A. Stouffer

13 The tricuspid valve, 163
David A. Tate and George A. Stouffer

14 Hemodynamic findings in pulmonic valve disease, 171
Cynthia Zhou, Anand Shah and George A. Stouffer

Part III: Cardiomyopathies

15 Hypertrophic cardiomyopathy, 185
Jayadeep S. Varanasi and George A. Stouffer

16 Heart failure, 200
Geoffrey T. Jao, Steven Filby and Patricia P. Chang

17 Restrictive cardiomyopathy, 212
David P. McLaughlin and George A. Stouffer

Part IV: Pericardial disease

18 Constrictive pericarditis, 221
David P. McLaughlin and George A. Stouffer

19 Cardiac tamponade, 234
Siva B. Mohan and George A. Stouffer

20 Effusive–constrictive pericarditis, 248
Eric M. Crespo, Sidney C. Smith and George A. Stouffer

Part V: Hemodynamic support

21 Hemodynamics of intra-aortic balloon counterpulsation, 255
Richard A. Santa-Cruz and George A. Stouffer

22 Hemodynamics of left ventricular assist device implantation, 266
Brett C. Sheridan and Jason N. Katz

Part VI: Coronary hemodynamics

23 Coronary hemodynamics, 279
David P. McLaughlin, Samuel S. Wu and George A. Stouffer

24 Fractional flow reserve, 288
Paul M. Johnson, Shriti Mehta, Prashant Kaul and George A. Stouffer

Part VII: Miscellaneous

25 Right ventricular myocardial infarction, 301
Robert V. Kelly, Mauricio G. Cohen and George A. Stouffer

26 Pulmonary hypertension, 310
Lisa J. Rose-Jones, Daniel Fox, David P. McLaughlin and George A. Stouffer

27 Hemodynamics of arrhythmias and pacemakers, 321
*Rodrigo Bolanos, Kimberly A. Selzman, Lukas Jantac
and George A. Stouffer*

28 Systematic evaluation of hemodynamic tracings, 341
George A. Stouffer

Index, 357

List of contributors

Rodrigo Bolanos MD
BayCare Medical Group
Winter Haven, FL

Thomas G. Caranasos MD
Assistant Professor of Surgery
University of North Carolina
Chapel Hill, NC, USA

Patricia P. Chang MD
Associate Professor of Medicine
University of North Carolina
Chapel Hill, NC, USA

Mauricio G. Cohen MD
Associate Professor of Medicine
University of Miami
Miami, FL, USA

Frederick M. Costello MD
Idaho Cardiology Associates
Meadowlake Building
Meridian, ID 83642, USA

Eric M. Crespo MD, MPH
Hartford Hospital Cardiology Dept
Hartford, USA

Eron D. Crouch MD
Medical Associates of Navarro County
Corsicana, UA

James E. Faber PhD
Professor of Cell Biology and Physiology
University of North Carolina
Chapel Hill NC, USA

Steven Filby MD
Reid Heart Center
Pinehurst, NC, USA

Daniel Fox MD
Critical Care, Pulmonary and Sleep
Associates
Lakewood, CO, USA

Chadwick Huggins MD
Cardiovascular Consultants
Savannah, GA, USA

Lukas Jantac MD
Sanford Cardiology
Sanford, NC, USA

Geoffrey T. Jao MD
Assistant Professor of Medicine
Division of Cardiology
Wake Forest Baptist Medical Center
Medical Center Boulevard
Winston-Salem, NC, USA

Paul M. Johnson MD
Division of Cardiology
University of North Carolina
School of Medicine
Chapel Hill, NC, USA

Jason N. Katz MD
Assistant Professor of Medicine
University of North Carolina
Chapel Hill, NC, USA

Prashant Kaul MD
Piedmont Heart Institute
Atlanta, GA, USA

Alison Keenon MD
Assistant Professor of Urology
University of Wisconsin School of Medicine
Madison, WI, USA

Robert V. Kelly MD
Beacon Consultants Concourse
Dublin, Ireland

J. Larry Klein MD
Professor of Medicine
University of North Carolina
Chapel Hill, NC, USA

David P. McLaughlin MD
Harrisonburg Medical Associates
Harrisonburg, VA, USA

Shriti Mehta MD
Division of Cardiology
University of North Carolina School of
Medicine
Chapel Hill, NC, USA

Siva B. Mohan MD
Southern Heart/Emory
Riverdale, GA, USA

Cassandra J. Ramm RN MSN
Structural Heart Program coordinator
University of North Carolina
Chapel Hill, NC, USA

Lisa J. Rose-Jones MD
Assistant Professor of Medicine
Division of Cardiology
University of North Carolina
School of Medicine
Chapel Hill, NC, USA

Richard A. Santa-Cruz MD
Agnesian Health Care
Fond du Lac, WI, USA

Kimberly A. Selzman MD, MPH
Associate Professor of Medicine
Division of Cardiology
University of Utah
Salt Lake City, UT, USA

Anand Shah BS
Duke University School of Medicine
Durham, NC, USA

Brett C. Sheridan MD
Sutter Health
Palo Alto Medical Foundation
San Francisco Cardiology
San Francisco, CA, USA

Sidney C. Smith, Jr. MD
Professor of Medicine
University of North Carolina
Chapel Hill, NC, USA

Vickie Strang RN
University of North Carolina Health Care
Chapel Hill, NC, USA

David A. Tate MD
Associate Professor of Medicine Emeritus
University of North Carolina
Chapel Hill, NC, USA

Jayadeep S. Varanasi MD
Cone Health Medical Group
Greensboro, NC, USA

John P. Vavalle MD
Assistant Professor of Medicine
University of North Carolina
Chapel Hill, NC, USA

Samuel S. Wu MD
Cardiovascular Associates of Virginia
Richmond, VA, USA

Michael Yeung MD
Assistant Professor of Medicine
University of North Carolina
Chapel Hill, NC, USA

Cynthia Zhou BS
Division of Cardiology
University of North Carolina School of
Medicine
Chapel Hill, NC, USA

PART I

Basics of hemodynamics

CHAPTER 1

Introduction to basic hemodynamic principles

James E. Faber and George A. Stouffer

Hemodynamics is concerned with the mechanical and physiologic properties controlling blood pressure and flow through the body. A full discussion of hemodynamic principles is beyond the scope of this book. In this chapter, we present an overview of basic principles that are helpful in understanding hemodynamics.

1. Energy in the blood stream exists in three interchangeable forms: pressure arising from cardiac output and vascular resistance, "hydrostatic" pressure from gravitational forces, and kinetic energy of blood flow

Daniel Bernoulli was a physician and mathematician who lived in the eighteenth century. He had wide-ranging scientific interests and won the Grand Prize of the Paris Academy 10 times for advances in areas ranging from astronomy to physics. One of his insights was that the energy of an ideal fluid (a hypothetical concept referring to a fluid that is not subject to viscous or frictional energy losses) in a straight tube can exist in three interchangeable forms: perpendicular pressure (force exerted on the walls of the tube perpendicular to flow; a form of potential energy), kinetic energy of the flowing fluid, and pressure due to gravitational forces. Perpendicular pressure is transferred to the blood and vessel wall by cardiac pump function and vascular elasticity and is a function of cardiac output and vascular resistance.

Total energy (TE) = potential energy + kinetic energy

TE = (perpendicular pressure + gravitational pressure) + kinetic energy

TE = $\left(P_{\text{Per}} + P_{\text{grav}}\right) + 1/2\rho V^2$

Cardiovascular Hemodynamics for the Clinician, Second Edition. Edited by George A. Stouffer.
© 2017 John Wiley & Sons Ltd. Published 2017 by John Wiley & Sons Ltd.

where V is velocity and ρ is density of blood (approximately 1060 kg/m³)

$$\mathrm{TE} = P_{\mathrm{Per}} + \left(\rho \times h \times g \right) + 1/2 \rho V^2$$

where g is gravitational constant and h is height of fluid above the point of interest.

Although blood is not an "ideal fluid" (in the Newtonian sense), Bernoulli's insight is helpful. Blood pressure is the summation of three components: lateral pressure, gravitational forces, and kinetic energy (also known as the impact pressure or the pressure required to cause flow to stop). Pressure is the force applied per unit area of a surface. In blood vessels or in the heart, the transmural pressure (i.e., pressure across the vessel wall or ventricular chamber wall) is equal to the intravascular pressure minus the pressure outside the vessel. The intravascular pressure is responsible for transmural pressure (i.e., vessel distention) and for longitudinal transport of blood through the vessels.

Gravitational forces are important in a standing person. Arterial pressure in the foot will exceed thoracic aortic pressure due to gravitational pull on a column of blood. Likewise, arterial pressure in the head will be less than thoracic aortic pressure. Similarly, gravitational forces are important in the venous system, since blood will pool in the legs when an individual is standing. Decreased ventricular filling pressure results in a lower cardiac output and explains why a person will feel lightheaded if rising abruptly from a sitting or supine position. In contrast, gravity has negligible effect on arterial or venous pressure when a person is lying flat. Gravitational pressure equals the height of a column of blood × the gravitational constant × the fluid density. To calculate hydrostatic pressure at the bedside (in mm Hg), measure the distance in millimeters between the points of interest, for example heart and foot, and divide by 13 (mercury is 13 times denser than water).

Kinetic energy is greatest in the ascending aorta where velocity is highest, but even there it contributes less than 5 mm Hg of equivalent pressure.

2. Blood flow is a function of pressure gradient and resistance

One of the properties of a fluid (or gas) is that it will flow from a region of higher pressure (e.g., the left ventricle) toward a region of lower pressure (e.g., the right atrium; Figure 1.1). In clinical practice, the patient is assumed to be supine (negating the gravitational component of pressure) and at rest. As already mentioned, kinetic energy is negligible compared to blood pressure at normal cardiac output and thus blood flow is estimated using the pressure gradient and resistance.

The primary parameter used in clinical medicine to describe blood flow through the systemic circulation is cardiac output, which is the total volume of blood pumped by the ventricle per minute (generally expressed in L/min). Cardiac

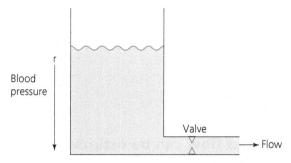

Figure 1.1 A simple hydraulic system demonstrating fluid flow from a high-pressure reservoir to a low-pressure reservoir. Note that the volume of flow can be affected by a focal resistance (i.e., the valve).

output is equal to the total volume of blood ejected into the aorta from the left ventricle (LV) per cardiac cycle (i.e., stroke volume) multiplied by the heart rate. This formula is important experimentally, but of limited used clinically because stroke volume is difficult to measure. Cardiac output is generally measured using the Fick equation or via thermodilution techniques, which are discussed in Chapter 6.

To compare cardiac output among individuals of different sizes, the cardiac index (cardiac output divided by body surface area) is used. Normalization of cardiac output for body surface area is important, as it enables proper interpretation of data independent of the patient's size (e.g., cardiac output will obviously differ widely between a 260-pound man and a 100-pound woman). Indexing to body surface area is also used for other measurements such as aortic valve area.

The relationship between blood flow, resistance, and pressure can be determined using a modification of Ohm's law for the flow of electrons in an electrical circuit:

$$\text{Flow}(Q) = \text{pressure gradient}(\Delta P) / \text{resistance}(R)$$

where ΔP is the difference in pressure between proximal and distal points in the system and R is the hydraulic resistance to blood flow between the proximal and distal points.

A useful clinical equation based on Ohm's law is:

$$\text{Mean arterial pressure}(\text{MAP}) - \text{central venous pressure}(\text{CVP})$$
$$= \text{cardiac output}(\text{CO}) \times \text{systemic vascular resistance}(\text{SVR})$$

Using this equation, we can calculate systemic vascular resistance knowing cardiac output, CVP, and arterial pressure. MAP is the average arterial pressure over time and is generally estimated using the following formula:

$$\text{MAP} = (1/3 \times \text{aortic systolic pressure}) + (2/3 \times \text{aortic diastolic pressure}).$$

This formula was developed for a heart rate of 60 beats per minute (bpm; at this heart rate, diastole is twice as long as systole) and becomes progressively more inaccurate as heart rate increases. In a patient in shock (i.e., low blood pressure and impaired tissue perfusion), measurement of CO and calculation of SVR can help identify the etiology (e.g., septic shock with high CO+low SVR or cardiogenic shock with low CO+high SVR).

3. Resistance to flow can be estimated using Poiseuille's law

Blood is not an "ideal fluid" and energy (and pressure) is lost as flowing blood encounters resistance to flow. Resistance to blood flow is a function of viscosity, vessel radius, and vessel length in a vessel without any focal obstruction (resistance to blood flow also occurs from focal obstruction such as seen with atherosclerotic disease of arteries). The relationship is known as Poiseuille's law (sometimes referred to as the Poiseuille–Hagen law) and is described by the following equation:

$$\text{Resistance} = 8 \times \text{viscosity} \times \text{length} / \pi \times \text{radius}^4$$

or, since flow = difference in pressure/resistance:

$$\text{Blood flow} = \pi \times \text{radius}^4 \times \text{difference in pressure} / 8 \times \text{viscosity} \times \text{length}$$

Since radius is raised to the fourth power, its importance in determining resistance is paramount. A 20% increase in radius leads to a doubling in flow if all other variables are constant. Or, as another example, resistance is 16 times greater in a coronary artery with a diameter of 2 mm (e.g., a distal obtuse marginal) than in a coronary artery with a diameter of 4 mm (e.g., the proximal left anterior descending).

Viscosity is also important in determining resistance (commonly abbreviated as η and with units of poise = dyne s/cm^2). It is difficult to measure directly and thus is commonly reported as relative to water. The viscosity of plasma is $1.7 \times$ viscosity of water and viscosity of blood is $3–4 \times$ viscosity of water, the difference being due to red blood cells and thus hematocrit.

It is important to note that Poiseuille's law only provides an approximation of resistance when used in blood vessels. The four important assumptions underlying the derivation of this equation are: (1) the viscosity of the fluid is unchanging over time or space; (2) the tube is rigid and cylindrical; (3) length of the tube greatly exceeds diameter; and (4) flow is steady, nonpulsatile, and nonturbulent. Many of these assumptions are violated when this equation is applied to blood flow in the body. Poiseuille's law is important, however, as it indicates the variables that are the determinants of resistance to flow.

In the mammalian circulation, resistance is greatest at the level of the arterioles. While the radius of a typical capillary (e.g., 2.5 microns) is smaller than the radius of the smallest arterioles (e.g., 4 microns), the number of capillaries greatly exceeds the number of arterioles, and thus the effective area is much larger. Also of importance is that arteriolar resistance can be regulated (capillaries have no smooth muscle and thus resistance cannot be regulated at that level; however, pericyte cells can constrict capillaries in certain specialized structures like the kidney's glomerulus). This enables rapid changes in vascular resistance to maintain blood pressure (e.g. in hypovolemic shock) and also enables regulation of blood flow to various organs (i.e., autoregulation). A general principle to remember is that reduction of arteriolar resistance in a tissue decreases SVR, resulting in increased cardiac output while simultaneously decreasing pressure proximal to the arterioles and increasing pressure distal to the arterioles.

4. Reynold's number can be used to determine whether flow is laminar or turbulent

Flow in blood vessels, as in any hydraulic system, is usually smooth and orderly because the fluid separates into an infinite number of concentric layers, with the highest velocity in the center and the lowest next to the vessel wall. When a fluid (such as blood) flows past a solid surface (such as the vascular wall), a thin layer develops adjacent to the surface where frictional forces retard the motion of the fluid (Figure 1.2). There is a gradient of frictional resistance (and thus velocity) between fluid in contact with the solid surface and fluid in the center of the stream. If the fluid elements travel along well-ordered, nonintersecting layers, this is termed laminar flow. The flow resistance in laminar flow is due entirely to viscous resistance of the fluid and the interactions between the fluid and the stationary wall. In laminar flow, the average velocity of a fluid is one half of the maximum velocity observed in the center of the stream.

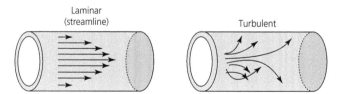

Figure 1.2 Schematic of laminar flow. Flow in straight, nonbranching tubes is usually smooth and orderly because the fluid separates into an infinite number of concentric layers with different velocities. When a fluid (such as blood) flows past a stationary surface (such as the vascular wall), a thin layer develops adjacent to the surface where frictional forces tend to retard the motion of the fluid. There is a gradient of frictional resistance (and thus velocity) between fluid in contact with the solid surface and fluid in the center of the stream. If the fluid particles travel along well-ordered, nonintersecting layers, this is termed laminar flow.

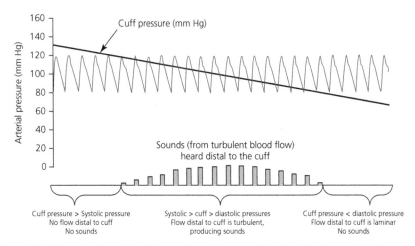

Figure 1.3 Schematic illustrating the use of transient transition from laminar to turbulent flow in measuring blood pressure.

In contrast, turbulent flow occurs when fluid elements from adjacent layers become mixed. Turbulent flow is chaotic and less efficient because of energy losses (these losses are termed inertial resistance). In turbulent flow, the relationship between pressure difference and flow is no longer linear, since the amount of resistance in the tube increases with flow. Thus, larger pressure differences are required to maintain flow. Turbulence, and associated loss of energy along with the narrowed radius, are two of the primary causes of the drop in pressure that occurs distal to a severe stenosis.

Turbulence is important for several reasons, one of which is that it creates noise (e.g., in a pipe when flow velocity is high), which is the cause of some cardiac murmurs and the Korotkoff sounds (used when measuring blood pressure; Figure 1.3). Another is that turbulence alters the relationship between flow and perfusion pressure, as already mentioned. Because of increased energy losses associated with turbulence, the relationship between perfusion pressure and blood flow is no longer linear (as described by the Poiseuille relationship) but rather, greater pressure is required to maintain adequate flow (Figure 1.4).

The transition from laminar to turbulent flow can be predicted by calculating the Reynold's number, which is the ratio of inertial forces ($V\eta$) to viscous forces (ρ/L):

$R = \text{diameter} \times \text{velocity} \times \text{density} / \text{viscosity}$

where viscosity (η) of blood at 37 °C is 0.0035 Pa·s (pascal-seconds; 3.5 centipoise), density (ρ) of blood is approximately 1060 kg/m^3, velocity (V) of blood is in m/s, and the diameter of the tube is in meters. Reynold's number is dimensionless.

In a given hydraulic system, a critical Reynold's number exists below which flow is laminar. At Reynold's numbers near this critical number, a transitional zone exists where flow is neither completely laminar nor turbulent. Higher Reynold's numbers are associated with turbulent flow. In a long, straight, nonbranching pipe

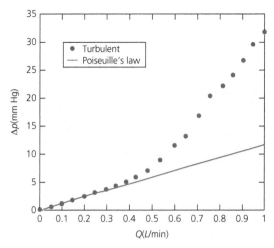

Figure 1.4 Transition from laminar to turbulent flow. Note that the pressure gradient required to increase flow increases markedly when flow transitions from laminar to turbulent.

with nonpulsatile flow, flow is generally laminar if $R < 2000$ and turbulent if $R > 2000$. It is important to note that the Reynold's number depends on the exact flow configuration and must be determined experimentally.

In the aorta, transition from laminar to turbulent flow generally occurs at a Reynold's number between 2000 and 2500. In atherosclerotic arteries and/or at branch points, the critical Reynold's number is much lower and there can be turbulence even at normal physiologic flow velocities. In severe stenoses, turbulence can be initiated at Reynold's numbers an order of magnitude less than in the theoretical, straight pipe.

The Reynold's equation is important for demonstrating variables important in determining whether flow is laminar or turbulent. As a simple approximation from this equation, we see that laminar flow is difficult to maintain in conditions of high velocity (e.g., stenotic artery) and large diameter. Vessel diameter is doubly important, for it is not only a direct variable in the equation but also influences velocity. Because of the continuity equation (see Principle 9 below), we know that velocity increases as diameter decreases. Thus, effects of blood vessel diameter on Reynold's number are magnified. Because both velocity and diameter decrease in the microcirculation, the flow there tends to be laminar.

5. Force developed by the ventricles is a function of preload or stretch—the Frank–Starling law

The three most important factors in the regulation of ventricular function (and thus cardiac output) are preload, afterload, and contractility. Preload for the ventricles is defined as amount of passive tension or stretch exerted on the ventricular walls (i.e., intraventricular pressure) just prior to the initiation of systole. This "load" applied to the ventricular wall determines end-diastolic sarcomere length and thus the force of

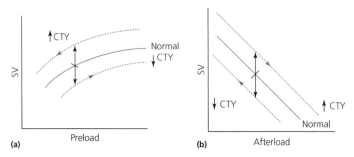

Figure 1.5 Frank–Starling principle. In panel (a), note that stroke volume (SV) increases as preload increases on any given line of contractility (CTY). Panel (b) demonstrates that stroke volume increases as afterload decreases.

contraction. The Frank–Starling law states that the passive length to which the myocardial cells are stretched at the end of diastole is a determinant of the active tension they develop when stimulated to contract. The Frank–Starling law is an intrinsic property of myocytes; that is, it is not dependent on nerve signals or hormones. The general principle is that increased preload causes increased force of contraction, which increases stroke volume and thus cardiac output (Figure 1.5). The Frank–Starling law (or mechanism) helps the heart match cardiac output to venous return.

The Frank–Starling law was derived from independent work by two investigators. In the 1890s, Otto Frank measured pressure developed by the isolated beating frog ventricle against an occluded aorta under varying preloading conditions. He found that as end-diastolic volume increased, ventricular systolic pressure and the maximum rate of pressure development (dP/dT_{max}) increased. Approximately 20 years later, Ernst Starling found similar results using a heart–lung preparation in an anesthetized dog in which he controlled heart rate, venous pressure, venous return, arterial pressure, and arterial resistance.

For any given heart, there is not just a single Frank–Starling curve. Rather, there is a family of curves, each of which is determined by the afterload and inotropic state (i.e., contractility) of the heart. While changes in venous return cause a ventricle to move along a single Frank–Starling curve, changes in contractility and afterload cause the heart to shift to a different Frank–Starling curve.

6. Wall tension is a function of pressure and radius divided by wall thickness—the Laplace relationship

Laplace's law describes the relationship between the transmural pressure difference and the tension, radius, and thickness of the vessel wall or ventricular chamber (Figure 1.6). A good approximation of wall tension in a vessel or chamber according to Laplace is:

Wall tension = pressure × radius / wall thickness

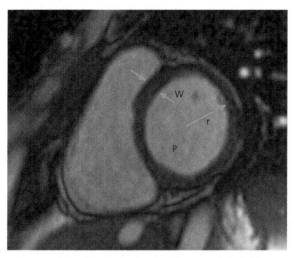

Figure 1.6 Magnetic resonance imaging (MRI) of a right ventricle and a left ventricle. The left ventricle is labeled to demonstrate Laplace's law: $t = (P \times r)/W$, where P is pressure; r is radius; W is wall thickness; and t is wall tension.

The pressure inside a blood vessel or ventricle exerts a distending force (tension) on the walls that is proportional to the magnitude of the pressure and radius. Thus, wall tension in the aorta is high. In chronic hypertension, aortic wall thickness increases as an adaptation to normalize wall tension. Similarly, LV hypertrophy develops in response to chronic elevations in ventricular pressure and/or dilatation, again as an adaptation.

There are several important implications of this relationship. One is that larger arteries must have stronger walls, since an artery of twice the radius must be able to withstand twice the wall tension at a given blood pressure. Similarly, the increased wall tension is thought to contribute to the development of aneurysms (and possibly to predict aneurysm rupture) in larger arteries. Another implication is that as the radius of the LV increases (e.g., in dilated cardiomyopathy), increased active wall tension must be developed during systole by the myocytes in order to create the same ventricular pressures for ejection. Thus, a dilated ventricle uses more adenosine triphosphate (ATP) and oxygen to generate the same stroke volume.

7. The normal venous system is a low pressure, large volume reservoir of blood which enables rapid increases in cardiac output

Approximately 60–80% of blood in the normal individual is in the venous system (with 8–10% being within the heart, 15–20% in arteries, and 5% in capillaries). There is a large capacitance in the normal venous system, and large veins are not

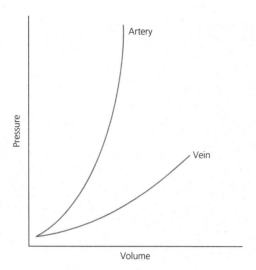

Figure 1.7 Pressure–volume relationship for arteries and veins.

fully filled but instead partially collapsed (elliptical). Thus, the venous system can absorb a large amount of volume with minimal increase in pressure. Once veins become fully distended, however, the pressure–volume relationship changes significantly (Figure 1.7). Veins have limited elasticity once they are fully distended, and at this point pressure increases rapidly with increased volume.

Since the cardiovascular system is a closed loop, venous return and cardiac output are closely coupled, and increased venous return to the heart is one of the primary mechanisms by which cardiac output is increased rapidly. For example, venous return (and cardiac output) can be rapidly augmented by increased sympathetic tone, which causes the smooth muscle in veins to contract. Similarly, skeletal muscular contractions during exercise reduce venous capacitance in the muscle beds by rhythmically compressing the veins and can markedly increase venous return.

8. The pressure and velocity of a fluid in a closed system are related

As we saw in Principle 1, Bernoulli derived the formula (now known as the Bernoulli equation) that relates the pressure, velocity, and height (i.e., gravitational forces) in the steady motion of an ideal fluid (i.e., a fluid with constant viscosity and in which there are no frictional losses during flow). The usual form is $TE = P_{Per} + (\rho \times h \times g) + 1/2\, \rho V^2$, where TE is the total energy, V is the blood velocity, P_{Per} the perpendicular pressure, ρ the blood density, g the gravitational constant, and h the height above an arbitrary reference level. It is based on the law of conservation of energy and states that the sum of potential and kinetic energy is the same at every point throughout a rigid tube.

The Bernoulli equation provides the theoretical foundation for the use of pulse wave and continuous wave Doppler to estimate pressures. While the actual derivation is more complex, for practical use in Doppler echocardiography the Bernoulli equation is simplified to $P_1 - P_2 = 4V^2$, where P is pressure and V is velocity (labeled the modified Bernoulli equation). Because of the relationship between velocity and pressure, Doppler-determined blood velocity can be used to estimate pressures within the heart and vasculature (e.g., estimating pulmonary artery pressures at the time of echocardiography by measuring the velocity of tricuspid regurgitation).

Derivation of the modified Bernoulli equation

Ignoring gravitational forces, the Bernoulli equation predicts that the relationship between pressures at two points (P1 and P2) within a system with a flowing fluid would be:

$P_1 + 1/2\rho V^2 = P_2$

Or, stated another way, the difference in pressure between the two points would be:

$P_2 - P_1 = 1/2\rho V^2$

Inserting units and blood density ($\rho = 1050$ kg/m³):

$\Delta P(\text{kg}/\text{ms}^2) = 1/2(1050\text{kg}/\text{m}^3)V^2(\text{m}^2/\text{s}^2)$

Since 1 mm Hg = 133.3 Pa = 133.3 kg/m²

$\Delta P \times 133.3 = 1/2(1050)V^2$

and thus we arrive at the formula we recognize:

$\Delta P(\text{mmHg}) = 3.938V^2$

commonly abbreviated to:

$\Delta P(\text{mmHg}) = 4V^2$

---

9. The velocity of blood increases and pressure decreases as the cross-sectional area of the blood vessel decreases

An important hemodynamic concept is the continuity equation, which is derived from the law of conservation of mass. This equation is based on the principle that flow at any given point in series in a closed hydraulic system will be equal to flow at any other point. Thus, since flow is constant, velocity is inversely proportional to the cross-sectional area (Figure 1.8):

$$Q = A_1 V_1 = A_2 V_2 = A_3 V_3$$

where A is area and V is velocity at any given point within the system. An implication of this equation is that velocity increases as the cross-sectional area decreases (e.g., at the site of an arterial stenosis). Similarly, blood velocity decreases as it

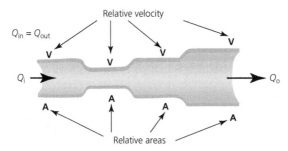

Figure 1.8 Relationship between blood velocity and cross-sectional area of blood vessels. Because of the law of conservation of mass, flow within any given major division of the circulatory system in a closed hydraulic system will be equal to flow within any other major division. Thus, velocity in a major division is inversely proportional to the aggregate vessel cross-sectional area in that division.

flows from the aorta into the capillary system (which, for the purpose of this discussion, can be thought of as "one very large vessel" in series with the aorta and vena cava), but then increases again as it coalesces from venules to veins to the vena cava. An average velocity of blood at any given point within the major divisions of the circulation (i.e., aorta, arteries, arterioles, capillaries, venules, veins, vena cava) can be estimated, knowing the volume of blood and the aggregate cross-sectional area of the blood vessels in a given division.

The continuity equation is used in the echocardiography laboratory to estimate aortic valve area. The cross-sectional area of the LV outflow tract is measured along with blood velocity at that point (using pulse wave Doppler) and then volumetric blood flow in the outflow tract is calculated. Using the continuity equation, the cross-sectional area of the valve can be calculated by dividing volumetric blood flow by the measured velocity at the valve.

10. Resistance increases when blood vessels are connected in series and decreases when blood vessels are connected in parallel

Poiseuille's equation estimates resistance to flow in a single vessel. The human cardiovascular system, however, includes complex circuitry with distinct blood vessels in series (connected one after another) and in parallel (arising from the dichotomous divisions of larger vessels into smaller branches). Blood ejected from the heart moves from aorta → large arteries → small arteries → arterioles → capillaries → venous system → heart. While the aorta is a single vessel, the rest of the circulatory system involves multiple vessels connected in parallel (e.g., the carotid arteries, renal arteries, and other major branches from the aorta form a parallel circuit).

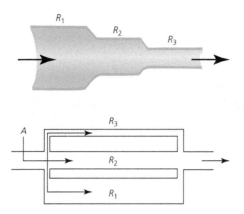

Figure 1.9 Circuits (or blood vessels) in series and in parallel.

For blood vessels connected in series, the total resistance of the system is equal to the sum of resistance in each vessel (Figure 1.9):

$$R_{\text{total}} = R_1 + R_2 + R_3$$

Thus, for blood vessels connected in series, the resistance of the system is always greater than resistance in any one vessel. Thus, for three vessels in series, each with resistance R, the total resistance of the system is $3R$.

For blood vessels connected in parallel, resistance is equal to the sum of the reciprocal of the resistance in each vessel:

$$1 / R_{\text{total}} = 1 / R_1 + 1 / R_2 + 1 / R_3$$

Thus, for blood vessels connected in parallel, resistance of the system is always less than resistance in any vessel. For three vessels in parallel, each with resistance R, the total resistance of the system is R/3.

An important principle is that more than 60% of the resistance to flow occurs within the arterioles. The diameter of the arterial system progressively decreases from aorta → arteriole. Energy losses (pressure drop) are minimized in the larger arteries, despite decreases in diameter, by having many arteries in parallel. The large pressure loss in arterioles is due to a dramatic decrease in diameter (Figure 1.10) without a correspondingly large enough increase in the number of arterioles in parallel. It goes without saying that the energy loss in arterioles serves many important functions, such as lowering pressure and velocity in capillaries to allow optimal transit time for red blood cells for diffusion of oxygen (O_2) and carbon dioxide (CO_2).

Since the greatest resistance occurs within the arterioles, systemic vascular resistance is very sensitive to changes in arteriolar diameter from constriction and dilation. Assuming constant cardiac output (keep in mind that cardiac output is a dynamic process and may increase or decrease by mechanisms other than changes

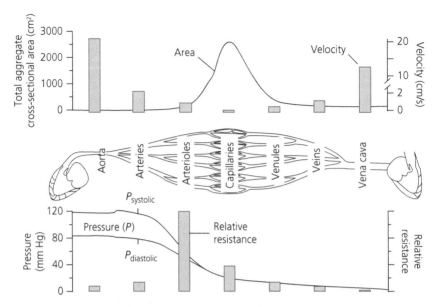

Figure 1.10 Pressure, velocity, and flow in various parts of the circulation.

in vascular resistance), agents that dilate arterioles in a tissue bed will decrease blood pressure (i.e., pressure proximal to the arterioles), but also increase pressures in the capillary bed. Similarly, vasoconstrictors increase blood pressure but reduce pressure within capillaries. In real life, cardiac output does not remain constant. The use of vasopressors to maintain blood pressure will increase vascular resistance but at a potential cost of decreased cardiac output (e.g., in the patient with cardiogenic shock) and/or organ failure due to increased vascular resistance (e.g., worsening renal function in patients on vasopressors).

CHAPTER 2

The nuts and bolts of right heart catheterization and PA catheter placement

Vickie Strang and George A. Stouffer

The pulmonary artery catheter

The pulmonary artery (PA) catheter (also known as the Swan–Ganz catheter or right heart catheter) was developed in the 1960s by Dr. Harold Swan, Dr. William Ganz, and colleagues [1]. The typical PA catheter is 100–110 cm long and has either 3 or 4 lumens (one lumen is used to inflate the balloon and thus there is one less port than the number of lumens). There is a proximal port approximately 30 cm from the tip that generally lies in the right atrium (RA) and can be used to transduce pressure or as an infusion port. The distal port is at the tip of the catheter and is used to measure PA pressure and pulmonary capillary wedge pressure (PCWP). Near the tip is a balloon that can be inflated and a thermistor to measure temperature (Figure 2.1).

The PA catheter provides information about ventricular preload (e.g., RA pressure is a reflection of right ventricular [RV] preload and PCWP is a reflection of left ventricular [LV] preload), afterload (systemic vascular resistance and pulmonary vascular resistance), and cardiac output. The PA catheter can be helpful in various clinical scenarios, including valvular heart disease, congestive heart failure, cardiomyopathy, pericardial tamponade, shock, renal failure, pulmonary edema, pulmonary hypertension, or cardiac structural abnormalities.

PA catheters are used primarily in three different settings: in the cardiac catheterization laboratory, in intensive care units (ICU), and in the operating room. Despite the tremendous theoretical benefits that could accrue from having the information obtainable from PA catheters, these catheters have never been shown to improve patient outcomes in either the operating room or intensive care unit (potential benefit has never been studied in the cardiac catheterization laboratory). In numerous studies examining various groups such as patients with heart failure, patients undergoing high-risk noncardiac surgery,

Cardiovascular Hemodynamics for the Clinician, Second Edition. Edited by George A. Stouffer.
© 2017 John Wiley & Sons Ltd. Published 2017 by John Wiley & Sons Ltd.

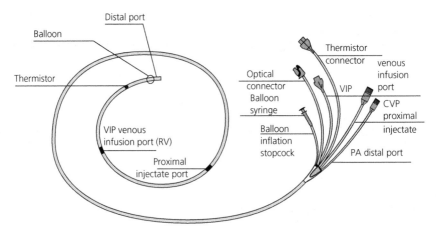

Figure 2.1 Schematic of PA catheter.

Table 2.1 Sample of trials that have examined the effect of PA catheter use on mortality in critically ill patients.

	Study population	N	Type of study	Mortality with PAC vs. without PAC
SUPPORT = [5]	Medical and surgical ICU patients	5735	Prospective cohort study	Increased mortality with PAC: odds ratio, 1.24; 95% confidence interval, 1.03–1.49
Sandham JD [6]	High-risk surgical patients	1994	Randomized controlled trial	No difference in mortality
Richard C [7]	Septic shock and/or ARDS	676	Randomized controlled trial	No difference in mortality
ESCAPE [8]	Heart failure	433	Randomized controlled trial	No difference in mortality; in-hospital adverse events were more common among patients in the PAC group
PAC-Man [9]	Intensive care unit patients	1041	Randomized controlled trial	No difference in mortality
Fluid and Catheter Treatment Trial (FACTT) [10]	Acute lung injury	1000	Randomized controlled trial with explicit management protocol	No difference in mortality, ICU days or time on ventilator

and patients with acute respiratory distress syndrome (ARDS), PA catheters have in general had no beneficial effects on survival with increased rates of complications (Table 2.1) [2,3,4]. These studies have been criticized for several reasons, including improper patient selection (e.g., including low-risk patients who would not be expected to benefit), study design (e.g., expecting a monitoring tool to affect outcomes without specified treatment protocols), and not controlling for operator experience in either insertion of the catheter or interpretation of data. Currently, there is no clear consensus on whether PA catheters are beneficial or harmful, with articulate proponents on both sides. PA catheters remain in widespread use presumably because they provide benefit to individual patients, but the studies sound a note of caution against indiscriminate use of these catheters.

The effectiveness of a PA catheter depends on accurate assessment of the information provided. Waveform analysis is crucial for proper interpretation of data from a PA catheter and is discussed in detail in Chapters 3, 4, and 5. Cardiac output is discussed in Chapter 6. In this chapter, we will concentrate on the following topics:

• Brief review of physiology relevant to right heart and PA catheterization
• Vascular access
• Right heart catheterization and placement of a PA catheter
• Ensuring that accurate data are obtained from a PA catheter
• Cardiac output
• Calculating vascular resistance
• SvO_2 monitoring
• Complications of PA catheters

Brief review of physiology relevant to right heart and pulmonary artery catheterization

Let us begin by looking at one mechanical cardiac cycle. While the ventricles are in systole the atria are filling, as blood flows continually from the venous system, with the inferior and superior vena cava emptying into the RA and the pulmonary veins emptying into the left atrium (LA). Meanwhile, the tricuspid valve and the mitral valve remain closed as long as the pressure in the ventricles exceeds the pressure in the atria.

Blood flow in the heart occurs due to pressure gradients. As ventricular pressure decreases during isovolumetric ventricular relaxation (Figure 2.2a), it reaches a point where atrial pressure is higher than ventricular pressure and the mitral and tricuspid valves open due to hydrostatic pressure. The ventricles now rapidly fill (rapid ventricular filling; Figure 2.2b). This rapid filling characterizes the first phase of diastole. During the second phase of diastole, the pressures in the atria and the ventricles are the same. During this time only a small amount of blood normally flows into the ventricles (slow ventricular filling). This is primarily blood returning to the atria from the great veins or pulmonic veins, which then passes into the ventricle. Near the end of diastole, the atria contract (atrial systole), which generates an increase in pressure in the atrium and enhances blood flow into the ventricles (Figure 2.2c).

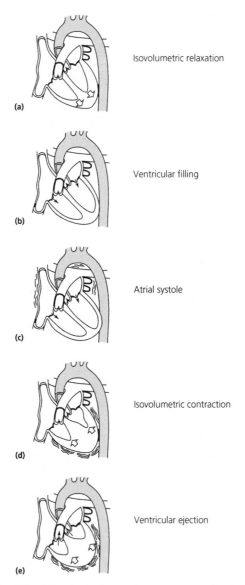

Isovolumetric relaxation

(a)

Ventricular filling

(b)

Atrial systole

(c)

Isovolumetric contraction

(d)

Ventricular ejection

(e)

Figure 2.2 Schematic of blood flow in the heart. Phases represented include isovolumetric ventricular relaxation (a), rapid ventricular filling (b), atrial contraction (c), isovolumetric contraction (d), and ventricular ejection (e).

Systole begins when electrical activation of the ventricles (QRS complex) leads to mechanical activation of the ventricles. Very shortly after onset of ventricular contraction, the pressure in the ventricle increases to the point where it exceeds atrial pressure and the mitral and tricuspid valves close (all four valves are now closed). As the ventricles contract (isovolumetric contraction; Figure 2.2d), right and left ventricular pressures increase until RV pressure exceeds PA pressure and LV pressure exceeds aortic pressure. At these points, the pulmonic and aortic valves open and ejection occurs (ventricular ejection; Figure 2.2e). At the end of systole, isovolumetric ventricular relaxation begins and ventricular pressures fall.

A point to remember is that as heart rate increases, myocardial oxygen consumption increases while supply decreases. This is because time in diastole decreases and time in systole increases as heart rate increases, while most coronary artery filling occurs during diastole, but oxygen consumption of the heart is maximal during systole. About 70–90% of blood flow in the left coronary artery and one-half of blood flow in the right coronary artery occur during diastole. During systole, intramural arteries and capillaries are compressed by the contracting heart muscle, which limits blood flow.

Vascular access

A PA catheter can be inserted via any vein that has uninterrupted access to the RA. The most commonly used insertion sites include subclavian veins, internal jugular veins, and femoral veins. The site is generally chosen based on patient preference and operator experience. All things being equal, the right internal jugular vein provides the shortest and straightest path to the heart. The use of ultrasound has been shown to increase success rates for venous access and to decrease complications. Complications associated with venous access include bleeding, hematoma, arterial puncture, infection, pneumothorax, and hemothorax (Table 2.2). Advantages and disadvantages of various access sites are listed in Table 2.3.

Table 2.2 Complications of PA catheters.

Complications associated with vascular access	Complications associated with PA catheter insertion or removal	Complications associated with indwelling PA catheters	Problems causing inaccurate data interpretation
Hematoma	Arrhythmias	Damage to tricuspid or pulmonic valve	Improper calibration Improper leveling of transducer
Bleeding	Damage to tricuspid or pulmonic valve	Infection	Air in tubing Interpretation without using ECG
Arterial puncture	Infection	Thromboembolic	Effects of respiration not noted
Pneumothorax	Pulmonary infarction Right bundle branch block	Pulmonary infarction	Inaccurate computation constant used to determine cardiac output
Hemothorax	Pulmonary artery rupture	Pulmonary artery rupture	Use of improper pressure scale

Table 2.3 Advantages and disadvantages of venous access sites.

Site	Advantages	Disadvantages
Subclavian vein	Patient mobility; sterility	Risk of pneumothorax (especially in patients with COPD or on positive pressure ventilation); noncompressible site
Internal jugular vein	Compressible site; patient mobility; easily accessible	Inadvertent puncture of carotid; catheter can be dislodged from pulmonary capillary wedge position with neck movement; risk of pneumothorax
Femoral vein	Compressible site; easily accessible	Patient must remain in bed; infection risk
Brachial vein	Right heart catheterization can be done at the same time as left heart catheterization via radial artery	Brachial vein is smaller than subclavian, internal jugular, or femoral vein. Inadvertent cannulation of cephalic vein can make right heart catheterization difficult

Right heart catheterization and placement of a PA catheter

A PA catheter can be positioned using either fluoroscopy or pressure monitoring. Fluoroscopy is preferred for femoral artery insertion and/or if there is significant hardware in the right heart (e.g., biventricular pacer). If continuous pressure monitoring is used, transduce the distal tip. Insert the PA catheter 20 cm and inflate the balloon with air. Central venous pressure (CVP) is initially obtained. As the catheter is being "floated" into the heart, it first enters the RA and then goes into the RV. Atrial waveforms consist of an A wave, a V wave, a C wave, and X and Y descents (Figure 2.3a). The A wave in the RA waveform coincides with atrial contraction and occurs simultaneously with the PR interval on the electrocardiogram (ECG), whereas the peak of the V wave in the RA waveform can be found near or at the end of the T wave. A further discussion of interpretation of atrial waveforms can be found in Chapter 5.

Entry of the catheter into the RV can be identified by the appearance of ventricular systole on the pressure tracing (Figure 2.3b). There will be a rapid upstroke reflective of ventricular contraction and a rapid decline reflective of ventricular relaxation. Diastole will be similar to the atrial tracing. A further discussion of interpretation of ventricular waveforms can be found in Chapter 3. Normal RV systolic pressure is approximately 25 mm Hg, with diastolic pressures ranging from 0–8 mm Hg. The only time you should see an RV tracing is when the PA catheter is being inserted or removed. An RV pressure tracing from the distal port of the catheter appearing on the monitor at any other time is an indication that the catheter is no longer correctly placed. With the tip of the catheter in the RV, the risk of ventricular tachycardia is markedly increased. Note that some continuous

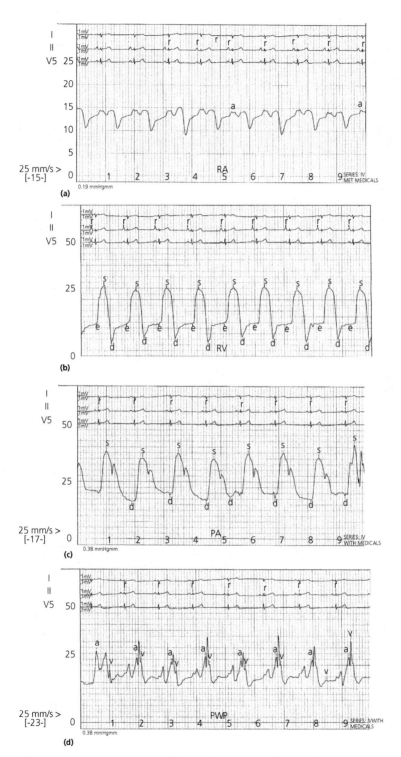

Figure 2.3 Pressure tracings encountered during the insertion of a PA catheter.

cardiac output catheters use a proximal port in the RV to monitor for correct positioning of the thermistor—the warning here is that if the pressure from the distal port of the catheter changes from PA to RV, that implies that the catheter tip is now residing in the RV.

As the catheter is advanced, it will leave the RV and enter the PA (Figure 2.3c). Remember that RV and PA systolic pressures are the same (both should coincide with the T wave on the ECG). Thus passage into the PA will be evident from diastolic pressures. If an RV waveform is still present approximately 20 cm after the initial RV pattern appears, the catheter may be coiling in the RV.

PCWP can be obtained by inflating the balloon on the catheter and advancing the catheter until it "wedges" (Figure 2.3d). When the balloon is "wedged," blood flow is stopped in that portion of the PA. Pressure equalizes in a nonflowing segment and, since there are no valves between the pulmonary arteries and pulmonary veins or between the pulmonary veins and the LA, pressure at the tip of the balloon is reflective of LA pressure. The A and V waves of the PCWP tracing will be delayed relative to RA tracing and ECG, with the A wave starting in or at the end of the QRS complex, and the V wave starting later in the T–P interval. This is because LA pressure is reflected back to the PA catheter via the pulmonary veins and through a static column of blood. PCWP is an important measurement since it is an estimate of LV end diastolic pressure and thus LV preload.

Tempe *et al.* [11] measured the distance to various chambers in 300 adult patients who had PA catheters placed via the right internal jugular vein. The right ventricle was reached at 25 ± 3 cm, the PA at 36 ± 4 cm, and the wedge position at 43 ± 6 cm. The length of catheter required was directly related to the height of the patient and was greater in patients with valvular heart disease.

In general, indwelling PA catheters rest in the PA (Figure 2.4), continuously giving a readout of PA systolic and PA diastolic pressure. Mean RA pressure can be obtained if the CVP port is transduced (but will often appear damped because the lumen is small).

Always deflate the balloon before withdrawing the PA catheter.

Ensuring that accurate data is obtained from a PA catheter

Remember the old saying: "Trash in equals trash out." The integrity of the data obtained from a PA catheter is dependent on the accuracy of the system. A few simple rules to start out with:
- The PA catheter needs to be "zeroed" at the level of the RA.
- Minimize the length of pressure tubing, the number of stopcocks, and the number of connections. Avoid narrow tubing, as the smaller the diameter of the tubing, the more pressure damping that occurs.

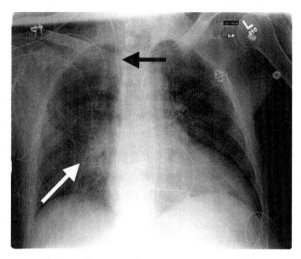

Figure 2.4 Chest X-ray showing placement of a PA catheter. The catheter was inserted via the right internal jugular vein. It passes through the superior vena cava (black arrow), RA, and RV. The tip rests in the right PA (white arrow).

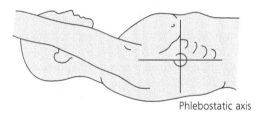

Phlebostatic axis

Figure 2.5 Phlebostatic axis.

- Eliminate any air bubbles in the pressure line.
- The proper pressure scale needs to be used
- Pressure tracings need to be interpreted in conjunction with an ECG tracing.
- The effects of respiration have to be identified.

It is essential that the PA catheter be properly "zeroed" at the level of the RA, which in the supine patient is assumed to be in the fourth intercostal space at the midaxillary line. Proper "zeroing" removes the effect of gravity on pressures. To locate the level of the RA, two imaginary lines are drawn (Figure 2.5) and the place where they intersect is called the phlebostatic axis. To locate the phlebostatic axis, locate the fourth intercostal space on the edge of the sternum, draw an imaginary line along the fourth intercostal space laterally, along the chest wall, and draw a second line from the axilla downward, midway between the anterior and posterior chest wall (i.e., the midaxillary line).

For every centimeter that the transducer is not correctly leveled, pressures will change by 0.75 mm Hg. If the transducer is too high, pressures will be falsely low. Alternatively, if the transducer is too low, pressures will be falsely high.

Pressure is transmitted from the catheter to the transducer via tubing filled with fluid, usually saline. Small changes in pressure in the PA are transmitted through the tubing and cause deflection of the transducer membrane, which converts these changes into electrical signals. Anything that hampers transmission of these small pressure changes to the membrane will distort pressure measurements and cause pressure "damping." Thus, it is important to use semirigid, noncompliant tubing, to minimize the length of tubing, and to make sure that there is no air in the pressure tubing. Other causes of pressure damping include long or compliant tubing, multiple stopcocks, transducer malfunction, loose connections, and partial occlusion of the port (e.g., with thrombus).

It is important that the proper scale be used when interpreting the pressure tracings. For example, when measuring LV pressure a scale of 0–200 mm Hg is useful. However, if this scale is used when examining RA pressure tracings, much of the information is lost about the "A" and "V" waves and "X" and "Y" descents that would be apparent if a scale of 0–25 mm Hg was used.

It is important that pressure tracings be interpreted in conjunction with an ECG recording. The most accurate method of obtaining hemodynamic data is to use a dual channel strip recorder, which will allow analysis of the waveform and ECG together.

When interpreting atrial pressure waveforms, emphasis should be placed on mean pressures or pressures obtained at end-expiration. In many intensive care units, all waveforms are read at end-expiration because this is when intrapleural pressures are negligible, which means that the waveforms are an accurate reflection of cardiac pressures.

In a spontaneously breathing patient, intrathoracic and thus intracardiac pressures will decline during inspiration and rise during expiration (Figure 2.6). The diaphragm pulls downward, creating a negative pleural pressure during inspiration, while the diaphragm relaxes and the elastic recoil of the lungs, chest wall, and abdominal structures compress the lung during expiration.

In patients who are mechanically ventilated, end-expiration is still used to record pressures. The difference is that pressures increase with inspiration and decrease with expiration. If the patient is not breathing over the ventilator, then interpretation is straightforward. If the patient is ventilated and also breathing spontaneously, then waveform interpretation becomes more difficult, as inspiration can be associated with decreases in pressure (spontaneous respiration) and increases in pressure (ventilator). The spontaneous breath with pressure support will result in an initial decrease in pressure, which can be used to locate end-expiration (just prior to the inspiratory effort marked by the dip in pressure). In patients receiving intermittent mandatory ventilation, identifying

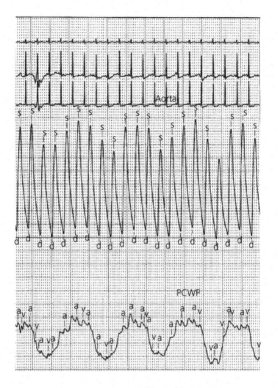

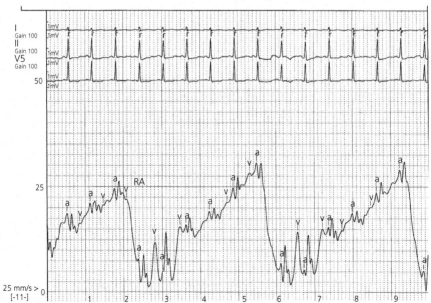

Figure 2.6 Effect of respiratory variation on RA and PCW pressures.

end-expiration can be a challenge. There are newer ventilators that show graphic respiratory waveforms that provide a means for accurately identifying end-expiration.

In the intensive care unit, manual interpretation of waveforms using a printed copy is necessary to ensure that pressures are interpreted at end-expiration, unless a monitor is available that displays the ECG, respiratory recording, and PA pressure waveforms on a single screen.

Cardiac output

A brief overview of cardiac output is presented here. For a more detailed discussion, see Chapter 6.

There are two primary methods used to calculate cardiac output when utilizing a PA catheter: thermodilution and assumed Fick. The thermodilution method requires that a substance that is cooler than blood (usually saline) be injected through the CVP port of the PA catheter. This injection should be smooth and take less than 4 seconds. The temperature in the PA is measured and the change over time, as the cooler injectate passes through the PA, is used to calculate cardiac output. The computer in the cardiac output machine uses the following formula:

$$CO = \frac{CC \times (Tb - Ti)}{\text{area under the curve}}$$

where CC is the computation constant, Tb the blood temperature, and Ti the injectate temperature.

A computation constant needs to be entered to provide the cardiac output computer with information on the amount and temperature of the injectate. Each PA catheter comes with an insert describing computation constants to be used under various conditions.

If you enter a computation constant that calls for 10 cc and you inject 9 cc, the measured cardiac output will be incorrect. Most of the time room-temperature saline is used as the injectate. If a different temperature injectate is used (e.g., iced saline), the computation constant must be changed.

The other method used to estimate cardiac output was first described by Adolph Fick in 1870. He postulated that the total uptake or release of a substance by an organ is the product of the blood flow through that organ and the arteriovenous difference ($A - VO_2$) of the substance. To directly measure oxygen consumption requires a Water's hood for the nonventilated patient or a metabolic cart for the ventilated patient. This is cumbersome and rarely used in daily practice. Instead, oxygen consumption is "assumed" (methods used to arrive at oxygen consumption are described in detail in Chapter 6).

The A – VO_2 gradient in the body is determined by comparing arterial oxygen saturation (measured directly or obtained via a pulse oximeter) with "mixed venous" oxygen saturation. Blood is considered "mixed venous" when it has circulated through the right side of the heart, to the PA. This mixing includes blood from the inferior and superior vena cava and the heart itself.

The formula used to estimate cardiac output using the assumed Fick approach is:

$$O_2 \text{ consumption} = CO\left(A - VO_2 \text{ difference}\right)$$

or

$$CO = \frac{O_2 \text{ consumption}}{A - VO_2 \text{ difference}}$$

$$CO = \frac{130 \times BSA}{1.36 \times Hgb \times 10 \times \left(SaO_2 - SvO_2\right)}$$

where BSA = body surface area; 130 mL/min = standard oxygen consumption; 1.36 = a gram of hemoglobin (Hgb) holds 1.36 mm of oxygen; Hgb = reported as grams per deciliter; 10 = to convert deciliters to liters you need to multiply the Hgb by this; SaO_2 = either from an ABG or from the pulse oximeter; SvO_2 = either from an oximetric PA catheter or by during oxygen saturation on a blood sample drawn from the PA port.

An example of calculating cardiac output using the assumed Fick method

The 'assumed oxygen consumption' is 130 mL/min

If BSA = 17; Hg = 12, SaO_2 = 0.98, and SvO_2 = 0.55

$$CO = \frac{130 \times 1.7}{1.36 \times 12 \times 10 \times \left(0.98 - 0.55\right)} = \frac{221}{70.1} = 3.48 \text{ L/min}$$

The cardiac index (CI) enables comparison of cardiac output between patients of different sizes. It is calculated by dividing cardiac output by BSA. The normal cardiac index is 2.5–4 L/min.

Calculating systemic vascular resistance and pulmonary vascular resistance

Vascular resistance is an indicator of ventricular afterload. Systemic vascular resistance (SVR) can be calculated using the following formula:

$$SVR = \frac{MAP - CVP}{CO} \times 80$$

Normal SVR is $800 - 1200 \text{ dynes / sec/ cm}^5$.

An example of calculating SVR

If MAP = 93 mm Hg, CVP = 3 mm Hg and CO = 5 L/min:

$$SVR = \frac{(93-3)*18}{18} = 1440 \text{ dynes/sec/cm}^5$$

The cardiac index (CI) enables comparison of cardiac output between patients of different sizes. It is calculated by dividing cardiac output by BSA. The normal cardiac index is 2.5–4 L/min.

Next, we will figure out pulmonary vascular resistance (PVR), which is an estimate of RV afterload. Normal PVR is in the range of 40–150 dynes/sec/cm^5. PVR can be calculated using the following formula:

$$PVR = \frac{\text{Mean PAP} - \text{PCWP}}{CO} \times 80$$

Mean pulmonary artery pressure (PAP) is calculated similar to mean arterial pressure:

$$\text{Mean PAP} = \left(\text{PA systolic pressure} + \left(2 \times \text{PA diastolic pressure}\right)\right)/3$$

An example of calculating PVR

If PAS = 30 mm Hg, PAD = 15 mm Hg, PWP = 10 mm Hg, and CO = 5 L/min :

$$PVR = \frac{20-10}{5} \times 80 = 2 \times 80 = 160 \text{ dynes/sec/cm}^5$$

Occasionally, PVR will be reported in Wood units (named after Paul Wood, a British cardiologist). It is the same formula as earlier, but the conversion factor of 80 is not used. To calculate PVR in Wood units, do the same calculation as earlier but do not multiply by 80 (i.e., PVR = 160 dynes/sec/cm^5 = 2 Wood units).

PVR is an important parameter in patients being evaluated for a heart transplant. If PVR is elevated, the right heart in the transplanted heart will not be able to generate enough pressure to maintain cardiac output. In general, survival in transplanted patients is better if PVR <3 Wood units.

SvO$_2$ monitoring

A full discussion of mixed venous oxygen saturation monitoring (SvO$_2$) is beyond the scope of this chapter; however, we will cover some of the basic concepts of SvO$_2$ monitoring.

The body maintains a balance between the oxygen delivered and the oxygen consumed. The supply side consists of cardiac output, oxygenation, and hemoglobin. The demand side is basal energy consumption plus anything that increases oxygen use, for example pain, shivering, infection, agitation, or any number of disease processes. Oxygen use is decreased by various factors, including anesthesia, hypothyroidism, paralyzing agents, sleep, and pain medication. SvO_2 is a function of oxygen delivered minus oxygen consumed. For example, assume that $1000\ mL/O_2/min$ of oxygenated blood is delivered to the tissues. Next, assume that the tissues use or consume $250\ mL/O_2/min$. This would leave $750\ mL/O_2/min$ to return to the lungs through the venous system. A total of $1000 - 250 = 750\ mL$ or 75% of the oxygenated blood is returned to the lungs. This 75% is the venous oxygen reserve.

If a healthy individual's oxygen consumption increases, the body will increase cardiac output and respiratory rate to ensure that demand is met and blood is kept fully oxygenated. In a critically ill patient, the situation is different and some patients are incapable of meeting even resting oxygen demands. When supply fails to meet demand despite maximal extraction of oxygen from the blood, anaerobic metabolism and lactic acidosis may occur.

SvO_2 can be measured continuously if the patient has an oximetric PA catheter in place. The oximetric catheter has fiberoptic technology that enables measurement of oxygen saturation of hemoglobin within the PA. Alternatively, if the patient does not have an SvO_2 catheter in place, oxygen saturation in PA blood can be measured via an oximeter by obtaining intermittent blood samples from the PA via the catheter. There are several uses of continuous oximetry, including measuring tissue oxygen consumption, obtaining real-time estimation of cardiac output, and monitoring responses to medications.

Important points about SvO_2 monitoring:
- Mixed oxygen saturation monitoring and arterial saturation monitoring may allow identification of an imbalance of oxygen supply and demand.
- Cardiac output is the largest determinant of oxygen supply.
- Normal SvO_2 is 60–80%.
- Oximetric catheters allow continuous monitoring of SvO_2.
- If the patient does not have an oximetric catheter in place, intermittent PA blood samples can be used to determine SvO_2. The disadvantage of this method is that you only know what the SvO_2 is at that specific time.
- SvO_2 may be high in sepsis because of impaired oxygen extraction. In this case, tissues are generally hypoxic despite high SvO_2. Some practitioners are using $ScvO_2$ (central venous oxygen saturation monitoring) in the patient with sepsis. The concept is the same, however the blood sample is taken from distal port of a triple lumen that has been placed in the right subclavian vein, therefore this saturation measurement does not include venous return from the heart.

Complications of pulmonary artery catheterization

There are several risks associated with PA catheter insertion that are independent of vascular access (Table 2.2). These include arrhythmias, transient right bundle branch block (RBBB) infection, pulmonary infarction, PA rupture, myocardial perforation, damage to the pulmonic or tricuspid valves, thromboembolic complications, air embolism, and knotting of the catheter.

Arrhythmias primarily occur during passage through the RV and are increased in patients with acute ischemia, hypocalcemia, hypokalemia, hypomagnesemia, hypoxemia, acidosis, shock, or digitalis toxicity. Atrial arrhythmias can also be precipitated by PA catheter placement.

RBBB can occur during passage of the catheter through the tricuspid valve. The right bundle is a fairly discrete and superficial structure in the septal wall and thus subject to trauma during the catheter advancement. RBBB is usually transient and does not cause any problems unless the patient has a preexisting left bundle branch block (LBBB), in which case complete heart block develops. In patients with LBBB, it is prudent to have a transcutaneous pacemaker readily available. In one series of 82 patients with LBBB, two episodes of complete heart block occurred. Both of these episodes occurred in patients with recent-onset LBBB and both occurred one day after the catheter had been inserted [12].

PA catheters have been associated with an increase in the risk of pulmonary embolus. In a randomized trial of PA catheters in 1994 high-risk surgical patients, there was a higher rate of pulmonary embolism in the catheter group than in the standard-care group (8 events versus 0 events, $P = 0.004$) [6]. One clue to the appearance of thrombus on the tip of a PA catheter can be pressure damping.

PA catheters have also been associated with valve damage and endocarditis. A study of autopsies from 55 patients who had undergone PA catheterization found that 53% had right-sided endocardial lesions. These included 22% with subendocardial hemorrhage, 20% with thrombus, 4% with hemorrhage and thrombus, and 7% with infective endocarditis. The pulmonic valve was the most common site of lesions (56%) followed by tricuspid valve (15%), RA (15%), right ventricle (10%), and PA (5%) [13].

There are two complications that can occur with wedging of the PA catheter: PA ischemia and/or infarction and PA rupture. As the PA catheter wedges it blocks blood flow in a branch of the PA and therefore can cause ischemia and/or infarction if the balloon is left inflated too long. Alternatively, the catheter can migrate into a small branch and occlude flow without balloon inflation (called "spontaneous wedge"). During the first few hours that the PA catheter is in place, it warms up and can migrate further into the distal lung vasculature.

The most feared complication of PA catheters is PA rupture. The presentation can be dramatic, with sudden onset of hemoptysis followed by cardiovascular collapse. It generally occurs when the balloon is inflated in a small nondistensible branch, but can also be caused by the tip of the catheter perforating the artery. Risk factors for PA rupture include pulmonary hypertension, age, female gender, anticoagulation, and frequent wedging. This complication is fatal approximately 50% of the time.

To avoid complications from wedging the PA catheter, inflate the balloon slowly with continuous waveform monitoring. If a PCWP tracing is obtained, stop inflating the balloon. If the PA catheter wedges with 0.5 cc of air or less, then it probably needs to be repositioned. A few other important points: try never to wedge longer than 2 respiratory cycles; never inflate the balloon with more than 1.5 cc of air; continuously monitor waveforms to ensure that the PA catheter does not spontaneously wedge; and never flush the catheter in a wedged position. When a PA catheter overwedges, the waveform usually goes straight up or down. If you see this waveform you should immediately let the air out of the balloon and obtain a chest X-ray to determine the location of the tip of the catheter.

If PA diastolic pressure and PCWP are closely related (a widely used rule of thumb is if they are within 6 mm Hg), there is no need to obtain wedge pressures repeatedly. PA diastolic pressure can be used to make clinical decisions.

One of the most common sources of errors when using PA catheters is inaccurate interpretation of data. Multiple studies have demonstrated inconsistent, incomplete, and improper data interpretation. It is important to obtain a complete understanding of how best to analyze the data obtained at the time of PA catheter placement in order to use the PA catheter optimally.

Case studies

1 You are working in surgical ICU caring for a 75-year-old male who was in a motor vehicle accident 36 hours ago. Despite adequate fluid resuscitation with a CVP reading of 10 mm Hg, he remains hypotensive, acidotic, and has a base balance of -3. Vital signs: HR 120 bpm, BP 90/40 mm Hg with MAP 56 mm Hg, urine output = 15 ml/hour. Ventilator settings are as follows: SIMV/PRVC, FiO_2 = 70%, TV 450 ml, Rate 14, PS 10 cm H_2O, PEEP 5 cm H_2O. He is not breathing over the ventilator.

   The decision is made to place a PA catheter to evaluate his cardiac status. His PA catheter numbers are CVP = 10 mm Hg, PA pressures = 40/20 mm Hg, PCWP = 16 mm Hg, CO/CI = 3.5/1.8 L/min.

   (a) What is his stroke volume (SV)?

   (b) What is his SVR?

   (c) Based on the PA numbers, would you change your therapy?

   (d) On his pressure waveforms, how will you identify end-expiration?

2 You are working in the medical ICU when a 69-year-old female is admitted with the diagnosis of severe dyspnea. There is no documented history of heart disease. Vital signs: HR = 130 bpm, BP = 80/30 mm Hg with MAP = 46 mm Hg, urine output = 10 ml/hour, Temp 35 °C orally, lactate = 4 mg/dl. Ventilator settings = SIMV/PRVC, FiO_2 = 100%, TV 400 ml, Rate 22, PS 10 cm H_2O, PEEP 10 cm H_2O. Initially she had a CVP of 2 mm Hg and an $ScvO_2$ of 65%. Despite an increase in CVP to 10 mm Hg after fluid resuscitation and the addition of two vasopressors, her blood pressure does not improve. Her chest X-ray shows diffuse pulmonary edema. To answer the question of whether the pulmonary edema is cardiogenic or noncardiogenic, a PA catheter is inserted and the following information obtained: CVP = 10 mm Hg, PA pressure = 25/15 mm Hg, PCWP = 12 mm Hg, SvO_2 = 60%, and CO = 8 L/min with CI = 3.5 L/min.

(a) Based on the information available, is the primary etiology of the pulmonary edema cardiogenic or noncardiogenic?

3 You are working in the coronary care unit (CCU) when a 62-year-old female is admitted with the diagnosis of cardiogenic shock. The patient became extremely fatigued 48 hours ago, but only recently came to the emergency room (ER) when she became very short of breath. The ECG shows Q waves in leads I, aVL, and V1–V6, consistent with a large anterolateral MI. Her vital signs are as follows: HR 120 bpm, BP 86/40 mm Hg with MAP 55 mm Hg, RR 32 times per minute. Pulse oximetery is reading 85% on room air. Temp = 36.5 °C.

A PA catheter is inserted to assist with her treatment and the following information is obtained: CVP = 15 mm Hg, PA pressure = 45/30 mm Hg, PCWP = 26 mm Hg, and CO = 3 L/min with CI = 1.7 L/min.

(a) What is her SV?

(b) What is her SVR?

(c) Based on the PA numbers, would you change your therapy?

(d) Would you use beta blockers to decrease the heart rate at this time?

4 You are working in the cardiac catheterization laboratory and a 33-year-old male is referred for evaluation for potential orthotropic heart transplant. He was well until 18 months ago when he developed severe LV dysfunction of unclear etiology, but thought to be a sequela of a viral syndrome. He has had a steady downward course during the past 3 months, during which his symptoms have progressed to Class III (i.e., he cannot walk across a room without having to stop to catch his breath). Ventriculography confirms severe LV dysfunction. Coronary angiography is normal. A right heart catheterization is performed and the following information obtained: RA pressure = 20 mm Hg, PA pressure = 78/41 (mean of 58 mm Hg), PCWP = 38 mm Hg, and cardiac output = 4.6 L/min.

(a) What is the PVR?

(b) What would you do next?

Nitroprusside infusion was begun and titrated until systemic systolic blood pressure was approximately 80 mm Hg. The following information was obtained from the PA catheter: PA pressure = 65/30 (mean of 46 mm Hg), PCWP = 24 mm Hg, and cardiac output = 7.9 L/min.

(c) What is the PVR now?

(d) Is the patient a candidate for heart transplantation?

Case study answers

1 (a) SV = CO/HR = 3500 ml/min/120 bpm = 29 ml.
   The patient's stroke volume is 29 mL.

(b) SVR = ((MAP − CVP) × 80)/CO = ((56 − 10) × 80)/3.5 = 1051 dynes/sec/cm^5.

(c) LV Preload is reflected by PCWP = 16 mm Hg with an afterload (SVR) of 1051 dynes/sec/cm^5. Cardiac output is low despite reasonable preload, suggesting LV dysfunction (possibly due to a cardiac contusion suffered at the time of the accident). An echocardiogram would be useful. Giving intravenous (IV) fluids to increase PCWP might increase cardiac output (at the risk of worsening oxygenation) and/or an inotrope such as dobutamine might be used to increase contractility.

(d) The patient is receiving positive pressure ventilation and thus inspiration is characterized by an increase in pressure on RA and PCWP waveforms. End-expiration will be just prior to the ventilator-stimulated increase. If the patient has any spontaneous respirations, remember to ignore the initial inspiratory dip in pressure—end-expiration will be just prior to this brief drop in pressure.

2 (a) A PCWP less than 18 mm Hg favors pulmonary edema of noncardiac origin rather than of cardiogenic origin. According to Schwarz and Albert [14], "acute lung injury (ALI) and ARDS (ALI/ARDS) are defined as follows: (1) an illness having an acute onset, (2) an arterial oxygen tension/inspired oxygen fraction ≤200 mm Hg (or ≤300 mm Hg for ALI), (3) the presence of bilateral infiltrates on frontal chest radiographs, and (4) a pulmonary artery occlusion pressure ≤18 mm Hg if measured, or no clinical evidence of left atrial hypertension when not measured." According to the Berlin Modification of the American-European Consensus Conference [15], ARDS can be divided into three categories of severity based on degree of hypoxemia: mild (200 mm Hg $< \text{PaO}_2/\text{FIO}_2 \leq$ 300 mm Hg), moderate (100 mm Hg $< \text{PaO}_2/\text{FIO}_2 \leq$ 200 mm Hg), and severe ($\text{PaO}_2/\text{FIO}_2 \leq$ 100 mm Hg).

3 (a) SV = CO/HR = 3000 ml/min/120 bpm = 25 ml.

(b) SVR = ((MAP – CVP × 80)/CO = ((55 – 15) × 80)/3 = 1067 dynes/sec/cm^5.

(c) Her preload is high (CVP = 15 mm Hg and PCWP = 26 mm Hg), her afterload is within the normal range, and her cardiac output is low. These numbers confirm the diagnosis of cardiogenic shock. Treatments might include pharmacologic diuresis to decrease preload and thus improve LV function according to the Frank-Starling curve. An IABP could be inserted to augment coronary artery perfusion, increase MAP, and decrease afterload. Some practitioners might also use dobutamine to improve LV contractility.

(d) No, as the heart rate is necessary to maintain blood pressure. The heart rate has increased in order to enhance cardiac output in the setting of a decreased stroke volume.

4 (a) PVR = (Mean PAP – PCWP)/CO = (58 – 38)/4.6 = 4.4 Wood units.

(b) In severe LV dysfunction, total PVR includes both a "fixed" component and a "dynamic" component, which is dependent on LA pressure. Following a heart transplant, LA pressure is less and the dynamic component of PVR is greatly reduced or eliminated. The fixed component of PVR persists, however, and the new RV must be able to maintain cardiac output against this resistance. In determining which patients are at risk for acute RV failure following heart transplantation, it is essential to quantify the fixed component of PVR. This can be done by measuring PA pressures, PCWP, and cardiac output during infusion of a vasodilator (e.g., prostacyclin, adenosine, or nitroprusside).

(c) The PVR is now (46 – 24)/7.9 = 2.8 Wood units.

(d) This level of PVR would not exclude the patient from receiving a heart transplant in most centers.

References

1 Swan HJ, Ganz W, Forrester J, Marcus H, Diamond G, Chonette D. Catheterization of the heart in man with use of a flow-directed balloon-tipped catheter. *N Engl J Med* 1970;**283**:447–451.

2 Shah MR, Hasselblad V, Stevenson LW, *et al.* Impact of the pulmonary artery catheter in critically ill patients: meta-analysis of randomized clinical trials. *JAMA* 2005;**294**: 1664–1670.

3 Marik PE. Obituary: pulmonary artery catheter 1970 to 2013. *Ann Intensive Care* 2013;**3**(1):38.

4 Rajaram SS, Desai NK, Kalra A, *et al.* Pulmonary artery catheters for adult patients in intensive care. *Cochrane Database Syst Rev* 2013;**2**.

5 Connors AF, Jr, Speroff T, Dawson NV, *et al.* for SUPPORT Investigators. The effectiveness of right heart catheterization in the initial care of critically ill patients. *JAMA* 1996;**276**:889–897.

6 Sandham JD, Hull RD, Brant RF, *et al.* A randomized, controlled trial of the use of pulmonary-artery catheters in high-risk surgical patients. *N Engl J Med* 2003;**348**:5–14.

7 Richard C, Warszawski J, Anguel N, *et al.* Early use of the pulmonary artery catheter and outcomes in patients with shock and acute respiratory distress syndrome: a randomized controlled trial. *JAMA* 2003;**290**:2713–2720.

8 Binanay C, Califf RM, Hasselblad V, *et al.* Evaluation study of congestive heart failure and pulmonary artery catheterization effectiveness: the ESCAPE trial. *JAMA* 2005;**294**:1625–1633.

9 The National Heart, Lung, and Blood Institute Acute Respiratory Distress Syndrome (ARDS) clinical trials network: pulmonary-artery versus central venous catheter to guide treatment of acute lung injury. *N Engl J Med* 2006;**354**:2213–2224.

10 Harvey S, Harrison DA, Singer M, *et al.*: Assessment of the clinical effectiveness of pulmonary artery catheters in management of patients in intensive care (PAC-Man): a randomised controlled trial. *Lancet* 2005;**366**:472–477.

11 Tempe DK, Gandhi A, Datt V, *et al.* Length of insertion for pulmonary artery catheters to locate different cardiac chambers in patients undergoing cardiac surgery. *Br J Anaesth* 2006;**97**(2):147–149.

12 Morris D, Mulvihill D, Lew WY. Risk of developing complete heart block during bedside pulmonary artery catheterization in patients with left bundle-branch block. *Arch Intern Med* 1987;**147**:2005–2010.

13 Rowley KM, Clubb KS, Smith GJ, Cabin HS. Right-sided infective endocarditis as a consequence of flow-directed pulmonary-artery catheterization. A clinicopathological study of 55 autopsied patients. *N Engl J Med* 1984;**311**:1152–1156.

14 Schwarz MI, Albert RK. "Imitators" of the ARDS: implications for diagnosis and treatment. *CHEST Journal* 2004;**125**(4):1530–1535.

15 ARDS Definition Task Force. Acute respiratory distress syndrome. *JAMA* 2012;**307**(23): 2526–2533.

CHAPTER 3

Normal hemodynamics

Alison Keenon, Eron D. Crouch, James E. Faber and George A. Stouffer

The mechanical events of the cardiac cycle as they occur in series are as follows: right atrium (RA) contracts, left atrium (LA) contracts, left ventricle (LV) begins contraction, mitral valve closes, right ventricle (RV) begins contraction, tricuspid valve closes, pulmonary valve opens, aortic valve opens, aortic valve closes, pulmonary valve closes, tricuspid valve opens, mitral valve opens. The events of the cardiac cycle superimposed on cardiac pressure tracings and an electrocardiogram (ECG) tracing, often called the Wiggers diagram after Dr. Carl Wiggers who first arranged data in this useful manner, is helpful in illustrating the relationship and timing of events in the cardiac cycle to hemodynamic phenomena (a stylized version of a Wiggers diagram is shown in Figure 3.1).

The cardiac cycle is often divided into systole (ventricular contraction) and diastole (ventricular filling; Figure 3.2). Systole can be further divided into four stages: isovolumetric contraction, rapid ejection, reduced ejection, and isovolumetric relaxation (Figure 3.3). The isovolumic phase of LV contraction is that time in which ventricular pressure is increasing, but is not sufficient to open the aortic valve (Figure 3.1). This phase ends when the aortic valve opens and blood is ejected (ejection phase). On an LV pressure tracing, the onset of ventricular contraction coincides with the R wave on the ECG and is indicated by the earliest rise in pressure after atrial contraction. During ventricular systole, the atrial pressure initially declines. This is thought to be due to stretch of the atria as the base of the heart descends. Following this brief period, atrial pressure progressively increases during the rest of ventricular systole as blood flow into the atria increases.

Diastole is the period during the cardiac cycle between aortic valve closure and mitral valve closure. A common mistake is to think of diastole as less important than systole, or more inaccurately as merely the absence of systole. Our appreciation of diastole has increased over the years as we have realized the importance of diastolic dysfunction in patients with congestive heart failure.

Cardiovascular Hemodynamics for the Clinician, Second Edition. Edited by George A. Stouffer.
© 2017 John Wiley & Sons Ltd. Published 2017 by John Wiley & Sons Ltd.

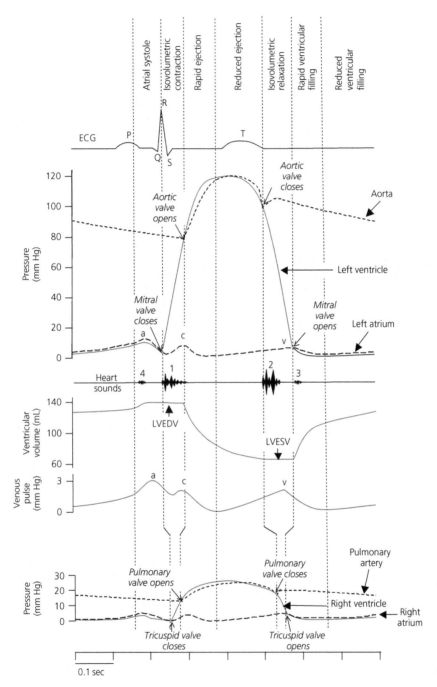

Figure 3.1 Wiggers diagram.

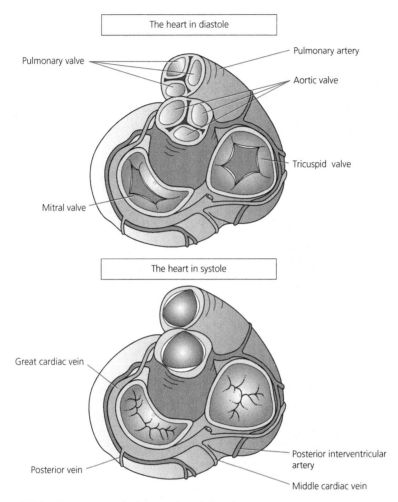

The heart in diastole

Pulmonary valve

Pulmonary artery

Aortic valve

Tricuspid valve

Mitral valve

The heart in systole

Great cardiac vein

Posterior vein

Posterior interventricular artery

Middle cardiac vein

Figure 3.2 Cardiac structures during systole and diastole.

Diastole is commonly divided into three components: rapid filling phase, slow filling phase, and atrial systole (Figure 3.3). A fourth phase of diastole, isovolumic relaxation, is sometimes utilized. This is the period between the closing of the semilunar valve and the opening of the atrioventricular (AV; = mitral and tricuspid) valve. It is very brief and dependent on the relaxation properties of the ventricle. Analysis of this phase is useful experimentally, but has limited application clinically.

The rapid filling period occurs immediately on opening of the AV valve. In normal individuals, this phase accounts for the majority of ventricular filling. This phase is characterized by the Y descent on atrial pressure tracings and by a

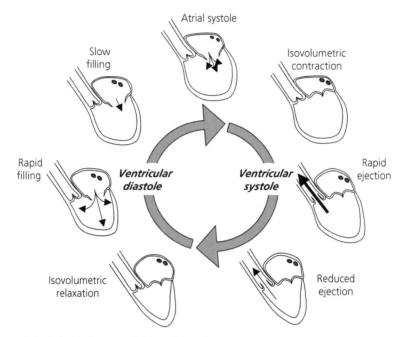

Figure 3.3 Mechanical events of the cardiac cycle.

rapid fall (because the ventricle is still relaxing) and then equally rapid rise in ventricular pressure. As the rate of ventricular filling declines, the slow filling phase is entered, following by diastasis (a period when ventricular filling ceases). During the slow filling period in a normal heart, the atrial and ventricular pressures are similar and continued filling of the ventricles is dependent on blood returning from the peripheral circulation (RV) or the lungs (LV). The slow filling period lasts longer than the rapid filling period in the normal heart. In patients with noncompliant ventricles, true diastasis may not occur. Rather, in the setting of elevated atrial pressure, passive blood flow from the atrium to the ventricle continues throughout diastole, with the rate of flow and increase in ventricular pressure dependent on the compliance of the diseased ventricle.

Atrial systole is the last phase of diastole. It occurs soon after the beginning of the P wave on the ECG and is concurrent with the A wave on the atrial pressure tracing. In the normal heart at rest, atrial systole contributes relatively little blood to the already filled ventricle. In the diseased heart, or in the normal heart during exercise, the contribution of atrial systole assumes a larger importance. In clinical practice, it is common to see patients with hypertrophied ventricles who do well until they develop atrial fibrillation. The rapid rate and the loss of atrial contraction can then precipitate congestive heart failure.

Cardiac chambers

Right atrium

Normal RA pressure is 2–8 mm Hg (Table 3.1) and is determined by central venous pressure (CVP), RA compliance, tricuspid valve function, and RV compliance (Figure 3.4). CVP, and thus RA pressure, is primarily influenced by blood volume, body position, reflex changes in venous tone, skeletal muscle contraction, and the respiratory cycle.

An examination of the RA pressure waveform in a patient in normal sinus rhythm reveals two major positive deflections, the A and V waves, and two negative deflections, the X and Y descents (Figure 3.5). A third minor positive deflection, the C wave, may be seen in some settings between the A and V waves. The A wave results from RA contraction and occurs immediately following the P wave on a surface ECG, with the peak of the A wave on the pressure tracing following the peak of the P wave on the ECG by approximately 60–80 milliseconds. Following RA contraction, the pressure declines, and this is manifested as the X descent. The X descent is caused by atrial relaxation as well as downward motion of the atrioventricular junction during early ventricular systole. The C wave, when seen, will interrupt the X descent, and is caused by tricuspid valve closure. The C wave

Table 3.1 Normal hemodynamic values.

Pressure measurement	Normal value (mm Hg)	Temporal relations of ECG to mechanical events
Right atrium (RA)		Onset of P wave to RA contraction is ~60–80 ms
Mean pressure	2–8	
Right ventricle (RV)		Onset of Q wave to RV contraction is ~65 ms
Peak-systolic pressure	17–32	
End-diastolic pressure	2–8	
Pulmonary artery		Onset of Q wave to RV ejection is ~80 ms
Mean pressure	9–19	
Peak-systolic pressure	17–32	
End-diastolic pressure	4–13	
Left atrium (PCWP)		Onset of P wave to LA contraction is ~85 ms.
Mean pressure	2–12	Onset of P wave on ECG to A wave on PCWP tracing will vary and may be >200 ms
Left ventricle (LV)		Onset of Q wave to LV contraction is ~52 ms
Peak-systolic pressure	90–140	
End-diastolic pressure	5–12	
Aorta		Onset of Q wave to LV ejection is ~115 ms
Mean pressure	70–105	

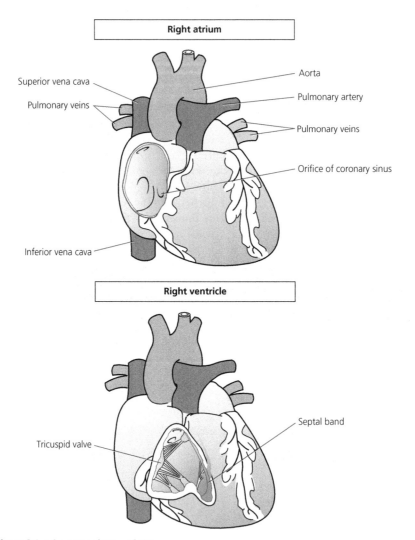

Figure 3.4 Schematic of RA and RV.

marks the onset of RV systole. It will be seen as a minor positive deflection immediately following the QRS complex, and will follow the A wave by a duration equal to the PR interval. After the peak of the C wave, the X descent continues (and is then called X prime; X′) as atrial relaxation occurs and the pressure declines. The V wave is seen following the nadir of the X descent and represents venous filling of the right atrium while the tricuspid valve is closed. The peak of the V wave occurs at the end of ventricular systole, just prior to tricuspid valve opening. V waves generally occur simultaneously with the T wave on a surface ECG. The Y descent follows the V wave and denotes the onset of RV diastole. This descent reflects the rapid fall of RA

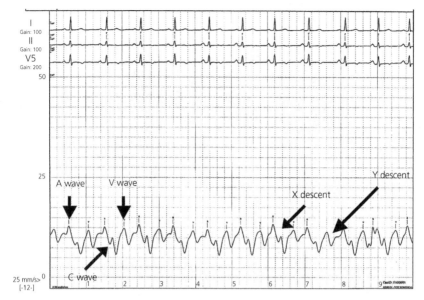

Figure 3.5 Right atrial pressure waveform.

pressure in conjunction with the exit of blood from the RA into the RV when the tricuspid valve opens (see Chapter 5 for a further discussion of atrial waveforms).

Right ventricle

Normal RV pressures are 2–8 mm Hg at the end of diastole and 17–32 mm Hg during systole. The pressure in the RV rises rapidly during systole, and when it exceeds the pressure in the RA, the tricuspid valve closes. Pressure rises further as contraction continues in the closed chamber, and when the pressure exceeds that in the pulmonary artery, the pulmonary valve will open. The waveform reflecting RV systole has a rapid upstroke and is rounded, and will occur with or immediately following the QRS complex (Figure 3.6). The peak of this waveform is the RV systolic pressure. As systole ends and ventricular relaxation occurs, pressure in the RV will rapidly fall to baseline, marking the onset of ventricular diastole. The pulmonary valve will close when the pressure in the RV falls below pressure in the pulmonary artery. When the pressure falls below that in the RA, the tricuspid valve will open.

RV diastole can be divided into three phases (Figure 3.7). The first phase comes with the opening of the tricuspid valve, and accounts for early filling of the ventricle, approximately 60–75% of total filling in the normal heart. The second phase is the slow filling period and accounts for 15–25% of RV filling. In some patients this phase will include a period of diastasis in which ventricular filling slows or ceases. Finally, the third phase occurs with RA systole, and accounts for 10–25% of total filling. At this point, the tricuspid valve is open, creating essentially one right-sided

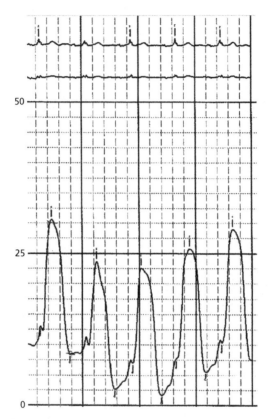

Figure 3.6 Ventricular pressure tracing.

chamber, so it follows that this waveform is simultaneous with and identical in morphology and amplitude to the A wave on the RA pressure tracing. The pressure at the end of this waveform represents RV end-diastolic pressure.

Left atrial pressure (pulmonary capillary wedge pressure)

Normal LA pressure ranges from 2–12 mm Hg, and is typically measured indirectly, via a balloon-tipped catheter placed in a distal branch of the pulmonary artery. Inflation of the balloon obstructs flow and allows pressure to equilibrate along the column of blood, thus giving an estimate of LA pressure. This pressure is called the pulmonary capillary wedge pressure (PCWP), or simply wedge pressure. LA mechanical events are transmitted retrograde through this column of blood in a wedge pressure tracing, thus the deflections on the wedge pressure waveform are often damped and delayed relative to events in the LA (and on the ECG). The LA (or PCWP) pressure wave, like an RA pressure wave, consists of positive A, C, and V waves, and negative X and Y descents.

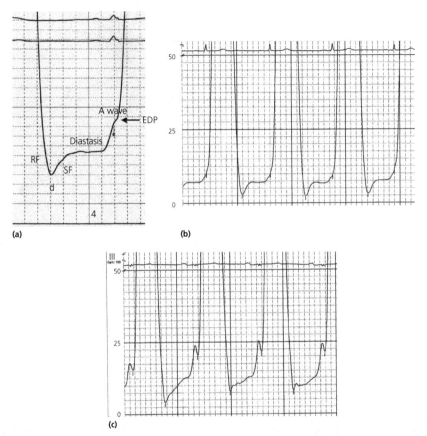

Figure 3.7 Ventricular diastole. The ventricular diastolic pressure waveform can be divided into three phases (a): the early or rapid filling (RF) phase occurs with the opening of the tricuspid valve. The slow filling (SF) phase follows and extends until the onset of right atrial systole (A wave). The nadir in pressure following the A wave is the right ventricular end-diastolic pressure (EDP). Left ventricular diastolic pressure is shown in a normal heart (b) and in a stiff, non-compliant ventricle (c). Note the elevated LVEDP, prominent A wave, and rapid rise in LV diastolic pressures with atrial contraction.

Left ventricle

Normal LV pressure is from 90–140 mm Hg during systole and 5–12 mm Hg during diastole. While the pressures in the LV are much higher than in the RV, the pressure waveform components are similar. LV systole leads to a rapid increase in pressure. The mitral valve closes when the pressure exceeds that in the LA (Figure 3.8). The pressure rises with continued contraction, and when it exceeds the pressure in the aorta, the aortic valve opens and ventricular ejection begins. LV pressure then continues to rise through the rapid ejection phase of systole, and peaks during the T wave of a surface ECG. Pressure in the LV then begins to decline through the reduced ejection phase of systole. When the pressure in the

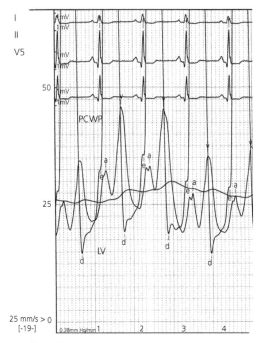

Figure 3.8 Simultaneous LV and PCWP tracings. The pressure tracing was taken from a 57-year-old male with severe ischemic cardiomyopathy. Note the large V wave and prominent A wave in the PCWP tracing.

LV falls below that in the aorta, the aortic valve closes and LV pressure continues to decline due to isovolumetric ventricular relaxation. When the pressure drops below that of the left atrium, the mitral valve opens and the left atrium empties into the LV. The mitral valve opening marks the onset of ventricular diastole. LV diastole, like RV diastole, consists of three phases.

Pulmonary artery

Normal pulmonary artery pressures range from 17–32 mm Hg during systole and from 4–13 mm Hg during diastole. The pulmonary artery waveform reflects the pressure seen during systole as blood is ejected from the RV into the pulmonary artery. Because of the pulmonic valve being open at this point, this waveform will be similar to the right ventricular systolic waveform. The pressure in the pulmonary artery and the RV declines as systole comes to an end. When the pressure in the RV falls below that in the pulmonary artery, the pulmonic valve closes, marked by a dicrotic notch on the downslope of the pulmonary artery pressure waveform. The dicrotic notch marks the end of ventricular ejection. The decline in pressure in the pulmonary artery continues gradually after closure of the pulmonic valve as blood flows through the pulmonary arteries and veins toward the left atrium. Note that the peak of the pulmonary artery waveform occurs within the T wave on a surface ECG.

Aorta

The shape of the pressure waveform generated in the aorta is similar to that generated in the pulmonary artery, with pressures significantly higher in the aorta. The upstroke of the aortic pressure waveform denotes the onset of left ventricular ejection, and occurs once the pressure in the left ventricle has exceeded the pressure in the aorta and the aortic valve has opened (Figure 3.1). In the absence of aortic valve or perivalvular pathology, the aortic systolic pressure will be equal to the left ventricular systolic pressure. Aortic and left ventricular pressures decline with reduced ejection and contraction, and when the ventricular pressure drops below that of the aorta, the aortic valve closes. This is sometimes apparent in the pressure waveform as a dicrotic notch in the downslope of the aortic pressure tracing.

The definition of hypertension has changed over time as the deleterious effects of even minor increases in blood pressure have been realized. The classification of normal blood pressure and hypertension is described in Chapter 5.

Left ventricular function

Myocardial contractile dysfunction is an important cause of morbidity and mortality and LV systolic function is an important determinant of survival in patients with cardiomyopathy and/or coronary artery disease. Despite its tremendous importance, clinical measurement of LV function is limited by the inability to assess myocyte performance directly. Instead, various surrogates such as ejection fraction are used. In interpreting these tests, it is important to remember that LV function is a dynamic process that varies not only with contractility, but also with preload and afterload.

Measurement of left ventricular preload

Preload for the ventricles is defined as amount of passive tension or stretch exerted on the ventricular walls (i.e., intraventricular pressure) just prior to the initiation of systole. This load determines end-diastolic sarcomere length and thus the force of contraction. The Frank–Starling law states that the passive length to which the myocardial cells are stretched at the end of diastole determines the active tension they develop when stimulated to contract. The Frank–Starling law is an intrinsic property of myocytes and is not dependent on extrinsic factors such as the autonomic nervous system or circulating hormones. The general principle is that increased preload causes increased force of contraction, which increases stroke volume and thus cardiac output.

In a given patient, elevated filling pressures do not differentiate primary diastolic dysfunction from primary systolic dysfunction, but do give an indication of the preload required to obtain a specific cardiac output.

Left ventricular preload as measured by LV end-diastolic pressure (LVEDP) is a common tool used clinically in assessment of LV performance. The LVEDP immediately precedes isometric ventricular contraction (Figure 3.6). This point, also known as the "Z" point, is located on the downslope of the LV "A" wave at the crossing over

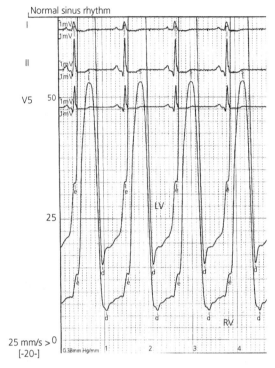

Figure 3.9 Abnormal EDP. Simultaneous RV and LV pressures from the 57-year-old male with severe ischemic cardiomyopathy depicted in Figure 3.8. Note that both LVEDP and RVEDP are elevated, demonstrating that both RV and LV are poorly compliant.

of LA and LV pressures and is coincident with the R wave on the surface ECG. Since the mitral valve is open during atrial contraction, the A wave is represented in the LV pressure tracing coincident with the A wave in the atrial tracing. Identification of the true LVEDP can at times be difficult, especially when using fluid-filled catheters.

LVEDP is influenced by ventricular compliance and intravascular volume status. LVEDP is normally <12 mm Hg, but may be elevated when the LV experiences volume (e.g., mitral regurgitation or aortic regurgitation) or pressure (e.g., hypertension or aortic stenosis) overload. Impairment of myocardial contractility also alters the diastolic pressure–volume relationship and shifts the end-diastolic pressure point upward (Figure 3.9).

Inspection of the waveform in diastole provides information about LV diastolic function that can supplement LVEDP. Myocardial relaxation abnormalities are suggested by the continuing decline of pressure during early diastole, with the pressure nadir occurring midway through the diastolic period. Alternatively, a stiff, poorly compliant ventricle is suggested by an abnormally tall A wave, resulting in a marked elevation of LVEDP, although the diastolic pressure prior to atrial contraction can be normal (Figure 3.10).

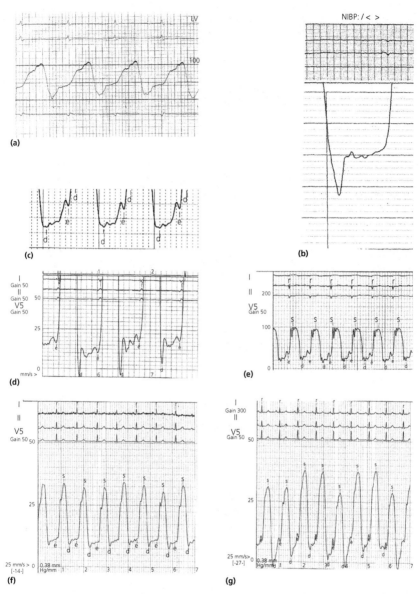

Figure 3.10 Examples of different ventricular diastolic waveforms. LV tracings taken from a patient with (a) aortic insufficiency (note the rapid rise in diastolic pressure); (b) constrictive pericarditis (note the dip and plateau configuration); (c) hypertrophic cardiomyopathy (note the elevated end-diastolic pressure and accentuated A wave); (d) restrictive cardiomyopathy (note the dip and plateau configuration); (e) ischemic cardiomyopathy (note the elevated end-diastolic pressure and accentuated A wave); and pericardial tamponade before (f) and after (g) pericardiocentesis.

Pressure–volume loops

A useful method of displaying the relationship between ventricular volume and pressure during the cardiac cycle is the pressure–volume loop (Figure 3.11). Stroke volume (change in volume) and stroke work (stroke volume × mean arterial pressure [MAP] or alternatively the area inscribed by the P–V loop) can be calculated using PV loops. Different pressure–volume loops are obtained following changes in preload, afterload, or contractility (Figure 3.12) and in different disease states (Figure 3.13).

Ventricular performance can be depicted by plotting LVEDP versus stroke volume or cardiac output (Figure 3.14). This curvilinear relationship is commonly called the LV function curve. Ventricular function curves are shifted upward by inotropes and downward by interventions impairing inotropic activity. Afterload may also significantly influence the elevation or decline of the ventricular function curve.

Indices of contractility

A completely satisfactory clinical index of contractility that is independent of preload and afterload has not been defined. The maximal rate of myocyte fiber shortening in the isolated heart correlates well and is little affected by preload or afterload, but is obviously of no use clinically. In the intact heart, contractility is best measured by the pressure–volume point as the aortic valve closes. Another index of contractility is dP/dt_{max}, which is the derivative of the maximal rate of

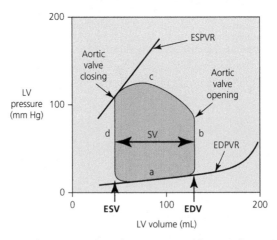

Figure 3.11 Schematic of pressure–volume loop in a normal heart. Following mitral valve opening, ventricular filling occurs with only a small increase in pressure despite a large increase in volume (a). The first segment of systole is isovolumic contraction (b). When the aortic valve opens, ejection begins and LV volume falls as LV pressure continues to rise (c). After closure of the aortic valve, isovolumic relaxation occurs (d). This point marks the end-systolic pressure–volume point on the curve. [EDPVR = end-diastole pressure–volume relationship; ESPVR = end-systole pressure–volume relationship.]

(A)

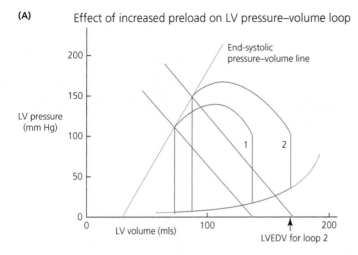

Effect of increased preload on LV pressure–volume loop

Loop 2 has an increased preload (increased LVEDV) as compared to loop 1.
Note: Loop 2 has a larger stroke volume than loop 1.

The afterload and contractility have remained constant. The afterload lines for the two loops are parallel so they have the same afterload. Both end-systolic points are on the same contractility line so the two loops have the same contractility.
(See discussion of contractility and afterload lines later in the chapter.)

(B)

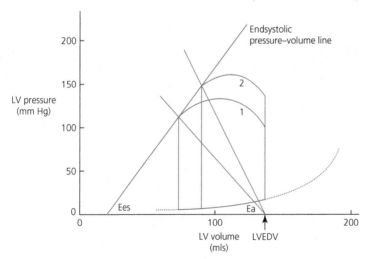

Effect of increased afterload on LV pressure–volume loop

Figure 3.12 Effect of changes in preload, afterload, and contractility on pressure–volume relationship.

(C)

Effect of increased contractility on LV pressure–volume loop

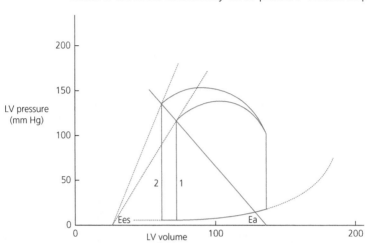

Note the increased stroke volume for loop 2 (which has the increased contractility).
- The increased slope of the end-systolic pressure–volume line is an index of the increased contractility.
- The end-systolic points of both loops lie on the same 'afterload line' so their afterload is the same for the two loops.
- The LVEDV is the same for the loops so the preload is the same.

Figure 3.12 (Continued)

ventricular pressure rise during the isovolumetric period. A complete discussion of indices of contraction is beyond the scope of this chapter.

Respiratory variation

The act of breathing influences hemodynamic measurements (Figure 3.15). Even in healthy patients, intravascular pressure in the thoracic aorta and vena cava (and thus preload and afterload) may be significantly altered by normal respiration. During normal, spontaneous respiration, intrathoracic pressure may drop from −3 to −4 mm Hg at end-expiration to −7 to −8 mm Hg during end-inspiration. With regard to cardiac chambers, this decreases transmural pressure in the normally compliant left atrium, resulting in an underestimation of wedge pressure. Conversely, during mechanical ventilation, intrathoracic pressure may increase to >10 mm Hg during end-inspiration. PCWP measurement is also particularly vulnerable to elevations in intrathoracic pressure, because elevated intrathoracic pressure blocks retrograde transmission of left atrial pressure events to the catheter tip, resulting in a significant underestimation of wedge pressure. In both cases, since end-expiration more closely resembles atmospheric pressure, intra-cardiac pressures should be recorded at end-expiration (Figure 3.16).

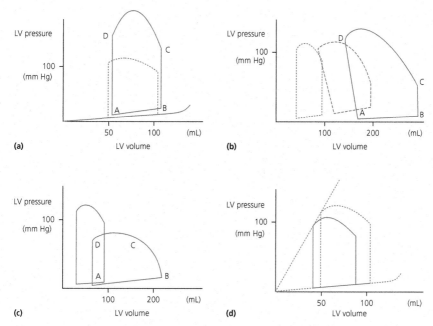

Figure 3.13 Schematics of pressure–volume loops in various disease states. (a) Aortic stenosis is characterized by a marked increase in afterload, minimal increase in preload, and increased contractility (dotted line is normal ventricle). (b) Aortic insufficiency (AI) is characterized by a marked increase in preload, with a smaller increase in afterload and decreased contractility. Acute aortic insufficiency manifests as increased preload with minimal change in afterload or contractility (dotted line, normal ventricle; dashed line, acute AI; full line, chronic AI). (c) Chronic mitral regurgitation is associated with a marked increase in preload, decreased afterload, and decreased contractility. (d) Mitral stenosis is primarily characterized by decreased preload.

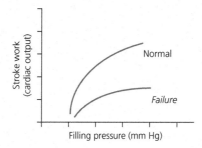

Figure 3.14 Ventricular function curve. Schematic of the relationship between filling pressure and cardiac output (or stroke volume) in a normal and in a failing left ventricle.

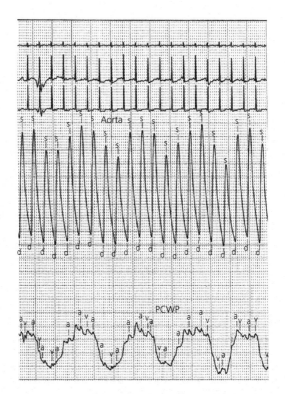

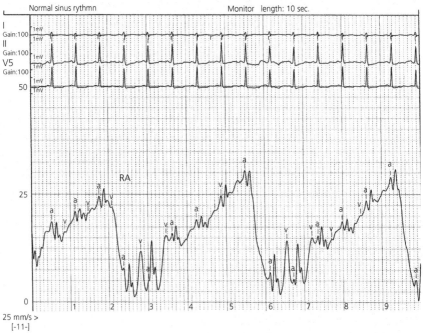

Figure 3.15 Respiratory variation. Aortic, PCWP, and RA pressure in a patient with large respiratory variation.

Normal respiration

No respiratory effort

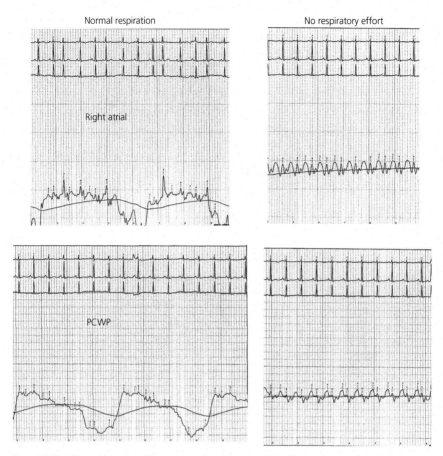

Right atrial

PCWP

Figure 3.16 Effect of breath hold on RA and PCW pressures (all pressures recorded on a 25 mm Hg scale).

CHAPTER 4

Arterial pressure

George A. Stouffer

Arterial blood pressure is one of the most fundamental measurements in hemodynamics. Because of the need to quantify pressure levels, emphasis is placed on mean, systolic, or diastolic values (see Table 4.1). These values, while tremendously useful, do not provide complete information to characterize the composite pressure wave, either within the aorta or as it undergoes significant changes during propagation within the arterial system.

The aortic pressure wave is not just determined by left ventricular mechanics, but rather results from hydraulic interactions between blood ejected from the contracting left ventricle and the systemic arterial system. The central aortic pressure wave is composed of a forward-traveling wave generated by left ventricular ejection followed by a backward-traveling wave reflected from the periphery. Ejection of blood into the aorta generates a pressure wave that is propagated to other arteries throughout the body at a given velocity (termed pulse wave velocity, PWV). At any discontinuity of the vascular wall, but mainly at the arteriolar branching points, the wave is reflected and comes back toward the heart at the same PWV. One way to think about reflected waves is to note that they would be absent if the aorta were an open tube rather than part of a closed system.

Pressure wave reflection in the arterial system serves two beneficial purposes. When normally timed, the reflected wave returns to the central aorta in diastole and therefore enhances diastolic perfusion pressure in the coronary circulation. Partial wave reflection also returns a portion of the pulsatile energy content of the waveform to the central aorta where it is dissipated by viscous damping. Thus, wave reflection limits transmission of pulsatile energy into the periphery where it might otherwise damage the microcirculation.

The velocity at which the outgoing and reflected waves travel is dependent on the properties (especially elasticity) of the arteries along which they propagate. PWV increases with stiffness and is defined by the Moens–Korteweg

Cardiovascular Hemodynamics for the Clinician, Second Edition. Edited by George A. Stouffer.
© 2017 John Wiley & Sons Ltd. Published 2017 by John Wiley & Sons Ltd.

Table 4.1 Definition of terms used to describe blood pressure.

Term	Definition
Systolic blood pressure	Maximum pressure (peak of arterial pressure wave)
Diastolic blood pressure	Minimum pressure (trough of arterial pressure wave)
Pulse pressure	Difference between systolic and diastolic pressure
Mean arterial pressure	Average pressure during the cardiac cycle

equation, $PWV = (Eh/2\rho R)$, where E is Young's modulus of the arterial wall (a measurement of elasticity), h is wall thickness, R is arterial radius at the end of diastole, and ρ is blood density. An important (although simplified) concept is that the longitudinal velocity of pressure waves traveling in distensible tubes is slowed by the extent that the vessel expands with each pulsation. In the normal arterial system, there is a steep gradient of increasing arterial stiffness moving outward from the heart. In a young adult, PWV is only 4–6 m/s in the highly compliant proximal aorta and increases to 8–10 m/s in the stiffer peripheral muscular arteries.

Disturbed reflection, for example with increased PWV, can cause the reflected waves to occur earlier, arriving in the central arteries during systole and not during diastole. Thus as aortic elasticity declines, transmission velocity of both forward and reflected waves increases, which causes the reflected wave to arrive at the central aorta earlier in the cardiac cycle and therefore augment pressure in late systole. This in turn contributes to an increase in systolic blood pressure and pulse pressure and a decrease in diastolic blood pressure [1]. These changes increase left ventricular afterload and decrease coronary perfusion pressure.

The concept of PWV was originally described early in the twentieth century, but recent advances in noninvasive technologies have greatly increased the interest in using PWV as a surrogate for vascular disease. There are many different ways to measure PWV, but the concept is similar in each. The time delay between arterial pulse wave arrival at a proximal artery (e.g., carotid) and a more distal artery (e.g., the femoral) is measured noninvasively. The distance traveled by the pulse wave is estimated (unless aortic imaging is available to enable direct measurement) and PWV is then calculated as distance/time (m/s). Measurement of PWV has been shown to correlate with aortic stiffness and, more importantly, to be predictive of clinical events [2,3]. Not surprisingly, PWV is increased in individuals with hypertension, diabetes mellitus (DM), tobacco use, atherosclerosis, and end-stage renal disease (CKD).

A simplified relationship to remember is stiffer arteries → increased PWV → earlier arrival of reflected waves → augmentation of systolic rather than diastolic pressure → increased pulse pressure.

Table 4.2 Recommendations for the management of hypertension by the Panel Members Appointed to the Eighth Joint National Committee (JNC 8).

	SBP (mm Hg)	DBP (mm Hg)
Patients <60 years	140	90
Patients >60 years	150	90
Patients with DM	140	90
Patients with CKD	140	90

Aortic pressure

The definition of hypertension has changed over time as more data have become available on the deleterious effects of different levels of blood pressure. Recommendations for levels of systolic blood pressure (SBP) and diastolic blood pressure (SBP) that would require treatment from the Report of the Eighth Joint National Committee (JNC 8) are described in Table 4.2 [4].

Aortic pressure is the primary determinant of the afterload against which the left ventricle (LV) must pump blood. Given constant preload and contractility, an increase in afterload will reduce cardiac output. The primary determinants of afterload are mean arterial pressure, aortic compliance (distensibility), and aortic valve resistance (the normal aortic valve presents minimal resistance to flow). Thus, hypertension, calcified arteries, and aortic stenosis all represent conditions of increased afterload.

Mean arterial pressure

The mean arterial pressure (MAP) is the average pressure during the cardiac cycle. Calculation of the true MAP requires integration of the arterial pressure over time. In clinical medicine, a useful approximation of MAP when the heart rate is 60 bpm can be obtained using the following formula:

$$MAP = DBP + 1/3(\text{pulse pressure})$$

where DBP is the diastolic blood pressure. This formula is only applicable at lower heart rates, because the relative amount of time spent in systole increases at higher heart rates.

The major determinant of systolic pressure is stroke volume. Lesser influences include diastolic pressure and aortic compliance. The major determinant of diastolic pressure is systemic vascular resistance (in turn, primarily determined by arteriolar resistance). Lesser determinants include systolic pressure, aortic compliance, and heart rate. The normal aorta is distensible and the diameter can increase up to 15%

during LV systole. During diastole, this stored potential energy is released as the aorta recoils, thus helping to maintain diastolic blood pressure (sometimes called the diastolic pump). With age, compliance of the aorta decreases as elastin and collagen change in both amount and properties. Systolic pressure, more so than diastolic pressure, tends to increase with age in individuals over 50 years old and this can be at least partially explained by changes in aortic stiffness. Diastolic pressure, largely determined by peripheral arterial resistance, increases until middle age and then tends to fall. In contrast, systolic pressure and pulse pressure, influenced more by the stiffness of large arteries, as well as peripheral pulse wave reflection and the pattern of left ventricular ejection, increase continuously with age.

Pressure waveform

A pressure waveform generated in the aorta has a characteristic waveform (Figure 4.1). When pressure in the LV exceeds aortic pressure, the aortic valve opens and blood flows rapidly from the LV into the aorta. The steep upstroke (or anacrotic limb) coincides with opening of the aortic valve and reflects the stroke volume ejected by the LV into the aorta (Figure 4.2). The rounded part at the top

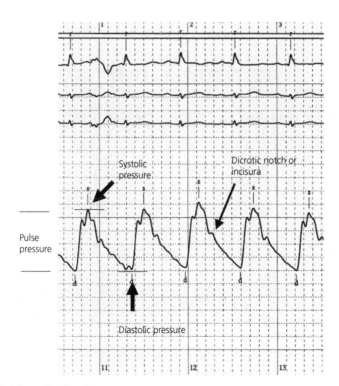

Figure 4.1 Schematic of aortic pressure.

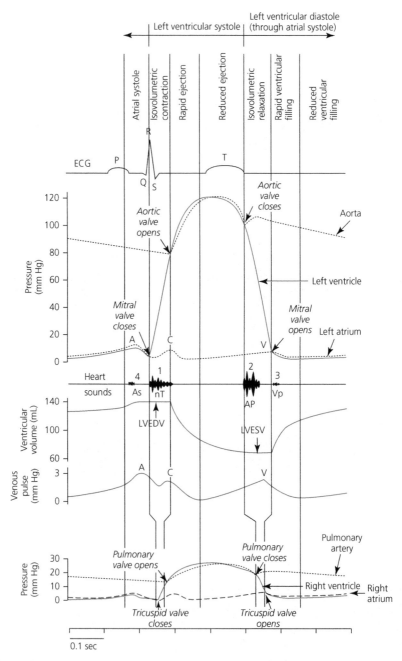

Figure 4.2 Wiggers diagram [LVEDV = Left Ventricular End Diastolic Volume; LVESV = Left Ventricular End Systolic Volume].

of the waveform (or anacrotic shoulder) reflects continued flow from the LV to the aorta, but at a reduced rate. The downslope of the pressure tracing (or dicrotic limb) is divided by the dicrotic notch (or incisura), which represents closure of the aortic valve. The location of the dicrotic notch varies according to the timing of aortic closure in the cardiac cycle and will be delayed in patients with hypovolemia (Figure 4.3).

Aortic and LV systolic pressures decline during the "reduced ejection" phase, which coincides with LV repolarization. When the ventricular pressure drops below that of the aorta, the aortic valve closes. This is represented in the pressure waveform as a dicrotic notch in the downslope of the aortic pressure tracing. This marks the end of LV ejection. Diastolic pressure declines gradually as blood flows from the aorta into the peripheral vessels.

The contour of the aortic pressure tracing can provide clues to various disease states (Table 4.3 and Figure 4.4): for example, aortic pressure that rises rapidly, dips, and then rises again (pulsus bisferiens) in hypertrophic obstructive cardiomyopathy or rises slowly (pulsus parvus et tardus) in aortic stenosis (Figure 4.5).

The augmentation index (AIx) is the proportion of central PP that results from arterial wave reflection and is a commonly used measure of arterial stiffness

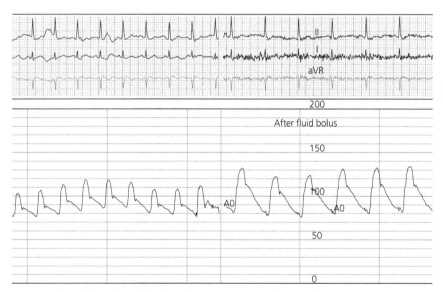

Figure 4.3 Aortic pressure in a hypovolemic patient. Aortic pressure tracings taken in a patient before and after an intravenous (IV) fluid bolus. The aortic waveform has a characteristic shape when left ventricular filling pressures are low. Aortic pressures are low, pulse pressure decreases, the dicrotic limb is steeper, and the dicrotic notch is delayed. The diastolic phase of the aortic pressure tracing gives an indication of peripheral runoff and may also be abnormal. In severe dehydration, there is a sudden descent in aortic pressure and then an almost flat diastolic phase.

Table 4.3 Disease states associated with various pulse characteristics.

Label	Characteristics	Disease states
Bounding	Large pulse pressure	Aortic insufficiency, hyperkinetic states (e.g., fever, thyrotoxicosis, anemia), AV fistula
Pulsus parvus et tardus	Slow and weak pulse	Aortic stenosis
Pulsus bisferiens	Two systolic peaks prior to dicrotic notch	Hypertrophic obstructive cardiomyopathy; more rarely in aortic insufficiency
Pulsus alternans	Alternating strong and weak pulses	Severe LV dysfunction
Pulsus paradoxus	Excessive decrease (>10 mm Hg) in systolic pressure with inspiration	Cardiac tamponade; less frequently it can be observed with acute aortic regurgitation (i.e., acute aortic dissection), elevated LVEDP, atrial septal defect, pulmonary hypertension, or right ventricular hypertrophy
Dicrotic pulse	Two systolic peaks with one occurring after dicrotic notch	Low cardiac output + low peripheral resistance; rare in patients >45 years old

(Figure 4.6). AIx is a function of the timing of the arrival of the reflected wave at the proximal aorta (determined mostly by large artery PWV) and the magnitude of the reflected waves. The magnitude of reflected waves is determined by the diameter and elasticity of small arteries and arterioles and is thus influenced by vasoactive drugs. AIx is positively correlated with age and blood pressure, and inversely correlated with height and heart rate.

Effects of respiration on aortic pressure

Changes in thoracic pressure with respiration will influence blood pressure. During normal, spontaneous respiration, intrathoracic pressure decreases during inspiration, which in turn causes a decrease in pericardial and right atrial pressures. This results in augmented systemic venous return to right-sided chambers and decreased venous return to left-sided chambers. It is thus normal to have a slight decrease in systolic blood pressure (approximately 5 mm Hg) with inspiration (Figure 4.7). Pulsus paradoxus is an exaggerated decrease in systolic pressure with inspiration and has been variously defined as a drop of >12 mm Hg, a drop of ≥10 mm Hg, or a drop of ≥9% during normal inspiration.

Not surprisingly, positive pressure ventilation causes an inversion in the normal relationship between respiration and blood pressure. Blood pressure will increase during inspiration (as thoracic pressure increases).

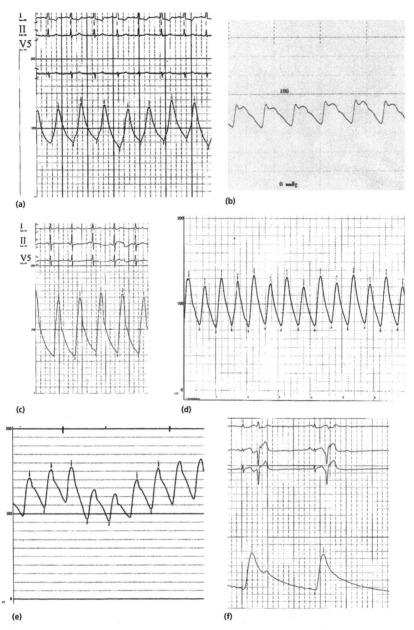

Figure 4.4 Arterial pressure tracings in various pathologic conditions. Aortic stenosis is characterized by slow upstroke (a). Bisferiens pulse, a name derived from Latin *bis* (= two) + *feriere* (= to beat), is characterized by an initial rapid rise in aortic pressure (spike), followed by a slight drop in pressure (dip), and then a secondary peak (dome), and is most commonly associated with hypertrophic obstructive cardiomyopathy (b). Severe aortic regurgitation is characterized by a wide pulse pressure (c). Pulsus alternans with beat-to-beat variability in systolic pressure is found in a patient with cardiomyopathy (d). Exaggerated decrease in systolic pressure with inspiration defines pulsus paradoxus (e). Bradycardia with hypotension and ineffective generation of systolic blood pressure during PVCs is apparent in a patient with inferior myocardial infarction (f).

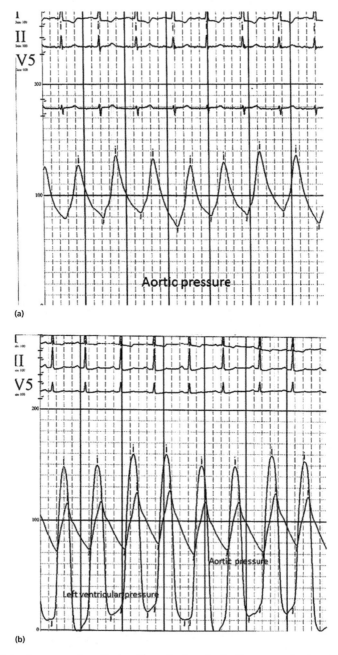

(a)

(b)

Figure 4.5 Aortic pressure in patients with aortic stenosis. Aortic pressure tracings taken in a 60-year-old male with aortic valve area of 0.4 cm^2 (a) and in a 58-year-old male with aortic valve area of 1.1 cm^2 (b). Note the delayed upstroke in the aortic pressure tracing during ventricular systole, especially in relation to the rise in left ventricular pressure (b).

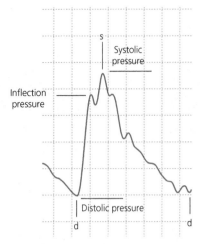

Figure 4.6 Augmentation index—the augmentation index (AIx) is given by $\text{AIx} = \pm \dfrac{P_s - P_i}{P_s - P_d}$ with P_s, P_d, and P_i indicating systolic, diastolic, and inflection pressure, respectively.

Peripheral amplification

Peripheral amplification is said to occur when systolic blood pressure is higher in peripheral arteries (e.g., femoral or brachial) than in the aorta (mean pressures will be the same). It is primarily observed in young individuals and is caused by the reflected pressure waves returning to the aorta during diastole (and to the peripheral arteries in late systole), making pulse pressure higher in peripheral than in central arteries (Figure 4.8).

Noninvasive measurement of blood pressure

Intra-aortic pressures are measured directly in the intensive care unit, operating room, and cardiac catheterization laboratory. Most clinical decisions are, however, based on noninvasive measurement of blood pressure. This introduces two potential problems: inaccuracies associated with noninvasive measurement of arterial pressure; and inaccuracies associated with the use of the brachial artery, rather than the aorta, as the site of measurement. Despite these limitations, there is a large amount of information including a study of more than 1,000,000 patients [5] demonstrating the usefulness of noninvasively determined brachial blood pressure in clinical decision making.

Determination of blood pressure by sphygmomanometer utilizes sounds that are thought to originate from a combination of turbulent flow and arterial wall oscillations. As the blood pressure cuff is deflated from a supraphysiologic pressure, flow through the brachial artery will begin once the systolic pressure is

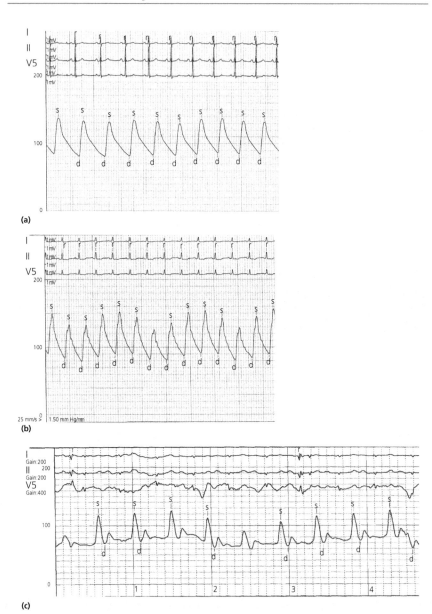

Figure 4.7 Effect of respiration on aortic pressure. The tracing in (a) is from a healthy 43-year-old female. Note the slight decrease (<10 mm Hg) in systolic pressure with respiration. The tracing in (b) is from a patient with pleural effusions. Note that the systolic pressure declines by 18–22 mm Hg with respiration. The tracing in (c) is taken from a patient in cardiac tamponade. Systolic pressure decreases by approximately 30 mm Hg with inspiration. Note also that the waveform is very abnormal with a steep dicrotic limb, narrow ejection phase, and flat diastolic phase. These findings are consistent with decreased stroke volume and vasoconstriction.

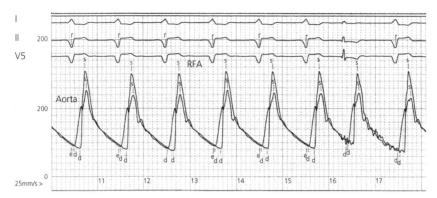

Figure 4.8 Peripheral amplification. Simultaneous aortic and right femoral artery pressures in a 49-year-old male with aortic insufficiency. Note that the systolic pressure is higher and the rapid increase phase narrower in the RFA.

reached. Turbulent flow (and arterial oscillation) ceases once cuff pressure falls below diastolic pressure.

In 1905, at a conference at the Imperial Medical Academy, Dr. Nicolai Korotkoff announced a new way to measure blood pressure. Since that time, the sounds heard by a stethoscope placed over the brachial artery during blood pressure cuff deflation have been called Korotkoff sounds and can be divided into five phases. Phase 1 occurs when the cuff pressure equals the systolic pressure and is characterized by a sharp tapping sound. As cuff pressure is lowered, phase 2 occurs, which is characterized by softer and longer sounds. Phase 3 is defined by a resumption of crisp tapping sounds, similar to those heard in phase 1. Phase 4 begins when there is an abrupt muffling of sound as turbulent flow decreases. Finally, phase 5 is when turbulent flow ceases and thus no sound is heard. There is agreement that the onset of phase 1 corresponds to systolic and that the disappearance of sounds (phase 5) corresponds to diastolic pressure. Although some investigators have advocated using phase 4 to define diastole, general practice now is to use phase 4 only in situations in which sounds are audible even after complete deflation of the cuff, such as in pregnancy, arteriovenous fistulas, and aortic insufficiency. No clinical significance has been attached to phases 2 and 3. It is important to note that using Korotkoff sounds to measure blood pressure tends to underestimate intra-arterial systolic pressure and overestimate intra-arterial diastolic pressure [6].

Oscillometric blood pressure devices

Automated oscillometric devices are commonly used to measure brachial artery blood pressure. These devices work by measuring the amplitude of pressure changes as the cuff is deflated. In general, oscillometric devices measure mean blood pressure (MAP) and calculate systolic SBP and DBP based on a proprietary algorithm that, for each manufacturer, is the same for all patients irrespective of age, height, sex, vascular disease, or other clinical variables. Oscillometric MAP correlates well with central aortic MAP, but the assumption that a common algorithm can be used to determine SBP and DBP for all patients may not be correct. Studies have shown that the accuracy of oscillometric pressure is dependent on height, gender, and age [7,8].

Fun fact: The ascending aortic pressure waveform in a kangaroo has a very large secondary wave that begins in late systole or early diastole and continues throughout most of diastole. The peak of this secondary wave is often greater than peak systolic pressure (similar to the aortic pressure waveform obtained in a patient with an intra-aortic balloon pump). The accentuated secondary wave in the kangaroo results from intense wave reflections in the large muscular lower body, which dominate the small wave reflections from the diminutive upper body (*Circulation Research* 1986;59:247–255).

References

1 Safar ME, Levy BI, Struijker-Boudier H. Current perspectives on arterial stiffness and pulse pressure in hypertension and cardiovascular diseases. *Circulation* 2003;**107**:2864–2869.

2 Blacher J, Asmar R, Djane S, London GM, Safar ME. Aortic pulse wave velocity as a marker of cardiovascular risk in hypertensive patients. *Hypertension* 1999;**33**:1111–1117.

3 Laurent S, Boutouyrie P, Asmar R, et al. Aortic stiffness is an independent predictor of allcause and cardiovascular mortality in hypertensive patients. *Hypertension* 2001;**37**:1236–1241.

4 James PA, Oparil S, Carter BL, et al. 2014 evidence-based guideline for the management of high blood pressure in adults: report from the panel members appointed to the Eighth Joint National Committee (JNC 8). *JAMA* 2014;**311**(5):507–520.

5 Lewington S, Clarke R, Qizilbash N, Peto R, Collins R. Age-specific relevance of usual blood pressure to vascular mortality: a meta-analysis of individual data for one million adults in 61 prospective studies. *Lancet* 2002;**360**:1903–1913.

6 Pickering TG, Hall JE, Appel LJ, et al. Recommendations for blood pressure measurement in humans and experimental animals. Part 1: blood pressure measurement in humans: a statement for professionals from the Subcommittee of Professional and Public Education of the American Heart Association Council on High Blood Pressure Research. *Circulation* 2005;**111**:697–716.

7 Alpert BS, Quinn D, Gallick, D. Oscillometric blood pressure: a review for clinicians. *J Am Soc Hypertens* 2014;**8**(12):930–938.

8 Bhatt SD, Hinderliter AL, Stouffer GA. Influence of sex on the accuracy of oscillometric-derived blood pressures. *J Clin Hypertens* 2011;**13**(2):112–119.

CHAPTER 5

The atrial waveform

David P. McLaughlin and George A. Stouffer

A fundamental understanding of the atrial waveform is extremely important for anyone applying hemodynamics to patient care. Data regarding volume status, valvular pathology, and ventricular compliance are contained within the tracings when examined carefully. The right atrial (RA) waveform is typically measured directly with a fluid-filled pressure catheter. The left atrial waveform can be measured directly by transseptal atrial puncture or more commonly indirectly via a balloon-tipped pulmonary artery catheter. In most cases, the pulmonary capillary wedge pressure (PCWP) accurately reflects mean left atrial (LA) pressure; however, the pressure wave deflections are delayed and damped on a PCWP tracing compared to LA pressures [1]. Similarly, the timing of the atrial waves and descents in reference to the electrocardiogram (ECG) will occur later in the PCWP tracing than the RA tracing, because of the delay in transmission of pressures from the left atrium through the pulmonary vein, capillaries, and pulmonary artery to the tip of the catheter.

The components of the atrial wave

In patients who are in sinus rhythm, the atrial waveform is composed of two positive and two negative deflections (Figure 5.1). The A wave is caused by atrial contraction and usually occurs 60–80 milliseconds after the onset of the P wave on the ECG. The A wave is delayed to about 200 milliseconds after the onset of the P wave when measured using PCWP, due to the time delay in transmission of the reflected wave. The A wave is absent in atrial fibrillation (because of the lack of atrial contraction) and is exaggerated in patients with a noncompliant ventricle or in the presence of tricuspid or mitral stenosis.

The decay of the A wave is the X descent, which is due to the decrease in atrial pressure as a consequence of atrial relaxation (Figure 5.1). In the RA the X descent

Cardiovascular Hemodynamics for the Clinician, Second Edition. Edited by George A. Stouffer.
© 2017 John Wiley & Sons Ltd. Published 2017 by John Wiley & Sons Ltd.

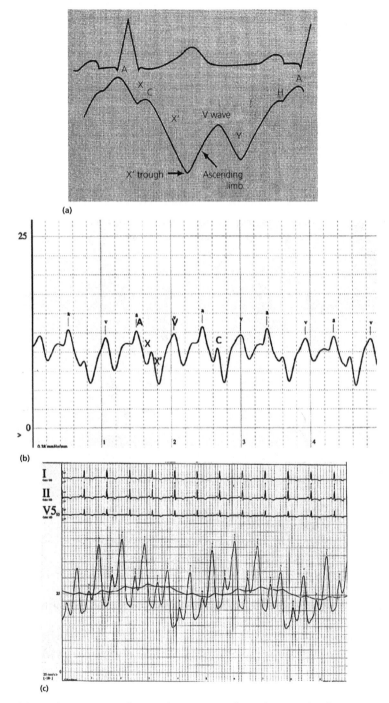

Figure 5.1 Atrial pressure waveforms. Schematic (a) and actual tracing (b) of RA pressure showing A and V waves and X and Y descents. Panel (c) is a PCWP tracing showing V > A. Source: Mark 1998. Reproduced with permission of Elsevier [2].

is often interrupted by a small positive deflection, and the C wave results from closure of the tricuspid valve during isovolumetric contraction of the ventricle. The C wave is more commonly seen in RA compared to PCWP tracings and is prominent in patients with prolonged PR intervals. Additional X descent after the C wave is referred to as the X' descent.

The second positive deflection in the atrial pressure tracing is the V wave, which represents rapid atrial filling during ventricular systole while the atrioventricular valve is closed. The peak of the V wave usually corresponds to the T wave on the ECG. The decay of the V wave is referred to as the Y descent (Figure 5.1). The Y descent corresponds to rapid ventricular filling in early diastole.

The waveforms are dependent on heart rate. Tachycardia reduces the duration of diastole and can abbreviate the Y descent, thus causing the V and A waves to merge. Bradycardia causes the waves to become more distinct and can elicit an H wave, a mid- to late-diastolic plateau that follows the Y descent and precedes the A wave.

The mean LA pressure is higher than the mean RA pressure in the normal heart. The A wave is usually higher than the V wave in the RA; in the LA either the V wave is greater than the A wave or the A and V waves are nearly equal. Also in the normal heart, mean atrial pressure falls with inspiration. The opposite effect, in which the mean RA pressure does not decrease with inspiration, is seen in constrictive pericarditis and occasionally other conditions (referred to as Kussmaul's sign).

It is important to remember that atrial pressure tracings represent pressure (and provide some indirect information on atrial volume) but not flow. Venous return to the RA is dependent on the pressure gradient between the venous system and the RA. Consequently, venous return to the RA is maximal during period of low pressure (X and Y descents).

Abnormalities in atrial pressures

Elevations in RA pressure are often a clue to cardiovascular pathology. Increased mean RA pressure is seen in valvular heart disease, constrictive pericarditis, restrictive cardiomyopathy, cardiac tamponade, fluid overload (e.g., renal failure), pulmonary hypertension, left to right shunts, pulmonary embolus, RV infarction, LV systolic or diastolic failure, and congenital heart disease. It is important to note that mean RA pressures may appear normal in patients with heart disease who are dehydrated.

The A wave is accentuated in patients with noncompliant ventricles and therefore can be increased in patients with ventricular ischemia, infarction, or hypertrophy from pressure or volume overload. A prominent RA A wave can occur in tricuspid regurgitation, pulmonic regurgitation, or stenosis as well as pulmonary embolus or cor pulmonale from any cause (Figure 5.2a and Tables 5.1 and 5.2). Intermittent cannon A waves can be seen in complete heart block or ventricular

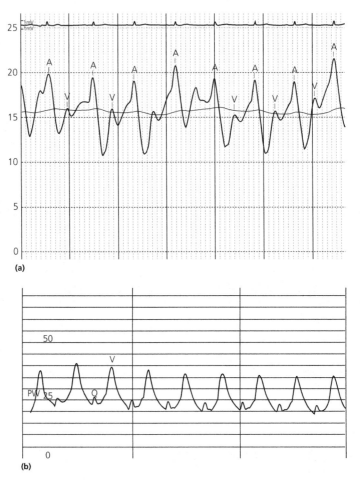

Figure 5.2 Examples of prominent A waves (a) and V waves (b).

tachycardia as the atria are contracting intermittently against a closed AV valve (Figure 5.2b). In patients with atrial flutter or atrial tachycardia, A waves may be present at an accelerated rate. Small A waves are rare in RA tracings but common in LA tracings (Figure 5.2c).

Abnormalities in the X descent are seen with severe tricuspid regurgitation (TR) or mitral regurgitation (MR) when the X descent and C wave can be interrupted by a prominent V wave.

The V wave reflects atrial pressures during ventricular systole and thus can be useful as a clue to the presence of AV valve regurgitation. In the RA a prominent V wave can be seen in patients with tricuspid regurgitation and the RA pressure tracing can take on a ventricularized character when TR is severe (Figure 5.3) [3]. Ventricularization of the RA pressure tracing is the most specific finding, but is

Table 5.1 Conditions associated with abnormal right atrial pressure tracings.

	Prominent	Blunted
A wave	A–V dissociation (e.g., complete heart block or ventricular tachycardia)	Atrial arrhythmia
	Decreased ventricular compliance	
	Tricuspid regurgitation or stenosis	
	Pulmonary stenosis or regurgitation	
X descent	Tamponade	Atrial arrhythmia
	RV ischemia (without RA involvement)	RA ischemia
	Atrial septal defect	Tricuspid regurgitation
V wave	Tricuspid regurgitation	Tamponade
	RV failure	Constrictive pericarditis
		Hypovolemia
Y descent	Constrictive pericarditis	Tamponade
	Restrictive cardiomyopathy	RV ischemia
	Tricuspid regurgitation	Tricuspid stenosis

found in a minority of patients with severe TR (see Chapter 13). In a study of 60 patients who had right ventriculography, Lingamneni *et al.* found that ventricularization of the right atrial pressure contour was present in only 40% of patients with severe TR [4]. Cha *et al.*, in their study of 59 patients with severe TR diagnosed on right ventriculography and/or at the time of surgery, found that a ventricularization pattern was present in 31%, and that prominent V waves (not further defined in the paper) and steep Y descents were present in an additional 37% of the patients [5]. In contrast, Pitts *et al.* reported that neither prominent right atrial V waves nor elevated mean right atrial pressures reliably predicted the presence of moderate or severe tricuspid regurgitation (as determined by echocardiography), but that the absence of right atrial V waves and elevated mean right atrial pressures were relatively specific for excluding significant tricuspid regurgitation [6]. For the purposes of their study, a "prominent" right-sided V wave was defined as (1) V wave >15 mm Hg, (2) a difference between V wave and mean RA pressure >5 mm Hg, or (3) a ratio of V wave to mean RA pressure >1.5.

Commonly, however, the left-sided V wave receives the most attention and that is what we will focus on in this section (examples are shown in Figure 5.4). The PA systolic pressure waveform and left atrial V wave are generated at the same time (assuming that the ventricles contract at the same time), however the V wave in the PCWP tracing will be seen later because of the delay in transmission of left atrial pressure to the catheter tip. Moore *et al.*, in their study of 13 patients

Table 5.2 Right atrial pressure tracing findings in various conditions.

	V wave	Y descent	A wave	X descent	RA mean pressure	Misc.
Normal	Atrial filling following ventricular contraction	Rapid ventricular filling phase	Atrial contraction		0–5	RA: A>V LV: V>A normal delay in pressure transmission from LA to pulmonary cap: 140–200 ms
Constriction		Prominent		Preserved	Elevated	Tracings can have M or W form; Kussmaul's sign
Tamponade		Small/absent		Preserved	Elevated	
Effusive constrictive		Prominent			Persistent elevation after pericardiocentesis	RA pressure remains elevated despite complete drainage (pericardial pressure=0)
Restriction		Prominent		Preserved	Elevated	RA tracings can have M or W form
RV infarct		Impaired			Elevated	RA intact: increased A wave and steep X descent RA infarct: decreased A wave and impaired X and Y descents

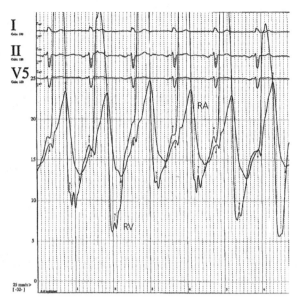

Figure 5.3 Pressure tracing from a patient with severe tricuspid regurgitation. Simultaneous RA and RV pressures are recorded in a 60-year-old male with severe TR. Note the ventricularization of the atrial pressure.

with large V waves, found that the onset of the V wave was approximately 110 milliseconds after the onset of the pulmonary arterial upstroke [7].

The V wave in the PCWP (or LA) tracing is dependent on the pressure–volume relationship of the left atrium and left atrial compliance as well as the volume of blood entering the atrium. A large V wave indicates a rapid rise in LA pressure during ventricular systole and can occur in setting of a noncompliant left atrium and normal flow (e.g., atrial ischemia) or a normally compliant left atrium with large flow (e.g., acute mitral regurgitation). Conversely, if the left atrium has a large capacitance then a prominent V wave may be absent even in the presence of severe mitral regurgitation.

In the left atrium or pulmonary capillary wedge pressure tracing, a prominent V wave suggests mitral regurgitation, but is neither sensitive nor specific. Some investigators have advocated using a grading system where a V wave that is twice the mean wedge pressure is suggestive of severe MR and a V wave maximum of three times mean wedge pressure is diagnostic of severe MR, but this has not been widely validated (Table 5.3). Although not typical, a prominent V wave can occasionally be observed in patients with mitral stenosis if the LA is relatively noncompliant, with limited ability to accept expanded filling volumes.

In patients with severe MR and a large V wave, mean PCWP can overestimate LV end-diastolic pressure. In a study by Haskell and French [8], mean PCWP pressure overestimated LVEDP by approximately 30% (in this study, a large

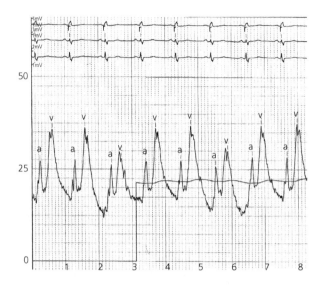

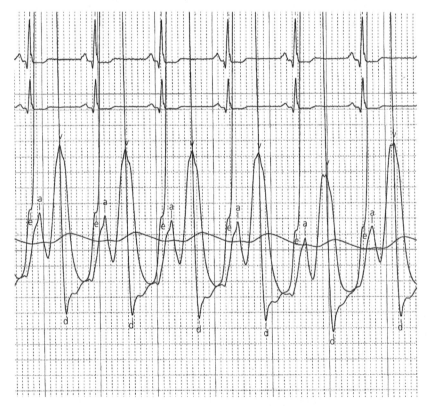

Figure 5.4 Examples of prominent V waves.

Table 5.3 Important points about V waves.

The V wave on PCWP tracing corresponds to (1) T wave on ECG and (2) descent of pressure tracing on LV recording

V wave >2x mean PCWP is suggestive of severe MR

V wave >3x mean PCWP is diagnostic of severe MR

Absence of significant V waves does not exclude significant MR

When large V waves are present, trough of Y descent is better predictor of LVEDP than is mean PCWP [8]

V waves are affected by arterial systolic blood pressure (i.e., ventricular afterload)

V wave was defined as being greater than the A wave by more than 10 mm Hg). A better estimate of LVEDP was obtained by using the trough of the X descent.

The Y descent or decay in the V wave occurs during the opening of the AV valve and represents rapid emptying of the atria into the ventricle (which results in a drop in pressure). It is a marker of passive ventricular filling and thus anything that prevents or enhances early diastolic filling affects the character of the Y descent. Conditions with high ventricular pressures during early diastole tend to be associated with blunted Y descents (e.g., tamponade or mitral stenosis). Y descents are usually blunted in cardiac tamponade but can become more prominent during inspiration; the Y descent becomes more apparent following pericardiocentesis. Conditions with low ventricular pressures during early diastole and prominent passive filling of the ventricle (e.g., constrictive pericarditis) tend to have large Y descents. Various examples of Y descents are shown: mitral stenosis can cause an attenuation or flattening of the terminal Y descent (Figure 5.5); venous pressures are elevated and Y descents are prominent in constrictive pericarditis (Figure 5.6); both X and Y descents are blunted in a case of right ventricular infarction (Figure 5.7); and Y descents are blunted, especially during expiration, in a case of cardiac tamponade (Figure 5.8). The Y descent can vary with the position of the patient in the rare instance of large atrial myxoma.

Physical exam

Physical examination of jugular venous pulse (JVP) provides valuable information to clinicians, as the JVP is a manometer of pressure in the right atrium. To determine JVP, sit the patient at 45° and turn his or her head slightly away from you. Use the internal jugular vein (not external jugular vein) medial to the clavicular head of sternocleidomastoid and measure JVP in centimeters above the sternal notch (vertical not diagonal distance). The venous pulse can usually be analyzed more readily using the right internal jugular vein, as the right innominate and jugular veins extend in an almost straight line from the superior vena cava.

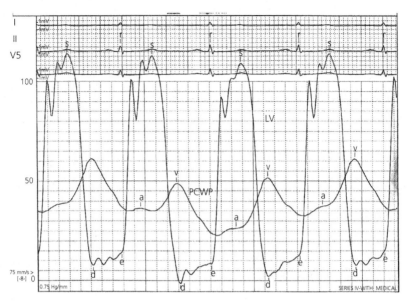

Figure 5.5 Example of simultaneous PCWP and left ventricular pressure tracings in a patient with mitral stenosis and mitral regurgitation. Note the persistent pressure gradient between the chambers throughout diastole. Note also that the PCW pressure is delayed relative to LV pressure, and that accurate determination of diastolic pressure gradient and mitral valve area requires shifting the PCWP tracing to the left. The V wave on the PCWP tracing should coincide with the downstroke (isovolumetric relaxation) of the LV tracing.

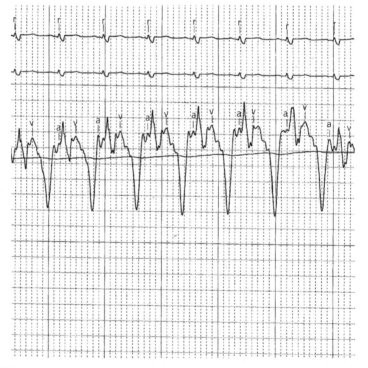

Figure 5.6 RA tracing in a patient with constrictive pericarditis. Constrictive pericarditis and restrictive cardiomyopathy are two hemodynamic states that cause significant abnormalities of the atrial wave with prominent Y descents. There are typically high atrial pressures and prominent early diastolic filling waves.

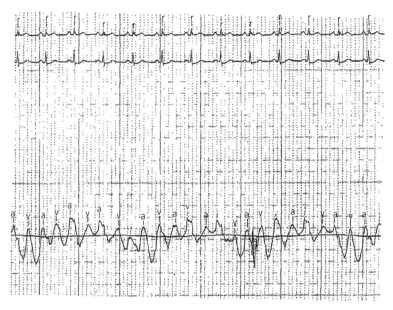

Figure 5.7 RA tracing in a patient with right ventricular myocardial infarction. RV infarction can occasionally cause a pattern of pseudoconstriction with a prominent X and Y descent. This occurs due to acute distention of the volume overloaded RV into a contained pericardial space.

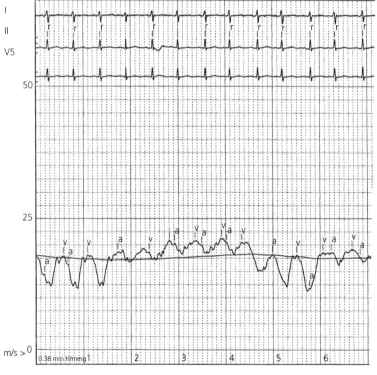

Figure 5.8 RA tracing in a patient with pericardial tamponade. Tamponade results in pandiastolic restriction of ventricular filling, as pericardial pressure exceeds RA pressure throughout diastole. This results in blunting of both the X and Y descents, which often return following successful pericardial drainage.

Sir Thomas Lewis in 1930 proposed a simple bedside method for measuring central venous pressure. He found that the catheter-measured CVP was equal to 5 cm plus the vertical distance of the JVP from the sternal angle and that this measurement was independent of the individual's position (e.g., supine, semiupright, or upright). Remember that CVP in cm of blood must be divided by 1.34 to get pressure in mm Hg. Also note that the distance between the sternal angle and the midportion of the RA, which Lewis estimated at 5 cm, varies considerably between individuals and is affected by age and anterior–posterior diameter of the chest [9].

JVP can be used to assess right heart filling pressures and the waveform can provide information suggestive of specific diagnoses. Raised JVP with normal waveform is suggestive of right heart failure and/or fluid overload. The lack of pulsations in a patient with elevated JVP would be suggestive of SVC obstruction. Various abnormalities of the A wave, V wave, X descent, or Y descent suggest diseases outlined in Tables 5.2 and 5.3. An increase in JVP with inspiration (Kussmaul's sign) is suggestive of constrictive pericarditis.

Important points

- The atrial waveform is composed of the positive atrial (A) and ventricular (V) waves and the X and Y descents.
- The A wave is prominent with abnormalities of RV and LV compliance (e.g., hypertrophy, ischemia).
- The V wave is accentuated in cases of atrioventricular valve regurgitation (RA V wave in TR, LA V wave in MR).
- The X and Y descents are diminished or absent in pericardial tamponade.
- The X and Y descents are accentuated in constriction and restrictive myocardial disease.

Historical anecdote

Karel Wenckebach described the arrhythmia that bears his name (also known as Mobitz type 1 AV block) in a paper entitled "On the analysis of irregular pulses" that was published in 1899, before the advent of clinical electrocardiography. He described the arrhythmia based on a careful examination of the arterial pulse and the A wave in the jugular venous waveform in a "forty-year old lady ... with a pulse that was small, soft and intermittent after 3 to 6 contractions" who had consulted him (more details can be found in *Ann Intern Med* 1999;**130**:58–63 or *Tex Heart Inst J* 1999;**26**:8–11).

References

1 Batson GA, Chandrasekhar KP, Payas Y, Rickards DF. Comparison of pulmonary wedge pressure measured by the flow directed Swan–Ganz catheter with left atrial pressure. *Br Heart J* 1971;**33**:616.

2 Mark JB. Atlas of cardiovascular monitoring. New York: Churchill Livingstone; 1998.

3 Rao S, Tate DA, Stouffer GA. Hemodynamic findings in severe tricuspid regurgitation. *Catheter Cardiovasc Interven* 2013;**81**(1):162–169.

4 Cha SD, Desai RS, Gooch AS, Maranhao V, Goldberg H. Diagnosis of severe tricuspid regurgitation. *Chest.* 1982;**82**:726–731.

5 Lingamneni R, Cha SD, Maranhao V, Gooch AS, Goldberg H. Tricuspid regurgitation: clinical and angiographic assessment. *Cathet Cardiovasc Diagn* 1979;**5**:7–17.

6 Pitts WR, Lange RA, Cigarroa JE, Hillis LD. Predictive value of prominent right atrial V waves in assessing the presence and severity of tricuspid regurgitation. *Am J Cardiol* 1999;**83**: 617–618, A10.

7 Moore RA, Neary MJ, Gallagher JD, Clark DL. Determination of the pulmonary capillary wedge position in patients with giant left atrial V waves. *J Cardiothorac Anesth* 1987;**1**: 108–113.

8 Haskell RJ, French WJ. Accuracy of left atrial and pulmonary artery wedge pressure in pure mitral regurgitation in predicting left ventricular end-diastolic pressure. *Am J Cardiol* 1988; **61**:136–141.

9 Seth R, Magner P, Matzinger F, van Walraven C. How far is the sternal angle from the mid-right atrium? *J Gen Intern Med* 2002;**17**:852–856.

CHAPTER 6

Cardiac output

Frederick M. Costello and George A. Stouffer

A key component of evaluating the hemodynamic status of a patient is a measurement of cardiac output. Cardiac output is the amount of blood moved per unit time from the venous system (i.e., the vena cava) to the arterial system (i.e., aorta). It is a dynamic process and tightly regulated so that the blood flow through the heart equals the perfusion needs of the body.

Cardiac output is primarily regulated by preload, afterload, heart rate, and myocardial contractility. Many factors have rapid effects on cardiac output, including metabolic demands, posture, volume status, adrenergic state, and respiratory rate (e.g., cardiac output increases with inhalation and decreases with exhalation or the Valsalva maneuver). Cardiac output decreases with age [1] and increases with exercise. For example, cardiac output can increase up to sixfold with exercise in trained athletes; oxygen extraction also increases with exercise and thus oxygen delivery to tissues can increase twelvefold to eighteenfold. Cardiac index is the cardiac output divided by the body surface area. A cardiac index $<1 \, \text{L/min/m}^2$ is generally incompatible with life.

Cardiac output is a measurement of the forward flow of blood in the vascular system and is equal to the heart rate × ventricular stroke volume (in the absence of valvular regurgitation). Measurement of the heart rate is easily attainable, but an accurate measurement of stroke volume is more challenging (see Table 6.1). Because of the difficulty in measuring left ventricular stroke volume, several methods have been developed that calculate blood flow through the right heart. In the cardiac catheterization laboratory or in the intensive care unit, cardiac output is primarily measured using either the Fick method or the indicator dilution method (e.g., thermodilution). Each of these techniques has advantages and pitfalls that are discussed in detail in this chapter (see Table 6.2).

Cardiovascular Hemodynamics for the Clinician, Second Edition. Edited by George A. Stouffer.
© 2017 John Wiley & Sons Ltd. Published 2017 by John Wiley & Sons Ltd.

Table 6.1 Important formulas involving cardiac output.

$$SVR \left(\text{in dynes s/cm}^5 \right) = \frac{(\text{mean arterial pressure} - \text{right atrial pressure}) \times 80}{\text{cardiac output}}$$

where SVR = systemic vascular resistance. Normal SVR = 700–1600 dynes s/cm^5

$$PVR \left(\text{in dynes s/cm}^5 \right) = \frac{(\text{mean PA pressure} - \text{PCWP}) \times 80}{\text{cardiac output}}$$

where PA = pulmonary artery, PCWP = pulmonary capillary wedge pressure, and PVR = pulmonary vascular resistance. Normal PVR = 20–130 dynes s/cm^5

$CO = SV \times HR$

where CO = cardiac output, SV = stroke volume, and HR = heart rate

Table 6.2 Comparison of Fick and thermodilution methods of determining cardiac output.

	Fick	Thermodilution
Underlying principle	Fick principle (conservation of mass): the uptake or release of a substance by an organ is the product of blood flow to the organ × difference in the concentration of the substance between blood entering and blood leaving the organ	Conservation of energy: that is, that there is no loss of cold injectate between the site of injection and detection Other underlying assumptions are that mixing of the indicator and blood is complete and that the temperature change elicited by injection of saline can be discriminated accurately from the fluctuations in baseline temperature in the pulmonary artery
Sources of error	Determination of oxygen saturations	Warming of injectate during transit through catheter
	Assumption of steady state	Irregular heart rates
	Assumed oxygen consumption values	Tricuspid regurgitation
		Temperature of blood in PA varies with respiratory and cardiac cycles
Advantages	More accurate than TD in low output states, tricuspid regurgitation, and irregular heart rates	More accurate than Fick in high output states
Variation under ideal conditions	10% when measuring oxygen consumption	5–20%

Fick method

In 1870, Adolph Fick described the first method to estimate cardiac output in humans. He postulated that oxygen uptake in the lungs is entirely transferred to the blood and therefore that cardiac output can be calculated knowing the oxygen consumption of the body and the difference in oxygen content between arterial and mixed venous blood. Cardiac output can be calculated using the Fick method knowing the oxygen saturation of arterial and mixed venous blood, the hemoglobin concentration, and the oxygen consumption based on this equation:

$$\text{Cardiac output} = \frac{\text{oxygen consumption}}{(\text{arterial} - \text{venous})O_2 \times \text{hemoglobin concentration} \times 1.36 \times 10}$$

The constant 1.36 is expressed in mL O_2/g hemoglobin.

Direct measurement of oxygen consumption is cumbersome and time consuming and requires a tight-fitting gas exchange system. An alternative approach, although less accurate, is to estimate the oxygen consumption based on the patient's weight. This method to determine cardiac output is commonly used today and is called the "assumed Fick." Since the assumed Fick method is used frequently, it is important to realize its limitations. The initial evaluation of the assumed Fick method was performed in young healthy adults. Subsequently, Krovetz and Goldbloom [2], LaFarge and Miettinen [3], and Bergstra et al. [4] derived empiric formulas to estimate VO_2, while others advocate taking oxygen consumption to be 125 mL/min/m² in adults with or without a correction for age. There is, however, large variability in oxygen consumption and thus use of assumed values can introduce errors. In a study of 108 patients (mean age 49 years) undergoing cardiac catheterization, Dehmer et al. found the mean oxygen consumption to be 126 mL/min/m², but with a large standard deviation of 26 mL/min/m² [5]. Oxygen consumption was not affected by age or sex, but varied with level of sedation. In a study of 80 patients, Kendrick et al. compared assumed (calculated using five different estimation methods) and directly measured values of oxygen consumption and found significant discrepancies, with over half the estimated values differing by more than 10% from directly measured amount and 35% differing by more than 25% [6]. Similarly, Wolf et al. directly measured oxygen consumption in 57 nonsedated patients (mean age 52 years) undergoing evaluation in a metabolic laboratory and found the mean to be 126.5 mL/min/m², but with large variation (71–176 mL/min/m²) [7]. Comparison with assumed values calculated using the LaFarge and Miettinen equation showed that there were large, unpredictable errors when assumed values were used.

The value ascribed to the assumption of oxygen consumption is generally the largest error in using the assumed Fick method; however, other sources of error exist including measurement of oxygen saturation (see Chapter 7 on intracardiac shunts for a more complete discussion of potential errors) and the assumption of steady state. Even under the best conditions, the error associated with measuring cardiac output using the assumed Fick method is generally 10–15%. Under less stringent conditions this variation can rise significantly.

In low output states, the Fick method is the most accurate measurement available. This is because the differences in oxygen saturations between arterial and mixed venous blood are large, which minimizes errors introduced in the measurement of oxygen saturation. It is also the most accurate method when the patient has an irregular rhythm such as atrial fibrillation or ventricular bigeminy.

Supplemental oxygen use during measurement of the cardiac output should be avoided. If oxygen is required, maintaining a steady state is imperative to obtaining the most accurate measurement.

Thermodilution method

The indicator dilution method was first used in 1897. In its simplest form, it involves injection (via either bolus or continuous infusion) of an indicator substance into the circulation and then measurement of this substance at a point in the circulation downstream of the injection. The amount of indicator that is measured downstream, per unit time after injection, will be a function of cardiac output. The substance must be nontoxic, capable of mixing completely with blood, not taken up from the blood stream, and capable of being accurately measured. Numerous indicators have been studied over the years, including indocyanine green, but currently saline is the substance most commonly used.

The thermodilution method involves injecting saline into the right atrium and then measuring the temperature of blood in the pulmonary artery. The typical technique involves placement of a right heart catheter with multiple ports into the pulmonary artery, then 10 mm of cold saline is injected into the right atrium and temperature changes are measured in the pulmonary artery. Accurate measurement requires that a "mixing chamber" be present between the injection site and the measurement site. Thus, the proximal port should lie in the right atrium and the distal tip of the catheter should be beyond the pulmonary valve.

Injection of saline into the right atrium will cause a small, transient decrease in pulmonary artery temperature and a thermodilution curve is generated by plotting the temperature of the pulmonary artery versus time. The curve generally has a smooth upslope and a gentler decline (Figure 6.1). The area under the thermodilution curve is inversely related to the cardiac output and can be used to calculate the cardiac output. The calculation of the area under the curve and calculation of cardiac output are performed by computer, but an estimate of the validity of the measurement can be obtained by checking the waveform of the thermodilution curve.

Significant tricuspid regurgitation is generally considered a contraindication to the use of thermodilution for measurement of cardiac output. An early study by Konishi et al. [8] did not find a significant difference in cardiac outputs measured using thermodilution or Fick in the presence of tricuspid regurgitation. Later studies, however, found that a high degree of tricuspid regurgitation was associated

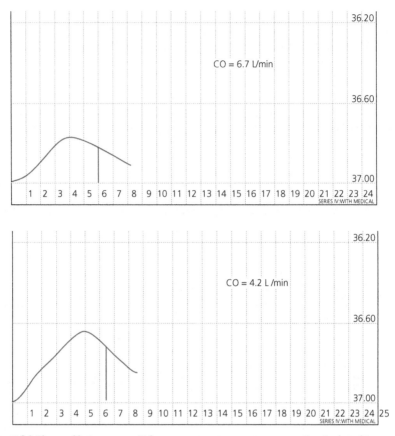

Figure 6.1 Thermodilution curves. Pulmonary artery temperature versus time is plotted in patients with thermodilution cardiac outputs (CO) of 6.7 L/min and 4.2 L/min. Note that the temperature curve is inverted so that a rise in the graph is indicative of a fall in PA temperature.

with underestimation of cardiac output by the thermodilution technique. Balik *et al.*, in their study of 27 patients undergoing cardiac surgery, reported a significant increase in the variation of cardiac output measurements with increasing degrees of tricuspid regurgitation [9]. Cigarroa *et al.* in their study of 30 patients (mean age 50 years) found excellent agreement between thermal dilution cardiac output and Fick or indocyanine green dye cardiac output in patients without tricuspid regurgitation [10], but results of thermodilution were consistently lower (by approximately 20%) than those obtained by the Fick or indocyanine green dye methods in the 17 patients with tricuspid regurgitation (see Table 6.2).

Of note is that mechanical ventilation can have an effect on cardiac output measurement with the thermodilution technique by causing or worsening tricuspid regurgitation. In a small study, Artucio *et al.* found that the use of positive end-expiratory pressure (PEEP) caused tricuspid regurgitation to develop or worsen in six out of seven patients studied [11]. Subsequently, Balik *et al.* [9] found that thermodilution underestimated cardiac output in 27 ventilated patients (using transesophageal echocardiographic cardiac output as the gold standard) and that inaccuracies increased proportional to the amount of tricuspid regurgitation.

For the sake of simplicity, room-temperature saline is often used, but this can lead to less accurate measurements. Berthelsen *et al.* reported a significant rise in variation and a loss of precision with the use of 20 °C saline versus the use of 0 °C saline [12]. They also noted, however, that if room-temperature saline was injected through a right heart catheter that had both proximal and distal thermistors, the variation was within an acceptable range. If ice-cold saline is used, careful attention must be paid to not allowing the saline to warm prior to injection. Iced injectate in a plastic syringe warms by 1 °C for every 28 seconds at room temperature. The rate of warming increases if the injectate is held in a gloved hand.

Potential sources of error in using thermodilution to measure cardiac output include "catheter warming" and temperature variation in the pulmonary artery. Catheter warming refers to the increase in temperature of the injectate as it passes through the catheter. Commercially available systems include an empiric constant that corrects for this warming. Variations in the temperature of blood in the pulmonary artery are generally minimal, except in cases of deep inspiration or positive pressure ventilation. In some cases, the variation in the temperature of the blood is enough to affect cardiac output determination. An additional limitation to thermodilution is the inaccuracy associated with determining accurate cardiac output with irregular heart rates or rhythms.

Thermodilution is most accurate when used in high output states, as the errors introduced by injectate warming are proportionally smaller. As cardiac output declines, the accuracy of thermodilution cardiac output declines (in contrast to the Fick method, in which accuracy increases with decreasing cardiac output). Van Grondelle *et al.* compared 57 cardiac output measurements by the thermodilution and Fick methods in 26 patients and found that thermodilution values were higher in all 16 cases in which Fick outputs were less than 3.5 L/min. In 10 cases where Fick values were less than or equal to 2.5 L/min, thermodilution and Fick measurements differed by an average of 35% [13]. They postulated that thermodilution is less accurate at low cardiac outputs because of warming of the injectate during conditions of low flow. Under ideal conditions, thermodilution can determine cardiac output within an error range of 5–20%.

Doppler echocardiographic measurement of cardiac output

Doppler echocardiography can also be used to determine cardiac output. The underlying principle is that the volume of flow can be determined by multiplying the velocity of flow by the area through which the blood is flowing. Thus, cardiac output can be calculated as the product of the heart rate, aortic time velocity integral, and the area of the left ventricular outflow tract (LVOT). This equation assumes that the area is constant and unchanging, and the LVOT is frequently used because it is the least dynamic. Because blood flow is pulsatile, a simple velocity cannot be used. Instead, a time velocity integral must be derived from Doppler measurements of flow.

This technique is very useful and can provide an accurate measurement of cardiac output, but as with all techniques, it too has pitfalls. The measurement of the time velocity integral using Doppler requires diligence. One must measure with pulse wave Doppler at the precise location where the LVOT diameter will be measured. Additionally, the pulse wave Doppler must be parallel to the flow. Any variance greater than 20° off the direction of flow will significantly change the calculated result. Another source of potential area is the measurement of the diameter of the LVOT. The area of the outflow tract is calculated by squaring the diameter and multiplying by 0.785. Even very small errors in the measurement of the LVOT will result in large variations in the area because the diameter is squared in this calculation.

Cardiac output measurement in intensive care units

One of the primary goals for patients in shock is to increase tissue perfusion. Clinical surrogates, such as blood pressure, pulse rate, central venous pressure, and arterial oxygen saturation have not consistently proven useful in guiding use of therapies to maximize cardiac output. In the absence of a measurement of cardiac output, volume resuscitation is often the first approach to treating shock. However, studies have shown that tissue perfusion does not increase in response to volume resuscitation in a significant number of hemodynamically unstable patients. In the nonresponsive patients, volume resuscitation does not improve stroke volume and carries some risk of harm. Therefore, there is a large interest in developing methods to measure cardiac output continuously and accurately in critically ill patients. This would enable accurate fluid administration and optimal use of inotropic agents and vasopressors to maximize tissue perfusion [14].

Traditionally, continuous cardiac output monitoring has been accomplished using a pulmonary artery catheter. Because of the well-known limitations of PA catheters and the lack of evidence that they improve outcomes in critically ill patients, several new technologies have been developed to measure cardiac output continuously. An invasive method that is useful only in ventilated patients involves using an esophageal Doppler probe to measure velocity and diameter continuously in the descending aorta. Newer noninvasive methods include pulse contour analysis, bioimpedance systems, CO_2 partial rebreathing technique, and various noninvasive devices employing Doppler technology.

The concept of pulse contour analysis is based on the relationship between stroke volume, blood pressure, arterial compliance, and systemic vascular resistance (SVR). Stroke volume, and thus cardiac output, can be calculated from the arterial pressure waveform if arterial compliance and SVR are known. Bioimpedance systems measure the resistance to flow of electric current through the thorax. This resistance is referred to as impedance (Zo), which in the thorax includes impedance due to tissues that do not change over time (such as lung, muscle, bone, and fat) and impedance due to the amount of blood in the thorax. Thus Zo varies in proportion to the amount of fluid in the thorax and the instantaneous rate of the change of Zo is related to instantaneous blood flow in the aorta. The limitations of bioimpedance systems are many and include being sensitive to the placement of the electrodes on the body, variations in body size, and other physical factors such as temperature and humidity that have an impact on electric conductivity. Newer technologies have been developed, including bioreactance, which is used to measure the phase shift in voltage across the thorax. Pulsatile ejection of blood leads to instantaneous changes in the phase of Zo; phase shifts in Zo can thus be used as a surrogate for aortic flow. The CO_2 partial rebreathing technique uses the modified Fick equation to estimate pulmonary capillary blood flow (a surrogate for cardiac output that assumes the absence of any shunting) based on a comparison of end-tidal carbon dioxide partial pressure obtained during a period of no rebreathing with that obtained during a subsequent period of rebreathing.

References

1 Brandfonbrener M, Landowne M, Shock NW. Changes in cardiac output with age. *Circulation* 1955;**12**:557–566.
2 Krovetz LJ, Goldbloom S. Normal standards for cardiovascular data. I. Examination of the validity of cardiac index. *Johns Hopkins Med J* 1972;**130**:174–186.
3 LaFarge CG, Miettinen OS. The estimation of oxygen consumption. *Cardiovasc Res* 1970;**4**:23–30.
4 Bergstra A, van Dijk RB, Hillege HL, Lie KI, Mook GA. Assumed oxygen consumption based on calculation from dye dilution cardiac output: an improved formula. *Eur Heart J* 1995;**16**:698–703.
5 Dehmer GJ, Firth BG, Hillis LD. Oxygen consumption in adult patients during cardiac catheterization. *Clin Cardiol* 1982;**5**:436–440.
6 Kendrick AH, West J, Papouchado M, Rozkovec A. Direct Fick cardiac output: are assumed values of oxygen consumption acceptable? *Eur Heart J* 1988;**9**:337–342.
7 Wolf A, Pollman MJ, Trindade PT, Fowler MB, Alderman EL. Use of assumed versus measured oxygen consumption for the determination of cardiac output using the Fick principle. *Cathet Cardiovasc Diagn* 1998;**43**:372–380.
8 Konishi T, Nakamura Y, Morii I, Himura Y, Kumada T, Kawai C. Comparison of thermodilution and Fick methods for measurement of cardiac output in tricuspid regurgitation. *Am J Cardiol* 1992;**70**:538–539.
9 Balik M, Pachl J, Hendl J. Effect of the degree of tricuspid regurgitation on cardiac output measurements by thermodilution. *Intensive Care Med* 2002;**28**:1117–1121.
10 Cigarroa RG, Lange RA, Williams RH, Bedotto JB, Hillis LD. Underestimation of cardiac output by thermodilution in patients with tricuspid regurgitation. *Am J Med* 1989;**86**:417–420.

11 Artucio H, Hurtado J, Zimet L, de Paula J, Beron M. PEEP-induced tricuspid regurgitation. *Intensive Care Med* 1997;**23**:836–840.

12 Berthelsen PG, Eldrup N, Nilsson LB, Rasmussen JP. Thermodilution cardiac output. Cold vs room temperature injectate and the importance of measuring the injectate temperature in the right atrium. *Acta Anaesthesiol Scand* 2002;**46**:1103–1110.

13 van Grondelle A, Ditchey RV, Groves BM, Wagner WW, Jr, Reeves JT. Thermodilution method overestimates low cardiac output in humans. *Am J Physiol* 1983;**245**:H690–H692.

14 Marik PE. Noninvasive cardiac output monitors: a state-of the-art review. *J Cardiothorac Vasc Anesth* 2013;**27**:121–134.

CHAPTER 7

Detection, localization, and quantification of intracardiac shunts

Frederick M. Costello and George A. Stouffer

In the normal circulation, blood passes from the venous system through the right heart, into the pulmonary circulation, then into the left heart, and finally into the systemic circulation in a continuous, unidirectional manner. In certain conditions, however, oxygenated blood is shunted from the left heart directly to the right heart, as in the case of atrial septal defects (ASD; Figure 7.1) or ventricular septal defects (VSD; Figure 7.2), or from the aorta to the pulmonary artery (patent ductus arteriosus, PDA). More rarely, unoxygenated blood can be shunted from the right heart to the left heart (e.g., Eisenmenger's syndrome). Intracardiac shunts can be either congenital (Figures 7.1 and 7.2) or acquired (e.g., VSD as a complication of myocardial infarction).

Intracardiac shunting of blood results when there is an opening between the right and left heart chambers and a pressure difference to drive flow between the connected chambers. Because pressures (both systolic and diastolic) on the left side of the heart are generally higher than on the right side, most shunts are predominantly left to right, although right to left and bidirectional shunts are seen (predominantly in Eisenmenger's syndrome). Of note is that arterial-to-venous shunts can exist outside of the heart (e.g., intrapulmonary, intrahepatic, AV malformation) and affect oxygen saturations. We will not address these shunts in this chapter, but rather concentrate on intracardiac shunts.

Detection of an intracardiac shunt

The presence of a shunt can be determined either invasively or noninvasively (e.g., radionuclide studies, magnetic resonance imaging [MRI], or Doppler echocardiography). In current practice, many shunts are suspected based on physical exam or electrocardiogram (ECG), diagnosed at echocardiography and then quantified using right heart catheterization.

Cardiovascular Hemodynamics for the Clinician, Second Edition. Edited by George A. Stouffer.
© 2017 John Wiley & Sons Ltd. Published 2017 by John Wiley & Sons Ltd.

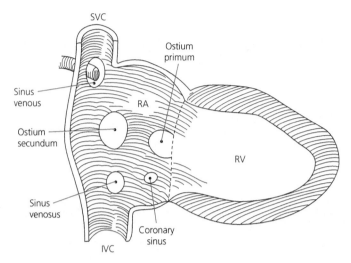

Figure 7.1 Schematic showing the location of various types of atrial septal defects.

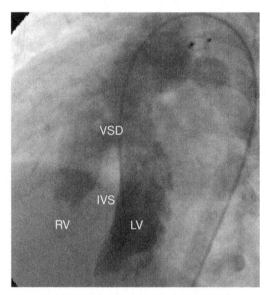

Figure 7.2 Ventriculogram in an LAO projection showing efflux of dye from the left ventricle into the right ventricle via a VSD. [IVS = intraventricular septum; LV = left ventricle; RV = right ventricle; VSD = ventricular septal defect.]

There are several methods by which an intracardiac shunt can be detected, localized, and quantified in the catheterization laboratory. The indicator dilution method is of historical interest, but is rarely used outside of research studies. It involves injecting a substance, such as indocyanine green, into the venous systems or a right heart chamber and monitoring its appearance in the systemic circulation. Dye curve measurements are very accurate, but are slow and require specialized equipment that is rarely available in modern catheterization laboratories. Contrast angiography, in which contrast dye is injected into the higher pressure chamber of a suspected shunt (e.g., left ventricle), is occasionally used to identify a VSD or PDA. It has limited ability to diagnose ASD and is a poor tool for quantifying the size of a shunt.

Oximetry, or measurement of the oxygen saturations in various locations in the venous system and the right heart ("oxygen saturation run"), is the most frequently used invasive technique due to its simplicity and reliance on readily available equipment.

Oxygen saturation run

The oxygen saturation run is performed as a catheter is passed through the venous system, right heart, and pulmonary circulation. The samples need to be acquired with the patient breathing room air or a gas mixture containing no more than a maximum of 30% oxygen [1]. Saturation data may be inaccurate in patients breathing more than 30% oxygen, since a significant amount of oxygen may be present in dissolved form in the pulmonary venous sample. Dissolved oxygen is not factored into calculations when saturations are used and thus pulmonary flow will be overestimated and the amount of shunt exaggerated.

The oxygen saturation run includes saturations from the superior vena cava (SVC), inferior vena cava (IVC), right heart, pulmonary artery, and arterial circulation. Pulmonary capillary wedge and/or left atrial samples are also sometimes obtained. Samples can be obtained as the right heart catheter is advanced, although many clinicians choose to place the catheter in the pulmonary artery first and then obtain samples as the catheter is withdrawn. This latter technique can improve the speed of obtaining samples, which can become an issue if there is difficulty advancing the catheter into the pulmonary artery.

Blood samples should be taken from the locations listed in Table 7.1 and oxygen saturations determined. IVC saturation varies depending on where the sample is obtained, and the sampling site should be at the level of the diaphragm to ensure that hepatic venous blood is taken into account. An arterial blood sample should be collected at the same time as the venous samples are being obtained.

Multiple samples may have to be taken in various chambers to ensure accuracy; however, it is important to note that variability in oxygen saturation (in the absence of shunt) decreases as blood flows through the heart. Oxygen content varies by approximately 2 mL O_2/100 mL blood in the right atrium (RA), 1 mL O_2/100 mL blood in the right ventricle (RV), and 0.5 mL O_2/100 mL blood in the pulmonary artery (PA) [2]. These values were determined by direct measurement of oxygen content in the days prior to the development of oximetry. Oxygen content can be approximated by the following formula:

$$\text{Oxygen content}(\text{mLO}_2/100 \text{ mL blood})$$
$$= \text{hemoglobin}(\text{g/dL}) \times 1.36(\text{mLO}_2/\text{g of Hg}) \times \text{percent saturation}$$

Table 7.1 Sites from which oxygen saturation should be measured when quantifying intracardiac shunts.

Superior vena cava just above the junction with the right atrium
Inferior vena cava just below the diaphragm
Low right atrium
Mid-right atrium
High right atrium
Right ventricle
Left, right and/or main pulmonary artery
Pulmonary capillary wedge (or left atrial)
Left ventricle and/or arterial

In a patient with a hemoglobin of 15 mg/dL, a difference in saturation of 5% is approximately equal to a difference in oxygen content of 1 mL O_2/100 mL blood.

The goal of the oxygen saturation run is to measure differences in oxygen saturation in various chambers of the heart. There are several practical factors that must be kept in mind to ensure accurate results:

- The oxygen saturation method assumes that the body is in a steady state during the collection of samples. To ensure that the results are as accurate as possible, the samples must be collected as close in time as good technique permits. For this reason, many physicians perform a retrograde oxygen saturation run in which they begin with the catheter in the PA.
- Blood samples should not be withdrawn into the syringe too rapidly. Matta *et al.* found that rapid aspiration increased oxygen saturations [3].
- Complete mixing of blood is assumed in all chambers.
- There has to be adequate flushing of the catheter between samples.

Limitations of using oximetry to detect and quantify intracardiac shunts

Using the saturation "step-up" method to detect and quantify intracardiac shunts has some limitations that should be noted. First, because of the inherent variability in determining oxygen saturations, the oximetry method of quantifying shunts loses accuracy when determining small shunts or in the presence of high cardiac output (which decreases AVO_2 difference). Second, the magnitude of the step-up varies with the oxygen-carrying capacity of blood and the cardiac output. Saturation step-ups are increased if hemoglobin concentration is low or cardiac output is low. As Shepherd *et al.* [4] note, a 5% step-up occurs with a shunt flow of 3400 mL/min when systemic blood flow is 7.5 L/min, a shunt flow of

1300 mL/min when systemic blood flow is 5 L/min, and a shunt flow of only 285 mL/min if systemic blood flow is 2.5 L/min.

Third, the relationship between the magnitude of step-up and the shunt flow is nonlinear and, with increasing left-to-right shunting, a given change in shunt flow produces less of a change in the saturation step-up. In contrast, quantification of shunt size using Q_p/Q_s is not affected by hemoglobin concentration and the relationship between Q_p/Q_s and shunt flow is linear. Q_p/Q_s is sensitive to cardiac output and some investigators advocate using exercise in patients with low cardiac output to improve accuracy.

Diagnosis of intracardiac shunts at right heart catheterization

Patients are often referred for cardiac catheterization to confirm and quantify a shunt that has been detected by physical exam and/or imaging. Occasionally, however, a patient will have a shunt that is unsuspected prior to right heart catheterization. These patients can be identified by routinely measuring oxygen saturation in the PA and the RA. Hillis *et al.* found that the difference (mean ± SD) between RA and PA saturations in 980 patients without intracardiac shunts was 2.3% ± 1.7%. In this same population, the difference (mean ± SD) between SVC and RA saturations was 3.9% ± 2.4%. Using threshold values of 8.7% between SVC and RA and 5.7% between RA and PA as "cut-offs" (mean + 2 SD) to identify patients with intracardiac shunts had excellent sensitivity and specificity [5]. Similarly, differences in oxygen saturation of 8% between SVC and PA and 5% between RV and PA can be used to detect intracardiac shunts.

Quantifying a left-to-right shunt

Quantifying a left-to-right shunt is generally done in two ways. The ratio of pulmonary blood flow versus the systemic blood flow can be calculated, termed the Q_p/Q_s, where Q_p is the pulmonary blood flow and Q_s is the systemic flow. Alternatively, the actual flow of the shunt can be calculated. This is the difference between the pulmonary blood flow and the systemic blood flow (these two are equal in a normal heart).

The pulmonary (Q_p) and systemic (Q_s) blood flows are calculated using the Fick method of estimating cardiac output (Table 7.2). The only difference between the pulmonary flow equation and the systemic flow equation is in the arterial and venous saturations used. The Q_p and Q_s equations are shown as well.

Cardiac output

$$= \frac{\text{oxygen consumption}}{\left(\text{arterial } O_2 - \text{venous } O_2\right) \times \text{hemoglobin concentration} \times 1.36 \times 10}$$

Table 7.2 Important formulas in quantifying shunts.

$$Q_P = \frac{\text{Oxygen consumption (mL / min)}}{\text{Oxygen content in pulmonary veins} - \text{oxygen content in pulmonary artery (mL / L)}}$$

$$Q_S = \frac{\text{Oxygen consumption (mL / min)}}{\text{Oxygen content in systemic artery} - \text{oxygen content in mixed venous sample}}$$

Simplified formula for calculating Q_P/Q_S in patients with left-to-right shunts.

$$\frac{Q_P}{Q_S} = \frac{(\text{arterial sat} - \text{mixed venous sat})}{(\text{pulm vein sat} - \text{pulm artery sat})}$$

• Pulmonary vein samples are rarely obtained. Instead, pulmonary capillary wedge samples or left atrial samples can be used. Alternatively, arterial saturation (in the absence of right-to-left shunt) can be substituted or an assumed value of 98% may be used

• Left ventricular may be substituted for arterial saturation, provided that there is no right-to-left shunt

• For PDA, use RV sample to determined mixed venous O_2

• For VSD, use RA sample to determined mixed venous O_2

• For ASD, calculate using mixed venous $O_2 = 3(SVC) + IVC/4$ (see Table 7.3 for a more complete discussion of calculating mixed venous O_2 from SVC and IVC samples)

For right-to-left and bidirectional shunts:

Calculate Q_P, Q_S, and Q_{EP} (the amount of oxygenated blood delivered to the body) using the following equations:

Constant to use in all calculations = oxygen consumption (either measured or estimated in mLO_2/min)/ hemoglobin (g/dL) × 1.36 (mL O_2/g)

$$Q_P = \frac{\text{oxygen consumption}}{(PVO_2 - PA\ O_2) \times \text{hemoglobin concentration} \times 1.36 \times 10}$$

where PVO_2 is the pulmonary venous oxygen saturation and PAO_2 is the pulmonary artery oxygen saturation

$$Q_S = \frac{\text{oxygen consumption}}{(SAO_2 - MVO_2) \times \text{hemoglobin concentration} \times 1.36 \times 10}$$

where SAO_2 is the systemic arterial oxygen saturation and MVO_2 is the mixed venous oxygen saturation.

These equations can be simplified to calculate Q_P/Q_S. The simplified equation is the difference of the systemic arterial oxygen saturation minus the mixed venous oxygen saturation divided by the pulmonary venous oxygen concentration minus the pulmonary arterial oxygen concentration. This equation is:

$$\frac{Q_P}{Q_S} = \frac{(SAO_2 - MVO_2)}{(PVO_2 - PAO_2)}$$

Since pulmonary veins are rarely entered during a cardiac catheterization, a pulmonary catheter wedge sample or left atrial sample (if the left atrium is entered via an ASD) can be used in its place. Alternatively, arterial saturation (in the absence of right-to-left shunt) can be substituted, or an assumed value of 98% may be used.

There are four factors that will help in using this simplified equation. The first is that the difference in the arterial–venous oxygen saturations is systemic over pulmonary, despite the fact that the ratio is Q_p/Q_s. This is somewhat counterintuitive, but a quick reference to the earlier flow equations will reveal the reason for this (i.e., cardiac output is inversely related to the difference in saturations).

The second factor is that the difference between the arterial and venous oxygen saturations in the Q_p equation is $PVO_2 - PAO_2$. This is because the difference is between oxygenated and unoxygenated blood. The anatomical pulmonary arteries carry unoxygenated blood and the pulmonary veins carry oxygenated blood, thus (oxygenated – unoxygenated) is equal to ($PVO_2 - PAO_2$).

The third factor is the mixed venous oxygen saturation (MVO_2) in the Q_s equation. Different values should be used depending on where the shunt is located. The MVO_2 should be from the chamber preceding the shunt, thus if there is a VSD the average of samples from the right atrium should be used. If there is an ASD, the MVO_2 is calculated from the superior vena cava (SVC) and the inferior vena cava (IVC). While theoretically coronary sinus blood flow contributes to mixed venous blood along with blood from IVC and SVC, the contribution is so small as to be safely ignored. The equation most frequently used is $(3 \times SVC + IVC)/4$. This is the most common, but certainly not the only calculation proposed as an appropriate estimate of the MVO_2. At least six different calculations have been suggested as ways to estimate MVO_2 (see Table 7.3).

Lastly, this equation can be used to calculate the ratio of pulmonary blood flow to the systemic blood flow, but should not be confused as a measure of the actual shunt blood flow. Shunt flow can be determined by calculating Q_p and Q_s; the shunt flow is the difference between the pulmonary and systemic flow, $Q_p - Q_s$. This can be useful in assessing the significance of the shunt.

Shunt management

Once a shunt has been detected, management varies depending on the severity and patient symptoms. Q_p/Q_s can be a very useful tool in making decisions about the need for repair of a shunt. The following numbers are generalizations about left-to-right shunts:

- A Q_p/Q_s of 1–1.5: observation is generally recommended.
- A Q_p/Q_s ratio of 1.5–2.0: significant enough that closure (either surgically or percutaneously) should be considered if the risk of the procedure is low.

Table 7.3 Determination of mixed venous oxygen saturation.

In the absence of an intracardiac shunt, the pulmonary artery provides a site of mixed venous blood. If there is a VSD, RA blood can be assumed to be mixed venous. In the presence of an ASD, mixed venous saturation needs to be estimated. In these cases, the formula most commonly used to determine mixed venous oxygen saturation is $MV = (3 \times SVC + IVC)/4$ (where MV = mixed venous, SVC = superior vena cava, and IVC = inferior vena cava). Formulas that have been advocated for estimating mixed venous oxygen saturation include:

First author	Year	Formula
Flamm	1969	$MV = (3 \times SVC + IVC)/4$
Iskandrian	1976	$MV = (2 \times SVC + IVC)/3$
Swann	1954	$MV = (SVC + 2 \times IVC)/3$
Barratt-Boyds	1957	$MV = (SVC + IVC)/2$
Miller	1974	$MV = IVC$
Goldman	1968	$MV = SVC$

- A Q_p/Q_s ratio of greater than 2: closure (either surgically or percutaneously) should be undertaken unless there are specific contraindications.

These recommendations are not absolutes and the entire clinical scenario should be considered along with these findings. Shunt flows can change over time. For example, left-to-right shunts via an ASD can increase with age as left atrial pressures rise in response to decreased left ventricular compliance. Alternatively, left-to-right shunts via an ASD can decrease in response to pulmonary hypertension.

Right-to-left shunting

Right-to-left shunting is unusual except in the case of Eisenmenger's syndrome. In right-to-left shunting, the effective pulmonary flow is reduced by the amount of the shunt (flow through the pulmonary valve + flow through the shunt = flow through the aortic valve). The amount of blood shunted as a percentage of cardiac output can be calculated using the Q_p/Q_s equation. In this case, the value will be less than 1. Other calculations that are useful in quantifying right-to-left shunts are shown in Table 7.2.

Sample case

The patient is a 50-year-old woman with hypertension and a known ASD. The ASD was detected 10 years ago and cardiac catheterization demonstrated a Q_p/Q_s ratio of 1.4:1. The ASD was not closed and the patient was lost to follow-up. She now returns with complaints of exertional dyspnea and paroxysmal atrial fibrillation and is referred for repeat cardiac catheterization to quantify the shunt. The following oxygen saturations were obtained:

SVC 69%
IVC 64%
RV 82%
PA 84%
FA 98%

Using the equations discussed in this chapter, we can determine the Q_p/Q_s ratio for this patient. The equations and calculations are shown here. Because the shunt is at the level of the atrium, the MVO_2 is calculated from the SVC and IVC saturations:

$$MVO_2 = \left[(3 \times SVC) + (1 \times IVC)\right]/4$$
$$MVO_2 = \left[(3 \times 69) + (1 \times 64)\right]/4$$
$$MVO_2 = (207 + 64)/4$$
$$MVO_2 = 271/4$$
$$MVO_2 = 67.75$$

With the MVO_2 calculated, the other variables are obtained directly from the collected oxygen saturations:

$$\frac{Q_p}{Q_s} = \frac{(SAO_2 - MVO_2)}{(PVO_2 - PAO_2)}$$

$$\frac{Q_p}{Q_s} = \frac{(98 - 68)}{(98 - 84)}$$

$$\frac{Q_p}{Q_s} = \frac{(30)}{(14)}$$

$$\frac{Q_p}{Q_s} = 2.2$$

This case illustrates an ASD with a significant left-to-right shunt developing over the course of many years. The magnitude of left-to-right shunting is determined primarily by the relative compliance of the two ventricles. Because of this individual's hypertension and the aging process, her left ventricular compliance decreased over time, resulting in increased left-to-right shunting.

References

1 Wilkinson JL. Haemodynamic calculations in the catheter laboratory. *Heart* 2001;**85**:113–120.
2 Dexter L, Haynes FW, Burwell CS, Eppinger EC, Seibel RE, Evans JM. Studies of congenital heart disease. II. The pressure and oxygen content of blood in the right auricle, right ventricle, and pulmonary artery in control patients, with observations on the oxygen saturation and source of pulmonary capillary blood. *J Clin Invest* 1947;**26**:554–560.

3 Matta BF, Lam AM. The rate of blood withdrawal affects the accuracy of jugular venous bulb. Oxygen saturation measurements. *Anesthesiology* 1997;**86**:806–808.

4 Shepherd AP, Steinke JM, McMahan CA. Effect of oximetry error on the diagnostic value of the Q_p/Q_s ratio. *Int J Cardiol* 1997;**61**:247–259.

5 Hillis LD, Firth BG, Winniford MD. Variability of right-sided cardiac oxygen saturations in adults with and without left-to-right intracardiac shunting. *Am J Cardiol* 1986;**58**:129–132.

PART II
Valvular heart disease

CHAPTER 8

Aortic stenosis

David P. McLaughlin and George A. Stouffer

The basic function of the aortic valve is to separate the aorta from the left ventricle cavity during diastole. At peak left ventricular (LV) ejection the aortic valve opens briskly to an average area of 4 cm². In rare conditions there can be obstruction of forward flow that can occur either at the subvalvular level (e.g., subaortic membrane or hypertrophic obstructive cardiomyopathy) or supravalvular (e.g., Noonan's syndrome). However, the overwhelming majority of cases are due to valvular stenosis. Pathologic thickening and fusion of the aortic valve leaflets results in restricted leaflet mobility and a decrease in the effective aortic valve area, leading to aortic valve stenosis (in this chapter, we will use the abbreviation AS to refer to aortic valvular stenosis).

The etiology of aortic valve disease in developed countries has changed dramatically in the last few decades. With the aging of the population and concurrent decrease in rheumatic fever, degenerative calcific AS is now by far the most common cause of AS. There is evidence that AS has similar histological findings to atherosclerosis with lipid infiltration and inflammation, but statin drugs have been largely ineffective in slowing the progression of AS in clinical studies. A congenitally malformed (bicuspid) aortic valve is one of the most common congenital cardiac defects and is currently the second most common underlying lesion in AS.

As aortic valve disease progresses and the valve orifice narrows, resistance to blood flow increases. In order to maintain stroke volume, the velocity of blood exiting the LV increases and a pressure gradient develops from the LV to the aorta (Figure 8.1). This leads to elevations in left ventricular systolic pressure and this "pressure overload" of the LV leads in turn to compensatory concentric LV hypertrophy. This adaptation allows the LV to generate the necessary pressure to maintain cardiac output, but can lead to abnormalities in diastolic LV function, coronary perfusion, and eventually LV systolic dysfunction.

Progressive increase in the pressure gradient across the aortic valve and cardiac (mal)adaptation explain the stages of hemodynamic findings that patients go

Cardiovascular Hemodynamics for the Clinician, Second Edition. Edited by George A. Stouffer.
© 2017 John Wiley & Sons Ltd. Published 2017 by John Wiley & Sons Ltd.

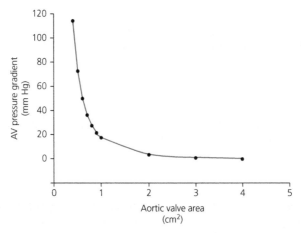

Figure 8.1 AV pressure gradient versus aortic valve area in a hypothetical patient with cardiac output = 5 L/min, HR = 80 bpm, and SEP = 0.33 seconds.

through as AS progresses. In mild AS, intracardiac pressures and cardiac output will appear normal. As the valve becomes more stenotic, the patient may have normal hemodynamic findings at rest, but may be unable to increase cardiac output during exercise. Progressive narrowing of the valve leads to decreased stroke volume and cardiac output, even at rest. In moderate to severe AS, patients may develop elevated filling pressures to compensate for the increase in LV end-diastolic pressure. In a minority of patients LV systolic failure also occurs, which may lead to further elevation in intracardiac pressures. It is important to remember that the pressure gradient across the aortic valve increases exponentially (not linearly) with decreasing aortic valve area. Thus, in patients with severe AS, small changes in aortic valve area can lead to large changes in hemodynamics (Figure 8.1).

Adaptive mechanisms of the LV and circulation allow most patients to remain asymptomatic until advanced narrowing of the aortic valve orifice occurs. The prognosis of patients with asymptomatic severe AS is good, with a sudden death rate of less than 0.5% per year. The onset of symptoms, however, heralds a marked change in the natural history of AS, with poor outcomes unless the patient undergoes aortic valve replacement. The classic clinical presentation of severe AS is typically an insidious onset of any of the triad of effort angina, exertional syncope, or dyspnea [1]. The average survival in untreated patients with severe AS is classically thought to be 2, 3, or 5 years after the onset of heart failure, syncope, or chest pain, respectively. Importantly, many patients report being asymptomatic, although careful questioning reveals that they have gradually decreased their level of activity and would, in fact, be symptomatic at their previous level of exertion. Extensive questioning, often involving a family member, is imperative. Occasionally, careful exercise treadmill testing can be useful in the nominally "asymptomatic" patient.

Physical exam

The physical examination of patients with AS can often be helpful in predicting which patients have hemodynamically severe disease. A low volume, late onset arterial pulse, referred to as parvus et tardus, is often present in severe AS. This finding can be appreciated on palpation of the carotid upstroke and radial artery. It may not be manifest in the elderly owing to a noncompliant vasculature. Other physical findings include a systolic murmur that is crescendo–decrescendo in intensity. The duration will vary with the severity of disease, but the murmur always begins after S1 and ends prior to S2. The timing of the loudest portion of the murmur correlates with the severity of AS, with late-peaking murmurs being more common in critical AS. The murmur is generally heard best in the right second intercostal space and can radiate to the carotid arteries. A diminished aortic component of the second heart sound is not uncommon and the second heart sound can also split paradoxically in severe AS (delayed aortic component with narrowing of the splitting with inspiration). Elderly patients with heavily calcified valves may develop systolic murmurs that radiate prominently to the apex (Gallavardin's phenomenon). Physical exam findings that are suggestive of severe AS include diminished carotid pulses, late-peaking systolic murmur, and absent aortic component of the second heart sound; however, it is important to realize that even in experienced hands the physical exam can be unreliable in terms of quantifying AS severity (see Table 8.1).

Echocardiographic hemodynamics

Echocardiographic evaluation of aortic valve disease has greatly facilitated the management of these patients [2]. Two-dimensional (2D) echo provides important information about valve morphology (Figure 8.2) and LV function as well as important prognostic ancillary findings, such as degree of left ventricular hypertrophy, presence of mitral regurgitation, and pulmonary artery pressures.

Table 8.1 Physical examination of severe AS.

• Parvus et tardus pulse (low amplitude, delayed upstroke)

• Sustained LV impulse

• Late-peaking systolic murmur (although murmur can be absent)

• Diminished or absent aortic component of the second heart sound

• Parodoxical splitting of the second heart sound

• Prominent fourth heart sound

• Gallavardin's phenomenon (radiation of murmur to apex in the elderly)

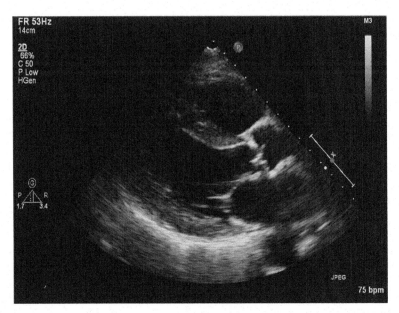

Figure 8.2 2D echocardiographic still frame in the parasternal long axis in a 73-year-old male with severe AS. Note the calcified aortic valve and left ventricular hypertrophy.

Flow through a stenotic AV is well approximated by flow through a convergent orifice (e.g., a nozzle), which causes acceleration of blood velocity as it passes from the LV outflow tract (LVOT) through the stenotic valve. The point of maximum velocity is termed the vena contracta (VC) of the jet and the area of the flow jet at the VC is known as the effective orifice area (EOA). Doppler evaluation enables the noninvasive measurement of blood flow velocity with estimation of aortic valve gradient and valve area. The LV–aortic pressure gradient is estimated by measuring blood flow velocity across the aortic valve and then using the Bernoulli equation to determine pressure gradient.

The primary hemodynamic parameters measured by echocardiography in patients with AS are (a) maximum systolic velocity across the aortic valve measured using continuous-wave Doppler; (b) mean aortic valve pressure gradient; and (c) aortic valve area as determined by continuity equation. Maximum systolic velocity should be measured using multiple views, a time scale on the x-axis of 100 mm/s, and a gray scale that allows visual separation of noise from the true velocity signal. In severe AS, the continuous-wave Doppler curve is generally more rounded, reflecting a high gradient throughout systole. A few additional caveats: (a) it is essential to measure velocity parallel to blood flow, as significant deviation results in velocity underestimation (underestimation is 5% or less if the intercept angle is within 15° of parallel); (b) avoid recording the continuous-wave Doppler signal of an eccentric mitral regurgitation jet; and (c) be careful of interpreting maximum velocity in the setting of irregular rhythms.

Mean transaortic pressure gradient is the average difference in pressure between the LV and aorta during systole. Peak velocity and mean gradient provide independent information regarding AS severity, with the relationship depending on the shape of the velocity curve. The mean gradient is calculated by averaging the instantaneous gradients over the ejection period followed by calculation of pressure from velocity using a simplification of the Bernoulli equation:

$$\Delta P = 4v^2$$

The mean transaortic gradient is easily measured with current echocardiography technology, but it is important to remember that the assumptions in the simplified Bernoulli equation include that (a) viscous losses and acceleration effects are negligible; (b) there is an approximation for the constant that relates to the mass density of blood; and (c) the proximal velocity can be ignored, a reasonable assumption only when the proximal velocity is <1.5 m/s and the aortic velocity is ≥3.0 m/s. Also the effects of pressure recovery, the conversion of kinetic energy into potential energy with a corresponding increase in pressure distal to a stenosis, are ignored, but these are generally small unless aortic diameter is <3 cm.

Maximum velocity and mean pressure gradients across a stenotic aortic valve are both flow dependent. In contrast, aortic valve area is independent of the conditions in which it is measured (at least in theory). When using echocardiography, aortic valve area is calculated based on the continuity equation, which was derived based on the assumption that the stroke volume flowing through the LVOT and the stenotic aortic valve are the same (Figure 8.3). Because volume flow rate at

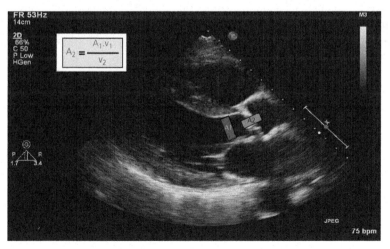

Figure 8.3 The image from Figure 8.2 is used to show the underlying assumption for the continuity equation: the amount of blood flowing through area 1 = the amount of blood flowing through area 2.

any point in the LVOT is equal to the cross-sectional area times velocity over the ejection period (the velocity time interval of the systolic velocity curve), the equation can be solved for aortic valve area:

$$AVA = \frac{CSA_{LVOT} \times VTI_{LVOT}}{VTI_{AV}}$$

$$CSA_{LVOT} = \pi \left(\frac{D}{2}\right)^2$$

where
CSA = cross-sectional area; D = diameter; VTI = velocity time integral.

In practice, determination of aortic valve area by the continuity equation requires measurement of velocity across the aortic valve by continuous-wave Doppler, LVOT diameter, and LVOT velocity by pulse-wave Doppler. There are several important caveats to keep in mind: (a) LVOT diameter and velocity measurements should be made at the same distance from the aortic valve; (b) the LVOT becomes progressively more elliptical (the equation assumes that the LVOT is circular) near the valve in many patients; and (c) this method assumes laminar flow in the LVOT, which may not be valid if there is dynamic subaortic obstruction, a subaortic membrane, or significant aortic regurgitation. Despite these limitations, continuity equation valve area calculations have been well validated [2,3].

A simplified continuity equation can be used, although there tends to be more variability when using maximum velocities rather than velocity time integral (VTI). The simplified equation assumes that the shape of the velocity curve in the outflow tract and aorta are similar, so that the ratio of LVOT VTI to aortic valve VTI is identical to the ratio of the LVOT maximum velocity to aortic valve maximum velocity:

$$AVA = \frac{CSA_{LVOT} \times V_{LVOT}}{V_{AV}}$$

Determination of severity of AS by echocardiography

Echocardiography grading of AS severity is based on maximum velocity, mean gradient, and valve area. General guidelines for determining mild, moderate, and severe AS as set forth by the American College of Cardiology/American Heart Association (ACC/AHA) are listed in Table 8.2. Other hemodynamic measurements of AS such as energy-loss index, AV resistance, valvuloarterial impedance, and LV stroke loss are less commonly used.

Table 8.2 Quantification of AS severity based on echocardiographic measurements as delineated in the AHA/ACC guidelines.

	Mild	Moderate	Severe
Aortic jet velocity (m/s)	2.6–2.9	3.0–4.0	>4.0
Mean gradient (mm Hg)	<20	20–40	>40
AVA (cm²)	>1.5	1.0–1.5	<1.0
Indexed AVA (cm²/m²)	>0.85	0.60–0.85	<0.6

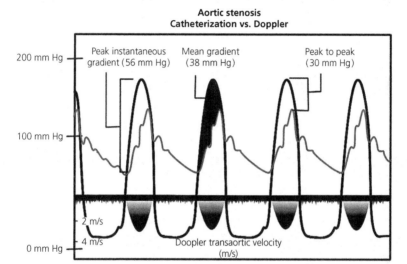

Figure 8.4 Comparison of invasive and echocardiographically derived hemodynamics in a hypothetical patient with AS. Source: Courtesy of Jatin Joshi.

Comparison between invasive and echocardiographic measurements of hemodynamics

It is common for different aortic valve pressure gradients to be reported by the echocardiographic laboratory and the cardiac catheterization laboratory in the same patient (Figure 8.4) [4]. This has led to the common misconception that AV gradients vary depending on whether echocardiography or left heart catheterization is used and that there is a poor correlation between hemodynamics found in the catheterization laboratory and in the echocardiographic laboratory. This misconception is based on comparing apples to oranges. In the catheterization laboratory, gradients are commonly expressed as "peak to peak" (the difference between the maximum LV systolic pressure and the maximum aortic systolic pressure), whereas the echocardiographic laboratory reports peak instantaneous gradients (Figure 8.4). Maximum LV and aortic pressure do not occur at the same time and thus peak-to-peak gradient measured during cardiac catheterization is a nonphysiologic measurement that does not have any echo correlate. Another common misconception is that peak-to-peak pressure defines the maximum pressure difference; this is not the case, as the peak-to-peak difference is always less than the maximum instantaneous pressure difference. The Doppler-derived mean gradient obtained from the VTI correlates well with cardiac catheterization mean gradients. Likewise, the peak Doppler-derived gradient by echo correlates well with the peak instantaneous transvalvular gradient at cardiac catheterization (although this is rarely calculated or reported).

Invasive hemodynamics

Hemodynamic findings associated with AS include fixed outflow tract obstruction and diastolic dysfunction. In contrast to a dynamic outflow tract obstruction (e.g., hypertrophic obstructive cardiomyopathy), the aortic valve gradient will decrease with preload reduction and pulse pressure will increase after a PVC (negative Brockenbrough sign). Over time, the left ventricle in patients with AS hypertrophies in response to the pressure overload. Increased wall thickness causes the left ventricle to become stiffer and less compliant and thus higher end-diastolic pressures are required to maintain left ventricular filling. This, in turn, leads to higher left atrial pressures and elevated pulmonary capillary wedge pressures. PA pressures are normal or only mildly elevated early in the disease, but increase as LV failure (both systolic and diastolic) worsens.

In the catheterization laboratory, the calculation of aortic valve area is traditionally performed using the Gorlin formula. This formula was initially derived in the early 1950s in patients with mitral stenosis. Although the Gorlin formula is seemingly straightforward, there are a number of potential pitfalls and meticulous detail is necessary to obtain an accurate estimation of aortic valve area.

The Gorlin formula requires measurement of cardiac output, heart rate, systolic ejection period, and *mean* transvalvular gradient. The transvalvular gradient requires simultaneous LV and aortic pressure measurement (Figure 8.5). The cardiac

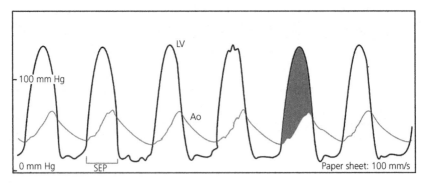

Figure 8.5 Simultaneous LV–aortic pressure tracings with systolic ejection period (SEP) and systolic transvalvular gradient (shaded area) indicated.

output can be obtained either by thermodilution or via the Fick method. The systolic ejection period extends from when the aortic valve opens (i.e., intraventricular pressure rises above aortic pressure) and ends with aortic valve closure.

Gorlin formula for estimating aortic valve area

$$AVA\left(cm^2\right) = \frac{CO/(SEP)(HR)}{44.3 \times \sqrt{mean\ pressure\ gradient}}$$

CO = cardiac output (mL/min); HR = heart rate; SEP = systolic ejection period (s/beat); 44.3 = constant.

Clinical pearl

Aortic valve area can be estimated in patients with severe AS by dividing the cardiac output by the square root of the peak-to-peak systolic pressure gradient measured in the catheterization laboratory. This is the so called Hakki formula [5,6]:

$$AVA\left(cm^2\right) = \frac{CO(L/min)}{\left(\sqrt{peak\ LV\ systolic\ pressure - peak\ aortic\ systolic\ pressure}\right)}$$

Common pitfalls

There are many common pitfalls in the estimation of aortic valve area in the catheterization laboratory:
- Peripheral amplification
- Aortoiliac stenosis
- Aortic regurgitation
- Low-gradient AS
- Poor-fidelity LV tracing

It is best to use simultaneous LV and ascending aortic pressures when determining the invasive hemodynamics of AS. If femoral artery pressure is used as a surrogate for central aortic pressure, obtaining the true LV–aortic gradient can be challenging in patients with peripheral amplification or with peripheral vascular disease. Peripheral amplification refers to the increase in peak systolic pressure and pulse pressure in peripheral arteries as compared to the central aorta (Figure 8.6; see also Chapter 4). It is important to account for peripheral amplification, because determination of AV gradient by comparing femoral artery and LV pressure will underestimate transvalvular gradient compared to a simultaneous recording of LV and aortic pressure.

In contrast, the presence of iliac artery disease causing decreased femoral artery pressures will result in overestimation of the severity of AV disease if comparison is made between femoral artery and LV pressure (Figure 8.7). It is

Peripheral amplification

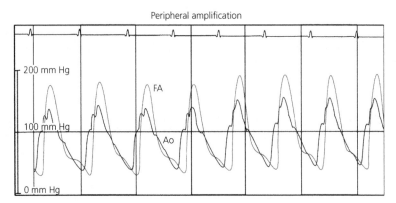

Figure 8.6 Simultaneous measurement of aortic and femoral artery pressure demonstrating peripheral amplification.

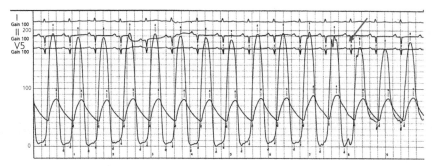

Figure 8.7 Simultaneous recording of LV and right femoral artery pressure followed by a pullback of LV catheter to aorta. The patient is a 65-year-old male with mild AS by echo. Note that there is a significant pressure gradient between LV and right femoral artery, but that most of the gradient persists even after the LV catheter is pulled back into the aorta (there is a ~20 mm Hg gradient between LV and aorta consistent with mild AS; shown by the arrow). This demonstrates that the pressure gradient is primarily due to an obstruction between the ascending aorta and right femoral artery. In this case, the patient had an 80% right common iliac artery stenosis.

essential to measure femoral artery and central aortic pressure simultaneously to confirm that there is no significant peripheral obstruction if femoral artery pressure is used to determine the severity of aortic valve disease. Potential pitfalls in utilizing femoral artery pressure to measure aortic valve gradient can be remedied by using either a pressure wire or a double lumen pigtail, thus allowing simultaneous measurement of left ventricular and central aortic valve pressure. Another approach is to use a long sheath that enables comparison of LV and distal aortic pressure.

Careful attention to detail and examination of the fidelity of the left ventricular waveform are imperative. It is not uncommon to find LV–aortic tracings in which the side holes of the pigtail catheter are in the aorta; this will lead to underestimation of the true valve gradient and overestimation of the valve area.

Another potential source of error is shown in figure 8.8. In this case, a pigtail catheter is "pulled back" from the LV to the aorta. Comparison of systolic pressures indicates a 40 mm Hg difference between the last beat in the LV and the first in the aorta (Figure 8.8). More careful examination, however, revealed that the heart rate had slowed. Within five beats, the aortic systolic pressure was the same as that observed in the LV. In general, catheter pullback across the aortic valve is a suboptimal way to measure aortic valve gradients.

Another potential mistake is illustrated in Figure 8.9. There appears to be a 40–50 mm Hg gradient between LV and femoral artery and on catheter pullback

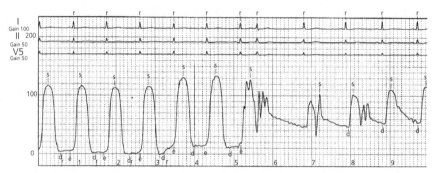

Figure 8.8 Pullback of pigtail catheter from LV to aorta.

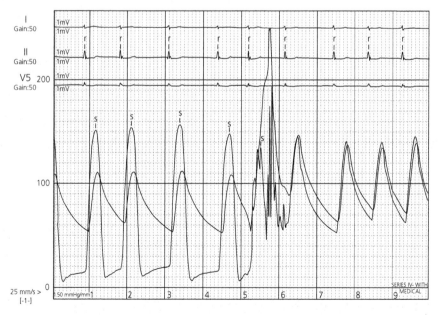

Figure 8.9 Pullback of pigtail catheter from LV to aorta while simultaneously measuring pigtail and femoral artery pressure.

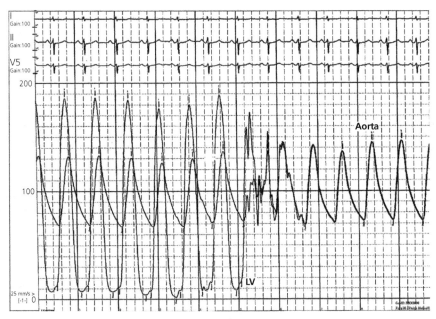

Figure 8.10 Carrabello's sign. Pullback of pigtail catheter from LV to aorta while simultaneously measuring aortic pressure in a 63-year-old male with severe AS (aortic valve area of 0.5 cm²). Note the small rise in aortic pressure when the catheter is removed from the LV.

the gradient resolves. Closer inspection, however, revealed that the femoral artery pressure increased following pullback and now corresponded with LV systolic pressure. The cause of the pressure gradient in this patient was an obstruction in the femoral artery sheath that was dislodged with manipulation of the catheter. Of note is that while aortic pressure can increase following removal of a catheter from the left ventricle in severe AS (Carrabello's sign; discussed in what follows and shown in Figure 8.10), it is never this dramatic and aortic systolic pressure will always be less than LV systolic pressure.

The challenge of low-gradient AS

In patients with low cardiac output and a small pressure gradient across the aortic valve, calculation of aortic valve area with the Gorlin formula can be problematic. The fundamental question in these patients is whether true severe AS coexists with secondary left ventricular systolic dysfunction, or alternatively whether the low gradient is due to a low cardiac output from the cardiomyopathy and the valve stenosis is minimal. Differentiating these two entities is critical, as the former may respond favorably to aortic valve replacement whereas the latter does not.

Increasing cardiac output pharmacologically (typically with dobutamine or nitroprusside), either in the catheterization laboratory or during echocardiography, can be helpful in this regard (Figure 8.11). Patients with true severe AS who will

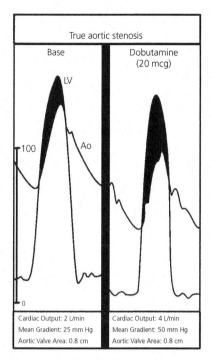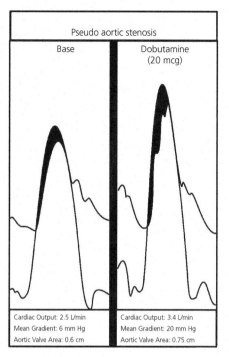

True aortic stenosis		Pseudo aortic stenosis	
Base	Dobutamine (20 mcg)	Base	Dobutamine (20 mcg)
Cardiac Output: 2 L/min	Cardiac Output: 4 L/min	Cardiac Output: 2.5 L/min	Cardiac Output: 3.4 L/min
Mean Gradient: 25 mm Hg	Mean Gradient: 50 mm Hg	Mean Gradient: 6 mm Hg	Mean Gradient: 20 mm Hg
Aortic Valve Area: 0.8 cm	Aortic Valve Area: 0.8 cm	Aortic Valve Area: 0.6 cm	Aortic Valve Area: 0.75 cm

Figure 8.11 Effects of dobutamine infusion in patients with and without valvular aortic stenosis.

likely improve with aortic valve replacement manifest contractile reserve (25% increase in stroke volume) and/or show an increase in their transvalvular gradient and cardiac output with no change or a decrease in the calculated aortic valve area. In contrast, patients with pseudo AS will not have contractile reserve, will not significantly increase their LV–aortic pressure gradient, and will often have an increase in calculated aortic valve area with dobutamine. These latter patients typically have myocardial disease as their primary lesion and "incidental" AS. They do not respond favorably to aortic valve replacement.

The challenge of estimating aortic valve area in patients with AS and significant AR

Another major challenge is accurate calculation of aortic valve area in patients with concurrent aortic regurgitation (AR). The problem lies in the numerator of the Gorlin equation; namely, the accurate determination of flow across the aortic valve. Commonly used ways to estimate cardiac output such as Fick and thermodilution measure effective and right-sided cardiac output, respectively, and thus will underestimate the flow across the aortic valve (flow across the aortic valve = cardiac output + regurgitant volume) and overestimate the severity of AS.

Case study

A 70-year-old man with 3 months of progressive chest pain presents with loss of consciousness while ascending a hill. Examination reveals a blood pressure of 136/80 mm Hg and a delayed carotid upstroke. The second heart sound is split paradoxically. There is a late-peaking systolic ejection type murmur heard best at the right upper sternal border radiating to the carotids. A poor quality 2D echo demonstrates a calcified trileaflet aortic valve with decreased leaflet mobility, normal left ventricular function, and severe LV hypertrophy. Doppler evaluation demonstrated an aortic velocity of 4 m/s corresponding to a peak instantaneous gradient of 64 mm Hg and a mean gradient of 50 mm Hg.

Invasive hemodynamics are shown in Figure 8.12. Note the large mean transvalvular gradient of 110 mm Hg and slow upstroke of the aortic tracing. A cardiac output of 4.2 L/min, with a systolic ejection period of 0.33 s/beat at a heart rate of 70 bpm, yields the following in the Gorlin equation:

$$AVA = \frac{(4200\,\text{mL}/\text{min})/(70\,\text{beats}/\text{min})(0.33\,\text{s}/\text{beat})}{44.3\sqrt{110}}$$

$$AVA = 0.4\,\text{cm}^2$$

This patient went on to aortic valve replacement and recovered fully.

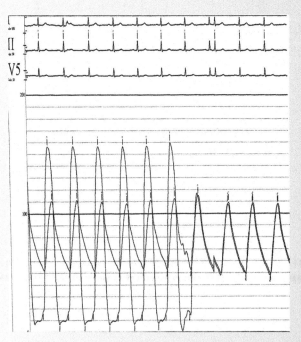

Figure 8.12 LV to aortic pullback of a pigtail catheter with simultaneous measurement of femoral artery pressure. Source: Courtesy of Cardiovillage.com.

Carabello's sign

In patients with AS, Carrabello's sign is defined as a rise in peak aortic systolic pressure by greater than 5 mm Hg when a catheter is removed from the left ventricle (Figure 8.10). This phenomenon occurs in the setting of a highly stenosed valve, because the additional occlusive effect of the catheter across the valve is enough to further decrease aortic pressure. Carrabello and colleagues found this sign in 15 of 20 patients with AVA <0.6 cm² and in none of 22 patients with AVA >0.7 cm² [7].

Subaortic membrane

Obstruction within the LVOT below the aortic valve can be either fixed or dynamic. Dynamic subvalvular stenosis is primarily due to hypertrophic cardiomyopathy (reviewed in Chapter 15). Fixed obstruction can be due to a thin membrane that is attached to the ventricular septum or completely encircles the left ventricular outflow tract (Figure 8.13). Rarely, subvalvular AS is due to a thick fibromuscular

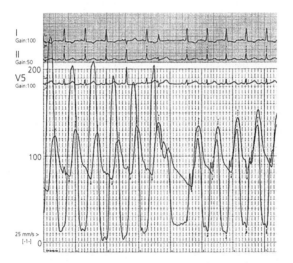

Figure 8.13 Subaortic membrane in a 31-year-old female with hypertension and tobacco abuse who was diagnosed with a possible subaortic membrane at the age of 2. She presented with exertional dyspnea and several episodes of near syncope. She had class III symptoms with dyspnea when walking across a room. This tracing is recorded as an endhole catheter is slowly pulled back from the apex of the LV to the aorta (with simultaneous continuous monitoring of aortic pressure). Note that there is a portion of the tracing when the systolic pressure decreases but there is still a ventricular waveform as the catheter is pulled back across the membrane. In the next portion of the tracing, the catheter is still in the LV but there is minimal systolic gradient between LV and aorta; this is the portion of the left ventricle between the membrane and the aortic valve.

ridge, diffuse obstruction, abnormal attachment of the mitral valve, or accessory endocardial cushion tissue. Clinically significant AS is rare in adults and is often found in patients with prior history of resection while in infancy or childhood.

References

1 Ross J Jr, Braunwald E. Aortic stenosis. *Circulation* 1968;**37**(suppl V):61–67.
2 Baumgartner H, Hung J, Bermejo J, *et al.* Echocardiographic assessment of valve stenosis: EAE/ASE recommendations for clinical practice. *Eur J Echocardiogr* 2009;**10**:1–25.
3 Nishimura RA, Otto CM, Bonow RO, *et al.* 2014 AHA/ACC guideline for the management of patients with valvular heart disease: executive summary: a report of the American College of Cardiology/American Heart Association Task Force on Practice Guidelines. *Circulation* 2014;**129**(23):2440.
4 Saikrishnan N, Kumar G, Sawaya FJ, Lerakis S, Yoganathan AO. Accurate assessment of aortic stenosis: a review of diagnostic modalities and hemodynamics. *Circulation* 2014;**129**(2): 244–253.
5 Hakki AH, Iskandrian AS, Bemis CE, *et al.* A simplified valve formula for the calculation of stenotic cardiac valve areas. *Circulation* 1981;**63**:150–1055.
6 Angel J, Soler-Soler J, Anivarro I, Domingo E. Hemodynamic evaluation of stenotic cardiac valves: II. Modification of the simplified formula for mitral and aortic valve area calculation. *Cathet Cardiovasc Diagn* 1985;**11**:127.
7 Carabello BA, Barry WH, Grossman W. Changes in arterial pressure during left heart pullback in patients with aortic stenosis: a sign of severe aortic stenosis. *Am J Cardiol* 1979;**44**(3): 424–427.

CHAPTER 9

Hemodynamics of transcatheter and surgical aortic valve replacement

John P. Vavalle, Michael Yeung, Thomas G. Caranasos
and Cassandra J. Ramm

Aortic valve replacement is the only definitive therapy for the treatment of severe aortic valve stenosis (AS). With the proportion of the US population over the age of 65 growing at the fastest rate, the prevalence of degenerative calcific aortic stenosis is growing rapidly [1]. The 2014 American College of Cardiology/American Heart Association (ACC/AHA) Guidelines list aortic valve replacement (AVR) as a class I therapy for the treatment of severe symptomatic aortic stenosis [2]. Indeed, AVR in patients with progressive symptoms, such as heart failure, angina, syncope, or left ventricular dysfunction, can not only dramatically improve a patient's quality of life, but is also a life-saving procedure. Contemporary data demonstrate the ineffectiveness of medical treatment of severe symptomatic AS with an average life expectancy of approximately one year for patients with heart failure due to severe AS in the absence of valve replacement [3].

For decades, the only option for AVR was open-heart surgery, usually through a median sternotomy incision requiring cardiopulmonary bypass. Unfortunately, many of the patients with severe AS are older and frail, with multiple comorbidities that make them high or even prohibitive risk for surgical AVR (SAVR). Thankfully, over the last decade a new therapeutic option, minimally invasive transcatheter aortic valve replacement (TAVR), has emerged as a viable alternative for these patients. Data from large randomized controlled trials comparing TAVR to SAVR demonstrated 1-year mortality rates with TAVR that are comparable to, or even lower than, those seen with surgery [4,5]. The uptake of TAVR as a treatment option for severe AS has been brisk due to favorable outcomes in patients who are at high risk or prohibitive risk for surgery. Currently, ongoing studies are looking at TAVR in the intermediate risk surgical population, and it is anticipated that the use of TAVR will eventually expand to this risk cohort as well.

Cardiovascular Hemodynamics for the Clinician, Second Edition. Edited by George A. Stouffer.
© 2017 John Wiley & Sons Ltd. Published 2017 by John Wiley & Sons Ltd.

Selection of appropriate patients

A successful outcome with TAVR starts with appropriate patient selection. The TAVR devices currently approved for use in the USA are designed to treat calcific AS and are less well suited to treating other forms of aortic valve disease. In particular, pure aortic valve insufficiency, bicuspid aortic valves, and disrupted aortic valves from ascending aortic aneurysms or dissections are best treated surgically, albeit with some exceptions.

In general, patients who are candidates for AVR are those who have symptoms attributable to AS and meet the criteria for severe AS, defined as having an aortic valve area (AVA) of $<1.0\,cm^2$ and either a mean aortic valve gradient above 40 mm Hg or jet velocity across the aortic valve of at least 4.0 m/s. The severity of AS can be determined by measuring simultaneous left ventricular and aortic pressure or by echocardiography, which uses Doppler to determine jet velocity across the stenotic valve as well as mean and peak aortic valve gradients.Further details on the hemodynamic assessment of AS are provided in Chapter 8.

Low flow–low-gradient aortic stenosis

An increasingly recognized form of AS is low-flow–low-gradient (LFLG) severe AS. This condition is characterized by a depressed left ventricular ejection fraction (LVEF), an aortic valve area $<1.0\,cm^2$, and a mean aortic gradient <40 mm Hg. Because the transvalvular aortic pressure gradient is dependent on flow across the valve squared, a low flow state (e.g., as seen in heart failure) can significantly diminish the pressure gradient despite the presence of severe AS. These patients often have a dilated left ventricle secondary to the aortic valve pathology and they represent approximately 5–10% of the total patients evaluated with severe AS [6]. A more comprehensive assessment of the severity of AS in these patients can be obtained by measuring pressure gradients during dobutamine administration, which results in increased cardiac output.

More recently, a "paradoxical" LFLG severe AS entity has been described, whereby patients have an aortic valve area $<1.0\,cm^2$ and a low transvalvular aortic gradient (<40 mm Hg), but normal left ventricular ejection fraction. These patients are analogous to their heart failure counterparts who have persistent symptoms despite a preserved LVEF, and are characterized by a small, restrictive LV cavity along with impaired diastolic filling. The criteria proposed to define this condition are a cardiac index $<3.0\,L/min/m^2$ or a stroke volume index $<35\,mL/m^2$. Currently, the most widely used measurement is the stroke volume index, since it is readily obtained by echocardiogram by taking stroke volume (SV) in mL divided by the body surface area (BSA) in m^2. This condition is often seen in elderly women with small body size [7]. It is estimated that up to 10–25% of patients undergoing severe AS may fall into this category [7].

Pseudo severe AS is a condition where there is minimal aortic valve disease in the setting of severe cardiomyopathy. Echocardiographic assessment reveals poor aortic valve leaflet mobility, which is primarily due to the myocardial disease and low flow state rather than inherent calcific aortic pathology. The decrease in aortic valve excursion is a function of the overall depressed cardiac state and is not due to AS.

Patients presenting with pseudo severe AS can be differentiated from LFLG severe AS by performing a dobutamine challenge during either echocardiography or cardiac catheterization. This is important, because patients with LFLG severe AS will generally benefit from AVR, whereas patients with pseudo severe AS will not. For those with truly severe AS, a dobutamine challenge will result in an increase in cardiac index and an increase in mean gradient across the aortic valve, with little to no change in the aortic valve area (AVA). A dobutamine challenge in a patient with pseudo severe AS will result in an increase in AVA with relatively no change in the transvalvular mean gradient.

A dobutamine challenge is also useful in order to assess for contractility and/ or flow reserve. This is defined as an increase in stroke volume by at least 20% from baseline. Contractile reserve has important prognostic implications, since its absence portends a poor prognosis regardless of valve replacement. However, this should not be used as a reason to withhold valve replacement therapy, since patients with no LV contractile reserve who undergo AVR still have a better survival rate compared to those managed medically, despite a higher perioperative risk.

Using hemodynamics to avoid pitfalls during TAVR

Increasingly, TAVR is the treatment of choice for severe AS when patients are at high risk or prohibitive risk for surgical intervention. TAVR requires a multidisciplinary heart team approach to achieve optimal outcomes. Invasive hemodynamics are an essential component of periprocedural patient monitoring as they help identify potential complications that may occur.

In the early stages of the TAVR procedure, a pigtail catheter is inserted into the left ventricle across the stenotic aortic valve. Simultaneous LV and aortic pressures are taken to confirm the severity of the aortic stenosis, but other hemodynamic parameters should also be assessed and noted (Figure 9.1). Left ventricular end diastolic pressure (LVEDP) and aortic diastolic pressure should be recorded. Often, these patients have stiffened calcified peripheral vessels and a low diastolic blood pressure is not an unusual finding. Noting this at the start of the procedure is helpful, because a significant reduction in diastolic blood pressure following valve deployment can be a sign of severe aortic valve insufficiency and/or paravalvular leak. An elevated LVEDP is also a common finding given the longstanding pressure overload of the ventricle from the stenotic aortic valve.

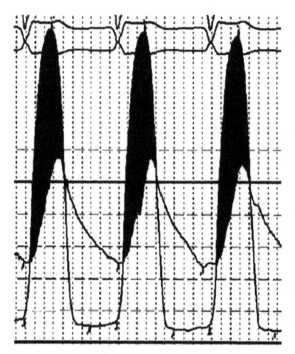

Figure 9.1 Simultaneous left ventricular and aortic pressure tracing showing severe aortic valve stenosis. The high transvalvular pressure gradient and delayed aortic pressure upstroke confirm the diagnosis. It is important during a TAVR procedure to note the starting left ventricular end diastolic pressure (LVEDP) and starting aortic diastolic pressure (DP).

Hypotension during a TAVR procedure can be due to many causes. In severe AS, placing a catheter across the aortic valve can result in a drop in aortic systolic blood pressure (a drop in aortic systolic blood pressure after a catheter is placed in the left ventricle is known as Carrabello's sign and is due to the occlusive effect of the catheter in very severe AS [8]). This can be remedied by balloon aortic valvuloplasty followed by TAVR. Less commonly, hypotension may be an ominous sign of a serious complication. Hypotension may indicate ventricular perforation with cardiac tamponade, severe mitral valve regurgitation due to catheter or wire entanglement into the mitral valve cords and leaflets, or serious vascular injury, usually at the site of vascular access. A pulmonary artery catheter and transesophageal echo, if available, can help quickly differentiate among these potential complications. Severe mitral regurgitation generally results in a large V wave on wedge tracing, while cardiac tamponade is associated with an elevated central venous pressure and equalization of diastolic pressures. Vascular trauma and hemorrhagic shock usually manifest with a low central venous pressure (Table 9.1).

During balloon aortic valvuloplasty or deployment of a balloon expandable TAVR valve, rapid ventricular pacing is performed to transiently diminish cardiac output and drop the forward flow across the left ventricular outflow tract. Typically, this requires rapid VVI pacing at 160–200 bpm to decrease the peak systolic aortic pressure to <50 mm Hg. Although self-expanding transcatheter valves may be deployed at lower pacing rates of 90–100 bpm, the concept of diminishing cardiac output remains paramount. Once this drop in pressure is achieved, valve implantation can safely occur without fear of the TAVR valve being ejected out of the aortic valve annulus due to LV systolic contraction (Figure 9.2).

Table 9.1 Differentiating between causes of hypotension during TAVR.

Potential intraprocedural causes of hypotension	Pulmonary artery catheter findings
Severe mitral regurgitation	Large V wave on PCWP
Cardiac tamponade	Elevated CVP and equalization of RV and LV diastolic pressures
Vascular trauma/hemorrhagic shock	Low CVP, tachycardia

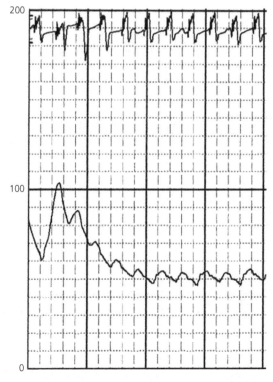

Figure 9.2 Aortic pressure tracing during of rapid ventricular pacing. The aortic systolic pressure should decrease below 50 mm Hg before inflating the aortic valvuloplasty balloon.

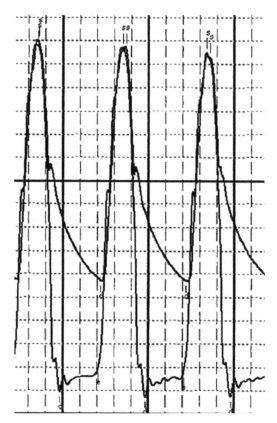

Figure 9.3 Hemodynamics after successful TAVR deployment on the same patient from Figure 9.1. There is no residual aortic stenosis and good separation between the aortic diastolic pressure and left ventricular end diastolic pressure.

Hemodynamic markers of successful valve deployment are minimal residual pressure gradient across the aortic valve and good separation of the aortic diastolic pressure and left ventricular end diastolic pressure (Figure 9.3).

Assessing aortic insufficiency

After deployment of the transcatheter aortic valve, assessment for paravalvular leak and aortic valve insufficiency is essential. Several studies have now demonstrated worse long-term outcomes with moderate or severe aortic insufficiency (AI) compared to mild or less AI [9,10]. A low diastolic aortic pressure with a wide pulse pressure may be the first indication of severe aortic valve insufficiency. Low diastolic blood pressures are not unusual in the TAVR population, especially while under anesthesia. However, a newly low diastolic blood pressure,

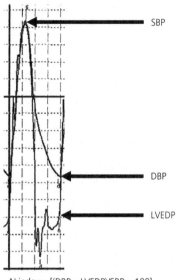

AI index = [(DBP − LVEDP)/SBP × 100]

Figure 9.4 Simultaneous aortic and left ventricular pressure tracing indicating significant aortic insufficiency. There is a wide pulse pressure (aortic systolic blood pressure [SBP] − aortic diastolic blood pressure [DBP]), low aortic diastolic blood pressure, high left ventricular end diastolic pressure, and low AI index (~18).

particularly in the presence of a high systolic pressure, may be due to hemodynamically significant AI. Additionally, an abrupt rise in left ventricular diastolic pressure may be an indication of severe AI (Figure 9.4).

An AI index can be calculated from simultaneous LV and aortic pressure measurements and has been correlated with both the severity of AI and long-term mortality. The AI index is calculated using the aortic diastolic blood pressure (DBP) minus the left ventricular end diastolic pressure (LVEDP) and dividing that by the peak systolic blood pressure (SBP) and multiplying by 100 (Figure 9.4). In one study, an AI index of <25 was associated with increased 1-year mortality (46%) as compared to those with an AI index ≥25 (16.7%); p <0.001 [11].

AI index = (DBP − LVEDP) × 100/SBP

Expected residual gradients after surgical valve replacement

After both TAVR and SAVR, some degree of residual transvalvular gradient is expected. With SAVR it is important to note the reference ranges of the estimated orifice area of the prosthesis to be implanted (Table 9.2) [12]. Residual pressure gradients tend to be higher after SAVR than TAVR, since most surgical valves have an integrated sewing cuff or region where the valve is implanted to the annulus

Table 9.2 Normal reference values of EOA for aortic prostheses.

	Prosthetic valve size, mm					
	19	21	23	25	27	29
Aortic stented bioprosthesis						
Mosaic	1.1±0.2	1.2±0.3	1.4±0.3	1.7±0.4	1.8±0.4	2.0±0.4
Hancock II	...	1.2±0.1	1.3±0.2	1.5±0.2	1.6±0.2	1.6±0.2
Carpentier-Edwards Perimount	1.1±0.3	1.3±0.4	1.50±0.4	1.80±0.4	2.1±0.4	2.2±0.4
Carpentier-Edwards Magna*	1.3±0.3	1.7±0.3	2.1±0.4	2.3±0.5	...	...
Biocor (Epic)*	...	1.3±0.3	1.6±0.3	1.8±0.4	...	...
Mitroflow*	1.1±0.1	1.3±0.1	1.5±0.2	1.8±0.2	...	...
Aortic stentless bioprosthesis						
Medtronic Freestyle	1.2±0.2	1.4±0.2	1.5±0.3	2.0±0.4	2.3±0.5	...
St Jude Medical Toronto SPV	...	1.3±0.3	1.5±0.5	1.7±0.8	2.1±0.7	2.7±1.0
Aortic mechanical prostheses						
Medtronic-Hall	1.2±0.2	1.3±0.2	...	...	...	...
Medtronic Advantage*	...	1.7±0.2	2.2±0.3	2.8±0.6	3.3±0.7	3.9±0.7
St Jude Medical Standard	1.0±0.2	1.4±0.2	1.5±0.5	2.1±0.4	2.7±0.6	3.2±0.3
St Jude Medical Regent	1.6±0.4	2.0±0.7	2.2±0.9	2.5±0.9	3.6±1.3	4.4±0.6
MCRI On-X	1.5±0.2	1.7±0.4	2.0±0.6	2.4±0.8	3.2±0.6	3.2±0.6
Carbomedics Standard	1.0±0.4	1.5±0.3	1.7±0.3	2.0±0.4	2.5±0.4	2.6±0.4

Note: EOA is expressed as mean values (cm^2) available in the literature.
* These results are based on a limited number of patients and thus should be interpreted with caution.
Source: Adapted from Pibarot 2009 [12].

after debridement. These sewing rings decrease the overall residual orifice area at the level of the annulus. Selection of a valve size that is too small for the annulus can lead to the phenomenon of patient–prosthetic mismatch (PPM). This occurs when gradients are higher than expected for that prosthesis. PPM is associated with lower survival and worse hemodynamic function.

With TAVR, the risk of PPM is decreased as the valve has no sewing cuff. Additionally, the valve sizing is performed prior to the procedure, which decreases the risk of undersizing the valve prosthesis. The data on postprocedure TAVR is striking, with low gradients and high effective orifice area (EOA), and residual gradients usually in the 5–12 mm Hg range and EOA in the 1.8–2.0 cm² range.

Contemporary data out to 5 years and longer show stable hemodynamics of transcatheter valves [10,13]. It is important to note that the transcatheter valve can deploy in an asymmetric shape due to the calcium burden at the annulus, thereby affecting the final EOA and gradient. However, the performance of these valves is impressive, with consistently low EOA and gradients with little to no PPM.

Long term follow-up after valve replacement

Currently there are no specific guidelines on the long-term follow-up for patients after TAVR. Much of the follow-up is extrapolated from surgical practice. Most surgical valves are evaluated intraoperatively with transesophageal echocardiogram (TEE). Usually a transthoracic echocardiogram (TTE) is obtained prior to discharge and then at 3–6 months. After noting no surgical complications, this surveillance may be extended to echocardiographic evaluations at 1–3-year intervals. With transcatheter valves, close surveillance is important as the rate of perivalvular leak is higher than with surgical valves and the true lifespan of the transcatheter valves is still unknown, due to the limited experience with this technology (although data from randomized trials show good durability of TAVR valve function now out to 5 years) [10,13]. Cardiac catheterization with crossing of the valve for measurement of pressure gradients should be reserved only for interrogating a failing valve or when echocardiography is unable adequately to diagnose a suspected valvular issue.

References

1 United States Census Bureau. 2010 census shows 65 and older population growing faster than total US population. 2011. https://www.census.gov/newsroom/releases/archives/2010_census/cb11-cn192.html Accessed July 1, 2015.

2 Nishimura RA, Otto CM, Bonow RO, *et al.* and American College of Cardiology/American Heart Association Task Force on Practice G. 2014 AHA/ACC guideline for the management of patients with valvular heart disease: executive summary: a report of the American College of Cardiology/American Heart Association Task Force on Practice Guidelines. *J Am Coll Cardiol* 2014;**63**:2438–2488.

3 Leon MB, Smith CR, Mack M, *et al.* and Investigators. Transcatheter aortic-valve implantation for aortic stenosis in patients who cannot undergo surgery. *New Eng J Med* 2010;**363**:1597–1607.

4 Smith CR, Leon MB, Mack MJ, *et al.* and Investigators. Transcatheter versus surgical aortic-valve replacement in high-risk patients. *New Eng J Med* 2011;**364**:2187–2198.

5 Adams DH, Popma JJ, Reardon MJ, *et al.* and Investigators USCC. Transcatheter aortic-valve replacement with a self-expanding prosthesis. *New Eng J Med* 2014;**370**:1790–1798.

6 Connolly HM, Oh JK, Schaff HV, *et al.* Severe aortic stenosis with low transvalvular gradient and severe left ventricular dysfunction: result of aortic valve replacement in 52 patients. *Circulation* 2000;**101**:1940–1946.

7 Hachicha Z, Dumesnil JG, Bogaty P, Pibarot P. Paradoxical low-flow, low-gradient severe aortic stenosis despite preserved ejection fraction is associated with higher afterload and reduced survival. *Circulation* 2007;**115**:2856–2864.

8 Carabello BA, Barry WH, Grossman W. Changes in arterial pressure during left heart pullback in patients with aortic stenosis: a sign of severe aortic stenosis. *Am J Cardiol* 1979;**44**: 424–427.

9 Reardon MJ, Adams DH, Kleiman NS, *et al.* 2-year outcomes in patients undergoing surgical or self-expanding transcatheter aortic valve replacement. *J Am Coll Cardiol* 2015;**66**: 113–121.

10 Mack MJ, Leon MB, Smith CR, *et al.* and Investigators. 5-year outcomes of transcatheter aortic valve replacement or surgical aortic valve replacement for high surgical risk patients with aortic stenosis (PARTNER 1): a randomised controlled trial. *Lancet* 2015;**385**: 2477–2484.

11 Sinning JM, Hammerstingl C, Vasa-Nicotera M, *et al.* Aortic regurgitation index defines severity of peri-prosthetic regurgitation and predicts outcome in patients after transcatheter aortic valve implantation. *J Am Coll Cardiol* 2012;**59**:1134–1141.

12 Pibarot P, Dumesnil JG. Prosthetic heart valves: selection of the optimal prosthesis and long-term management. *Circulation* 2009;**119**:1034–1048.

13 Kapadia SR, Leon MB, Makkar RR, *et al.* and Investigators PT. 5-year outcomes of transcatheter aortic valve replacement compared with standard treatment for patients with inoperable aortic stenosis (PARTNER 1): a randomised controlled trial. *Lancet* 2015;**385**: 2485–2491.

CHAPTER 10

Mitral stenosis

Robert V. Kelly, Chadwick Huggins and George A. Stouffer

The cross-sectional area of the mitral valve is 4–6 cm^2 in healthy adults. Mitral stenosis (MS) occurs when this area decreases, resulting in increased resistance to flow from the left atrium (LA) to left ventricle (LV), resulting in increased LA pressure. The increased LA pressure is transmitted to the pulmonary circulation, resulting in elevated right heart pressures and in some cases elevated pulmonary vascular resistance (Figure 10.1).

Almost all cases of MS are rheumatic in origin. Isolated MS occurs in 40% of all adults presenting with rheumatic heart disease and women with MS outnumber men by approximately 2:1. Rheumatic mitral valve changes including thickening of the mitral valve leaflets, calcification, and commissural fusion, which occurs over the course of decades. Other rare causes of MS include systemic lupus erythematosis, rheumatoid arthritis, carcinoid, mucopolysaccharidosis, mitral annular calcification, and congenital valve deformity.

There are some rare conditions that cause increased LA pressure that can mimic MS. Examples include LA myxoma, pulmonary vein obstruction, and cor triatriatum (a thin membrane across the left atrium that obstructs pulmonary venous inflow).

MS is a progressive disorder with symptoms worsening as mitral valve area decreases. Symptoms do not usually appear until the mitral valve area is <2 cm^2. Initially, symptoms occur only with exertion, emotional stress, or pregnancy and consist primarily of dyspnea. Symptoms can progress over time and in severe cases eventually include dyspnea at rest, orthopnea, and paroxysmal nocturnal dyspnea. More rarely, there may be angina, palpitations, recumbent cough, and/or hemoptysis. Symptoms can occur more acutely if the patient becomes pregnant, develops a systemic illness, or goes into atrial fibrillation.

Patients with MS generally pass through four separate hemodynamic stages (Figure 10.2):
- Normal hemodynamics
- Normal filling pressures at rest but increased filling pressures with normal cardiac output during exercise

Cardiovascular Hemodynamics for the Clinician, Second Edition. Edited by George A. Stouffer.
© 2017 John Wiley & Sons Ltd. Published 2017 by John Wiley & Sons Ltd.

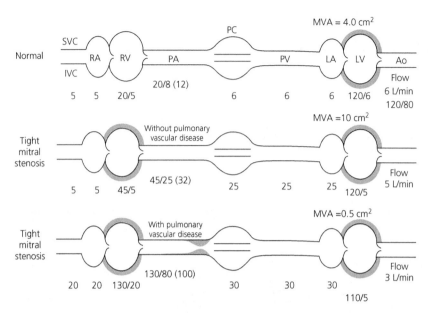

Figure 10.1 Hemodynamic changes of mitral stenosis. [LA = left atrium; LV = left ventricle; PA = pulmonary artery; PV = pulmonary veins; RA = right atrium; RV = right ventricle.]

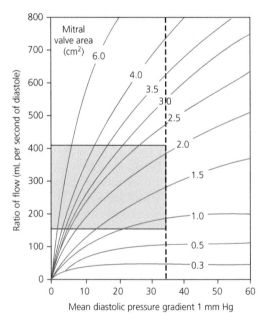

Figure 10.2 Hemodynamic effects of different degrees of mitral stenosis (calculations performed assuming HR × DFP = 32).

- Increased filling pressures at rest and inability to increase cardiac output with exercise
- Markedly increased filling pressures at rest

In addition to increasing resistance to flow, MS also increases transvalvular blood velocity and the ratio of turbulent to laminar flow across the mitral valve. For example, LV inflow velocity across the normal valve is approximately 1 m/s, but can reach 3 m/s in severe MS. The effects of accelerated velocity of blood are not completely understood.

Cardiac hemodynamics in patients with MS

The classic hemodynamic findings associated with MS include elevated LA pressure and a gradient between the LA and LV that persists throughout diastole (Table 10.1). There are several other findings that are discussed in the following in relationship to the cardiac chamber involved.

Left atrium

1 LA pressure is increased and there is a gradient between LA and LV during diastole (Figure 10.3).
2 Chronic LA hypertension causes LA dilatation over time in patients with MS. LA dilation is accelerated in patients with atrial fibrillation.
3 Passive LV filling is slowed, accounting for the decreased slope of the Y descent.
- Atrial contraction becomes more important in ventricular filling. This can lead to a prominent A wave on pulmonary capillary wedge pressure (PCWP) tracing (Figure 10.4).
- Atrial arrhythmias are poorly tolerated.
- Somewhat paradoxically, the contribution of active atrial contraction to transvalvular flow decreases as the severity of MS increases. Meisner *et al.* in a study of 30 patients with MS found that atrial contraction accounted for $29 \pm 5\%$ of filling volume in mild MS and only $9 \pm 5\%$ in severe MS. Computer modeling suggested that increased heart rate, rather than loss of atrial contraction, was the primary mechanism responsible for decompensation of patients with severe MS who develop atrial fibrillation [1].

Table 10.1 Findings at cardiac catheterization.

- Increased LA pressure
- Increased right heart pressures with exercise and/or at rest
- Prominent A wave on RA tracing
- Decreased slope of Y descent on RA tracing
- Gradient between LA and LV persists throughout diastole

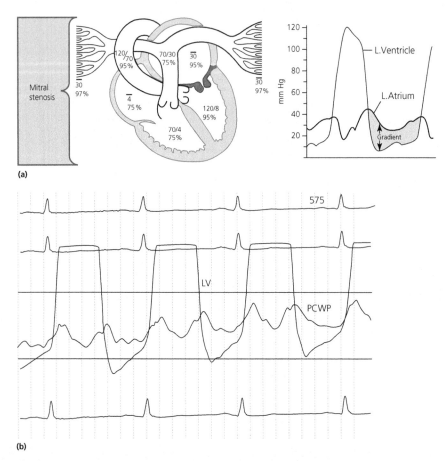

(a)

(b)

Figure 10.3 Transvalvular pressure gradient in a patient with MS. Schematic (a) and actual recordings (b) of simultaneous LV and PCWP pressures in a patient with MS. Note that in (b) the PCWP is delayed relative to LV and should be phase shifted prior to performing any calculations.

Pulmonary artery

In mild MS, pulmonary artery pressures may be normal or slightly elevated at rest but increase with exercise. In severe MS, pulmonary artery pressure will be elevated at rest. Pulmonary hypertension in severe MS can be caused by both elevated LA pressures and increased pulmonary vascular resistance due to pulmonary arteriolar constriction and obliterative changes in the pulmonary vascular bed. It has been speculated that the increased resistance in the pulmonary veins protects the patient from pulmonary edema.

Evidence for a reversible component of pulmonary vascular resistance was shown in a study of 18 women with MS and pulmonary hypertension. Inhaled nitric oxide reduced pulmonary artery systolic pressure by approximately 15%

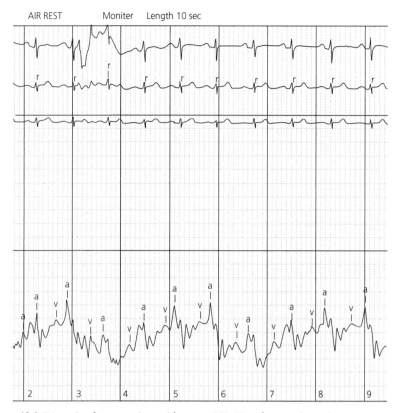

Figure 10.4 RA tracing from a patient with severe MS. Note the prominent A wave.

and pulmonary vascular resistance by 30% without having any effect on LV end-diastolic pressure, LA pressure, cardiac output, or systemic vascular resistance [2]. Following mitral valve surgery or percutaneous balloon mitral valvuloplasty (PBMV), pulmonary artery pressures decrease immediately due to decreased LA pressure. Over time, pulmonary artery pressures continue to decrease as pulmonary vascular resistance decreases. This was demonstrated in a study of 21 patients with severe MS and pulmonary hypertension undergoing PBMV. Mean PCWP decreased from 27 ± 5 (pre-procedure) to 15 ± 4 mm Hg (immediately post-procedure) and then remained constant at a mean follow-up of 1 year. Mean mitral valve gradient decreased from 18 ± 4 to 6 ± 2 mm Hg and then remained constant. Pulmonary artery systolic pressure decreased from 65 ± 13 to 50 ± 13 mm Hg to 38 ± 9 mm Hg. Pulmonary vascular resistance decreased from 461 ± 149 to 401 ± 227 to 212 ± 99 (dyn s/cm^5) [3].

Left ventricle

1 Filling is impaired and determined by degree of MS.
2 Passive LV filling is slowed, accounting for the delayed rise in LV diastolic pressure.

3 LV systolic function is generally normal in most patients with MS.

4 LV diastolic function may be abnormal and directly influences LA pressure.

In most patients with MS, the LV end-diastolic pressure (LVEDP) is normal. It is reduced in about 15% of cases. In the presence of heart failure or mitral regurgitation (MR), LVEDP can be elevated. Since flow across the mitral valve in MS is directly proportional to transvalvular pressure gradient, as LVEDP increases LA pressure must also increase to maintain the transvalvular pressure gradient. Also, reduced LV compliance from (a) displacement of the interventricular septum secondary to early filling of the right ventricle or (b) interstitial fibrosis from rheumatic fever may hinder LV filling during the second half of diastole.

Right ventricle

Right ventricular systolic pressures rise in line with the increases in pulmonary artery systolic pressures.

Cardiac output

1 The flow across the mitral valve during diastole can be approximated by flow = pressure gradient/resistance. As resistance increases (i.e., as MS becomes more severe), the transvalvular pressure gradient must increase to maintain flow. In most cases of MS, the primary mechanism to increase transvalvular gradient is via increased LA pressures. In mild to moderate MS, cardiac output is normal at rest, but increases in LV stroke volume (e.g., with exercise) are associated with further increases in LA pressures. This is why LA and pulmonary artery pressures can increase markedly with exercise. In severe MS, cardiac output can be decreased under basal conditions despite elevated LA pressures.

2 The length of the diastolic filling period is important in determining transvalvular flow. Tachycardia impairs LV filling, further increasing LA pressure, and can be worsened with atrial fibrillation and rapid ventricular response.

3 The flow across the mitral valve = cardiac output + amount of MR. Thus as MR increases, flow across the mitral valve during diastole must increase to maintain cardiac output.

Quantification of severity of MS

The severity of MS can be assessed by cardiac catheterization. The mitral valve gradient may be directly measured by comparing simultaneous pressures in the LV and LA (either by directly measuring LA pressures or using PCWP; Figure 10.5). Simultaneous LA and LV pressures are recorded and the gradients measured. For best results, the fastest paper recording speed (generally 100 mm/s) and a 0–50 mm Hg scale is used. The gradient across the mitral valve should be measured using an

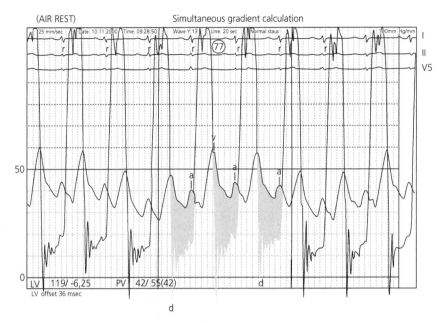

(AIR REST)   Simultaneous gradient calculation

Figure 10.5 Transvalvular gradient in a patient with MS. Simultaneous recording of LV and PCWP pressure tracings. The darkened portion represents transvalvular gradient.

average of five cardiac cycles in patients with normal sinus rhythm and ten cardiac cycles in patients with atrial fibrillation.

The severity of obstruction in MS can be quantified using mitral valve area, mitral valve resistance, or mitral valve gradient. Mitral valve area remains the standard used in most laboratories because it includes the three major hemodynamic variables: transvalvular pressure gradient, cardiac output, and diastolic filling period. By convention, a mitral valve area $<1\,\mathrm{cm^2}$ is considered severe MS, a valve area of $1-1.5\,\mathrm{cm^2}$ is moderate stenosis, and a valve area $1.5-2\,\mathrm{cm^2}$ is mild stenosis.

Mitral valve resistance is a useful research tool, although its clinical use lags behind mitral valve area. It is a measurement of the opposition to blood flow of the stenotic mitral valve and is computed by dividing pressure gradient by transvalvular flow. Mitral valve resistance has been advocated as being more accurate in patients with low cardiac output and low pressure gradients.

The degree of MS can also be defined by the gradient across the mitral valve. By convention, a mean gradient $>10\,\mathrm{mm}$ Hg at rest is severe MS, a mean gradient of $5-10\,\mathrm{mm}$ Hg at rest is moderate stenosis, and a mean gradient $<5\,\mathrm{mm}$ Hg at rest is mild MS. Transvalvular gradient will increase in direct proportion to flow across the valve and thus conditions that increase cardiac output (e.g., anemia, hyperthyroidism, anxiety, exercise, MR) will result in increased gradients.

Some patients may report significant exertional symptoms but have only a mild to moderate resting mitral valve gradient. In these patients, measuring

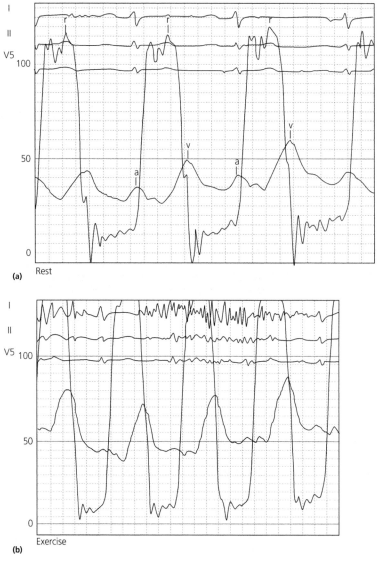

Figure 10.6 Exercise hemodynamics in a patient with MS. Transvalvular pressure gradient (simultaneous recording of LV and PCWP pressure tracings) at rest (a) and with exercise (b).

hemodynamic response to exercise can be very helpful. With exercise, blood flow across the mitral valve increases and this can dramatically change the gradient. If the mitral valve pressure gradient increases with exercise and symptoms develop, the patient's symptoms can be attributed to mitral valve disease (Figure 10.6).

Calculating mitral valve area

The Gorlin formula is the standard for mitral valve area calculation (see text box). It was derived by the Gorlins (father and son) based on Torricelli's law for flow across a round orifice [4]. An empiric constant was added (initially 0.7 and later changed to 0.85) to account for the difference between calculated and actual mitral valve areas.

Gorlin formula for calculating mitral valve area

MVA = (CO/DFP × HR)/(44.3 × 0.85 × square root of mean gradient)
MVA = mitral valve area (cm²)
CO = cardiac output (cm³/min)
HR = heart rate (bpm)
Mean gradient = average diastolic gradient across mitral valve (mm Hg)
DFP = diastolic filling period (s/beat) [measured between initiation of diastole (PCWP/LV crossover) and end of diastole (peak of R wave on ECG)] 44.3 × 0.85 = 37.7 is an empiric constant.

Potential sources of error in quantifying the severity of MS by using the Gorlin formula in the cardiac catheterization laboratory

1 Use of PCWP. To avoid a transseptal puncture, PCWP is commonly used in place of LA pressure. In this scenario, it is essential to ensure that an accurate wedge tracing is obtained. An oxygen saturation >95% helps ensure that the tracing is not a damped pulmonary artery tracing. Potential sources of error when using PCWP tracing include:
- Using damped PA tracing instead of PCWP.
- Inability to obtain PCWP in patients with severe pulmonary hypertension.
- Delay in transmittal of LA pressure to proximal PA, leading to alignment mismatch in PCWP/LV pressure tracing (in general, the pulmonary capillary wedge pressure is 40–120 ms delayed compared to LA pressure).
- PCWP does not approximate LA pressure in patients with venoocclusive disease or cor triatriatum.

Lange et al. compared PCWPs and LA pressures in 10 patients with MS. PCWP was measured using a Goodale–Lubin catheter and confirmed by oximetry. The mean and phasic LA pressure and PCWP were similar. Use of the PCWP with adjustment for time delay resulted in similar values for transvalvular pressure gradient and mitral valve area compared to use of LA pressure. In contrast, when PCWP was used without adjustment for time delay, the transvalvular pressure gradient and mitral valve area were significantly different from the values obtained with use of LA pressure [5].

More recently, Nagy et al. studied the correlation between PCWP (measured with a 6 F catheter) and LA pressure in 117 patients with pure mitral stenosis.

Exclusion criteria included significant aortic disease, more than mild (grade >1) MR, associated ischemic heart disease, systemic hypertension, or diabetes mellitus. The average age was 32 ± 9 years, 67% were female, and the average mitral valve area was $0.9 \, cm^2$. The authors found a very strong correlation between PCWP and LA pressure measurements (correlation coefficient = 0.97, mean bias $\pm$ CI, 0.3 ± -3.7 to 4.2 mm Hg). A statistical analysis showed that the 2 measurements demonstrated consistent correlation, independent of the value of PCWP. Multiple regression analysis found no association between the accuracy of PCWP and heart rate, left ventricular ejection fraction, cardiac output, right ventricular systolic pressure, systemic vascular resistance or pulmonary vascular resistance [6].

2 Measurement of cardiac output. See Chapter 6 for a discussion of the limitations of measuring cardiac output.

3 Atrial fibrillation. The Gorlin formula was developed based on sinus rhythm. It is commonly used in patients with atrial fibrillation, but mean transvalvular gradient will vary with differing diastolic filling periods, and thus it is important to average at least 10 consecutive heart beats.

4 Poor calibration of equipment.

5 Mitral regurgitation. This will increase flow across the mitral valve and can lead to an overestimation of the severity of MS if systemic cardiac output is used in the Gorlin equation. In patients with MR, blood flow across the mitral valve equals systemic cardiac output + regurgitant flow. Since the pressure gradient is dependent on flow across the valve, use of systemic cardiac output in patients with significant MR underestimates flow and thus overestimates the severity of stenosis.

Physical examination in MS

On physical exam, patients with severe MS may have "mitral facies" as a result of low cardiac output and systemic vasoconstriction. The amplitude of the arterial pulse will be small. Jugular venous pulse will be elevated and have a prominent A wave. In atrial fibrillation, this is absent and a CV wave predominates. Palpation of the apex may reveal a presystolic wave and a diastolic thrill may be felt in the left lateral position. An RV heave in the left parasternal area and a loud P2 in the left second intercostal space suggest pulmonary hypertension.

On auscultation, there is classically a loud S1, an opening snap (OS), and a diastolic rumble. The first heart sound may be lessened with a more calcified mitral valve. In addition, there may be a tricuspid regurgitation murmur, pulmonary regurgitation murmur (Graham Steel murmur), and an S4. An S3 may occur if MR or aortic regurgitation are present. In MS, the low-pitched rumbling diastolic murmur is best heard at the apex with the bell of the stethoscope and the patient in the left lateral position. It may radiate if loud. The intensity and duration of the diastolic rumble increase as the gradient across the mitral valve increases.

The murmur persists as long as the mitral valve gradient is more than 3 mm Hg. If a diastolic rumble is not heard, perform maneuvers to increase the patient's heart rate. The increased heart rate decreases the diastolic filling period and therefore causes the LA pressure to increase. Despite maneuvers, some patients with severe MS will not have an audible diastolic rumble due to body habitus.

The duration between A2 and the OS is indicative of the severity of MS. As the LA pressure increases, the A2–OS interval decreases. In mild MS, the A2–OS interval is >100–110 ms. In severe MS, the A2–OS interval is <60–70 ms.

In acute mitral valvulitis due to acute rheumatic fever, the Carey Coombs murmur can be heard. This is a soft early diastolic murmur that varies from day to day. It is also higher pitched than the classic MS murmur.

Echocardiography

Echocardiography is essential for diagnosing MS and can be quite helpful in assessing the severity of obstruction. In the parasternal long-axis view, the mitral valve has a "hockey-stick" deformity (Figure 10.7). In the short-axis view, the mitral valve area can be measured by planimetry. The mitral valve area may also be calculated using the pressure half-time method or continuity equation. The pressure half-time method may not be accurate in the setting of abnormal LA or LV compliance. In these situations, the continuity equation is preferred. The mean mitral valve gradient may be determined by Doppler examination in which an estimation of the diastolic pressure gradient is derived from the transmitral velocity flow curve using the simplified Bernoulli equation: $DP = 4v^2$ [7]. The Doppler gradient is usually assessed using the apical window, as that view is best for parallel alignment of the ultrasound beam and mitral inflow. For measuring maximal velocities, continuous-wave Doppler is preferred over pulse-wave Doppler. Maximal and mean mitral gradients are calculated based on the Doppler diastolic mitral flow waveforms.

Mean gradient is the most useful information, since maximal gradient is derived from peak mitral velocity, which is influenced by LA compliance and LV diastolic function. It is important to remember that mitral valve gradient is influenced by factors other than mitral valve area, such as cardiac output, heart rate, and MR. Other echocardiographic measurements can also be used to estimate mitral valve area, such as planimetry and pressure half-time ($T_{1/2}$). $T_{1/2}$ is the time interval in milliseconds between the maximum velocity and the point where the velocity is half the maximum. The decline of the velocity of transmitral flow during diastole is inversely proportional to valve area and MVA can be calculated using the empiric formula:

$$MVA = 220 / T_{1/2}$$

An echocardiographic grading system, based on 2D imaging of the valve and the subvalvular apparatus, is often used in decision making for mitral valve surgery

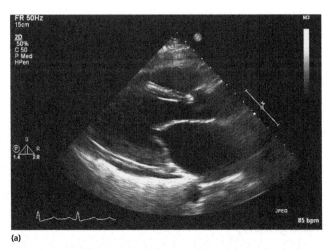

(a)

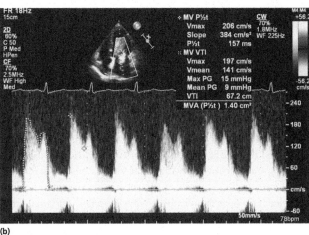

(b)

Figure 10.7 Echocardiographic findings in a patient with mitral stenosis. A 57-year-old female presented with worsening dyspnea on exertion. She was receiving home oxygen and carried a diagnosis of severe chronic obstructive pulmonary disease. Two-dimensional echocardiography (a) showed limited excursion of the mitral valve and continuous-wave Doppler (b) estimated a mean gradient of 9 mm Hg across the mitral valve.

versus PBMV. There are four categories: leaflet thickening, leaflet calcification, leaflet mobility, and subvalvular fusion. A score of 1–4 is assigned to each category, with 1 being least involvement and 4 being severe involvement. In general, a score ≤8 suggests a pliable, non-calcified valve in which PBMV may be technically possible. A full discussion of echocardiographic assessment of the mitral valve is beyond the scope of this book.

Hemodynamics of mitral valve surgery and percutaneous balloon mitral valvuloplasty (PBMV)

Two treatment options exist for MS: surgery and PBMV. In PBMV, a transeptal sheath is placed in the left atrium via a femoral vein. A balloon (most commonly an Inoue balloon) is placed in the mitral valve and inflated, resulting in fracture of the commissures. Class I indications include (a) symptomatic patients (New York Heart Association [NYHA] functional class II, III, or IV) with moderate or severe MS and valve morphology favorable for percutaneous mitral balloon valvotomy in the absence of left atrial thrombus or moderate to severe MR; and (b) asymptomatic patients with moderate or severe MS and valve morphology that is favorable for percutaneous mitral balloon valvotomy who have pulmonary hypertension (pulmonary artery systolic pressure >50 mm Hg at rest or >60 mm Hg with exercise) in the absence of left atrial thrombus or moderate to severe MR.

Among the surgical options are closed commisurotomy, open commissurotomy, and mitral valve replacement. Closed commissurotomy was developed prior to cardiopulmonary bypass. It involves a lateral thoracotomy and a splitting of the commissures with either a finger or a dilator. The success is limited by the amount of calcification present. An open commissurotomy utilizes cardiopulmonary bypass. The surgeon has direct visualization of the valve and is able to incise the commissures and perform subvalvular repair if needed. Mitral valve replacement is a third option. This option is often necessary in patients with heavily calcified valves.

Both PBMV and mitral valve surgery significantly improve mitral valve area, decrease transmitral pressure gradient, reduce pulmonary artery pressure, and increase cardiac output. In a multicenter registry of 290 patients undergoing PBMV, mitral valve area increased from 1.0 to 1.7 cm^2, mean LA pressure decreased from 24 to 19 mm Hg, transvalvular pressure gradient decreased from 13.4 to 6.1 mm Hg, mean pulmonary artery pressure decreased from 34 to 29 mm Hg, and cardiac output increased from 4.1 to 4.4 L/min immediately post-procedure [8].

References

1 Meisner JS, Keren G, Pajaro OE, *et al.* Atrial contribution to ventricular filling in mitral stenosis. *Circulation* 1991;**84**:1469–1480.
2 Mahoney PD, Loh E, Blitz LR, Herrmann HC. Hemodynamic effects of inhaled nitric oxide in women with mitral stenosis and pulmonary hypertension. *Am J Cardiol* 2001;**87**:188–192.
3 Fawzy ME, Mimish L, Sivanandam V, *et al.* Immediate and long-term effect of mitral balloon valvotomy on severe pulmonary hypertension in patients with mitral stenosis. *Am Heart J* 1996;**131**:89–93.
4 Gorlin R, Gorlin SG. Hydraulic formula for calculation of the area of the stenotic mitral valve, other cardiac valves, and central circulatory shunts. I. *Am Heart J* 1951;**41**:1–29.

5 Lange RA, Moore DM Jr, Cigarroa RG, Hillis LD. Use of pulmonary capillary wedge pressure to assess severity of mitral stenosis: is true left atrial pressure needed in this condition? *J Am Coll Cardiol* 1989;**13**:825–831.

6 Nagy AI, Venkateshvaran A, Dash PK, *et al.*. The pulmonary capillary wedge pressure accurately reflects both normal and elevated left atrial pressure. *Am Heart J* 2014;**167**: 876–883.

7 Baumgartner H, Hung J, Bermejo J, *et al.*; American Society of Echocardiography; European Association of Echocardiography. Echocardiographic assessment of valve stenosis: EAE/ASE recommendations for clinical practice. *J Am Soc Echocardiogr* 2009;**22**:1–23.

8 Feldman T. Hemodynamic results, clinical outcome, and complications of Inoue balloon mitral valvotomy. *Cathet Cardiovasc Diagn* 1994;**suppl 2**:2–7.

CHAPTER 11

Aortic regurgitation

George A. Stouffer

The aortic valve separates the left ventricle from the aorta. In normal hearts, it is pliable, opens widely, and presents minimal resistance to flow. The normal aortic valve is a trileaflet structure that is composed of three equal-sized bowl-shaped tissues that are referred to as cusps (left coronary cusp, right coronary cusp, and noncoronary cusp). The aortic valve serves an essential hemodynamic function in isolating the left ventricle from the arterial circulation and can fail in two ways. The valve can fail to open properly during systole, which thus inhibits ejection of blood from the left ventricle (aortic stenosis). Alternatively, the valve can fail by becoming incompetent, thus enabling back flow into the ventricle during diastole (aortic regurgitation) [1].

The hemodynamic changes associated with aortic regurgitation (AR) differ depending on the time–course of the valve dysfunction. If AR develops rapidly (i.e., acute or subacute AR), the left ventricle (LV) is unable to handle the pressure and volume overload, causing a rapid increase in LV pressures during diastole, markedly elevated pressures at end diastole, and premature closure of the mitral valve. Systemic diastolic pressures may be low, but generally there is a minimal increase in pulse pressure; in very severe cases of acute AR, cardiac output may fall, leading to hypotension. LV function can be further impaired by decreased coronary blood flow resulting from the combination of decreased aortic diastolic pressure and elevated LV diastolic pressures.

In chronic AR, stroke volume increases to maintain effective forward flow. This causes dilation of the LV, leading in some patients to the development of a massively dilated LV termed cor bovinum (the largest left ventricles are seen in patients with chronic AR). The body's adaptation to chronic AR results, at least in part, in the classic physical examination findings of a widened pulse pressure and low aortic diastolic pressure. If and when the regurgitant flow overwhelms the adaptive mechanisms, this leads to uncompensated chronic AR with signs and symptoms of heart failure.

Cardiovascular Hemodynamics for the Clinician, Second Edition. Edited by George A. Stouffer.
© 2017 John Wiley & Sons Ltd. Published 2017 by John Wiley & Sons Ltd.

Before the development of aortic valve replacement, severe AR had an ominous prognosis. The availability of surgical treatment has greatly reduced the mortality of this disease (currently there are few percutaneous options available for AR, but several transcatheter valves that could be used to treat AR are in the development stage). The important question now in treating patients with this disease is the timing of aortic valve replacement. An understanding of the hemodynamic changes associated with chronic AR can help in determining cardiac adaptation to the regurgitant flow, and also help determine the severity of AR in patients with moderate AR by angiography or echo but decreased ejection fraction.

Hemodynamic changes of chronic aortic regurgitation

Hemodynamic changes associated with chronic AR result from aorta to left ventricle blood flow during diastole, compensatory responses of the left ventricle to increased diastolic filling, and adaptations by the cardiovascular system to maintain systemic blood flow. In mild AR, increased ejection fraction and/or heart rate lead to an increase in cardiac output across the aortic valve, thus maintaining systemic blood flow. As the severity of AR increases, increases in LV stroke volume are necessary to maintain cardiac output and thus the left ventricle begins to remodel and dilate. This remodeling allows the maintenance of relatively normal filling pressures as left ventricular volumes increase. Left ventricular dilation progresses as the severity of AR worsens and patients with severe chronic AR, if untreated, often develop the largest end-diastolic volumes associated with any heart disease (cor bovinum). LVEDP will increase if the progression of the valve incompetence exceeds the rate of left ventricular remodeling (e.g., acute AR), if the limits of left ventricular remodeling are reached, or if systemic vascular resistance increases to such a degree as to increase regurgitant flow above the ability of the left ventricle to adapt.

Aortic pressures

The two most common blood pressure manifestations associated with chronic AR are a wide systemic pulse pressure and a low aortic diastolic pressure. The wide pulse pressure results from an increased stroke volume (which is needed to deliver enough blood to the aorta to maintain systemic blood flow despite large regurgitant fractions) and decreased peripheral vascular resistance. The low diastolic pressure results from a relatively low resistance to aortic diastolic flow: both backward flow into the LV and forward flow into the periphery. As the competence of the aortic valve decreases, resistance to flow from aorta to LV decreases, regurgitation increases, and aortic diastolic blood pressure drops. A widened and elevated systemic arterial pressure without a dichrotic notch is sometimes observed.

There are other, more subtle changes in arterial pressure that are associated with AR. Peripheral arterial pressures are generally higher than aortic pressures because of amplification due to summation of pressure wave reflections. In AR, because of the accelerated velocity of ventricular ejection, peripheral amplification is more profound than normal. This phenomenon may also lead to the appearance of a bisferiens systolic aortic pressure waveform, in which the first peak is due to ventricular emptying and the second peak to reflections propagated back from the arterial circulation.

Left ventricular pressures

The LV hemodynamic findings associated with chronic AR depend on the extent of ventricular remodeling. In mild to moderate AR, filling from the aorta enables the left ventricle to increase stroke volume by increasing LV end-diastolic volume (i.e., Starling's law). As the AR becomes more severe, the LV dilates in order to handle increased volumes with minimal changes in ventricular diastolic pressures. Thus patients with longstanding, severe AR may have very large hearts with normal diastolic pressures. In some patients with AR and dilated left ventricles, myocardial function begins to decline for reasons that are poorly understood. The development of LV dysfunction leads to increased LV diastolic pressures and eventually to development of pulmonary congestion and symptoms of dyspnea.

Hemodynamic findings in aortic regurgitation

Aorta
* Wide pulse pressure
* Low diastolic pressure
* Increased peripheral amplification

Left ventricle
* Increased LV end-diastolic pressure (LVEDP); in severe AR, LVEDP and aortic diastolic pressure will be equal
* Early closure of the mitral valve during diastole

Hemodynamic changes detected by physical exam

There are several physical findings associated with chronic AR. In the absence of left ventricular failure, patients generally have a wide pulse pressure (the diastolic pressure is usually less than one-half of the systolic pressure). This wide pulse pressure produces a variety of physical findings that are described in the text box. A low diastolic pressure is observed with Korotkoff sounds occasionally persisting to zero. On auscultation, there is a diastolic murmur that usually increases during maneuvers that increase peripheral resistance (e.g., handgrip, squatting). If the AR is heard best along the left sternal border, the etiology may be either valvular or from aortic root pathology, while AR heard best along the right sternal border is typically due to aortic dilation (Harvey's sign). The duration and intensity of the murmur correlate poorly with severity of AR. More subtle diastolic murmurs may be better appreciated with the patient sitting up and leaning forward. A systolic murmur (usually due to increased and/or turbulent flow across the aortic valve) may be present. A2 may be soft or absent and a blowing, high-pitched diastolic murmur may be heard along the sternal border.

A mid- to late-diastolic apical rumble that resembles the murmur of mitral stenosis may be heard in patients with AR (Austin Flint murmur). This murmur was initially thought to reflect rapid antegrade flow across a structurally normal mitral valve that is partially closed in response to rapid increases in LV diastolic pressures. More recent studies have suggested that the murmur is present in patients in whom the AR jet is directed at the anterior mitral valve leaflet. Shuddering of the MV causes vibrations and shock waves that distort the AR jet, leading to the murmur. Mitral stenosis may coexist in patients with AR (particularly in patients with rheumatic disease); the presence of a loud S1 and/or an opening snap are clues that the mitral valve is abnormal. Exercise, amyl nitrite inhalation, or any maneuver that decreases peripheral resistance intensifies the murmur of mitral stenosis while diminishing the murmur of aortic regurgitation and the Austin Flint murmur. Handgrip and other maneuvers that increase peripheral resistance will have the opposite effect.

In patients with chronic AR, cardiac palpation generally reveals that the apical impulse is hyperdynamic, diffuse, and displaced laterally and inferiorly. In patients with left ventricular systolic dysfunction, the precordial impulse may be less prominent and there may be findings of left-sided heart failure (e.g., pulmonary rales, S3).

Physical exam findings of chronic aortic regurgitation

- Wide pulse pressure
- Low diastolic pressure
- Blowing, high-pitched diastolic murmur ± a systolic murmur
- A2 may be soft or absent
- Austin Flint murmur, a mid- to late-diastolic apical rumble that resembles the murmur of mitral stenosis
- Apical impulse is hyperdynamic, diffuse, and displaced laterally and inferiorly

Classic findings described in patients with severe chronic AR

- de Musset's sign: head bobbing with systolic pulse
- Muller's sign: uvula bobbing with systolic pulse
- Corrigan's pulse: booming pulse with quick collapse
- Quincke's pulse: capillary pulsations seen in digits
- Traube's sign: pistol shot sounds heard over femoral artery during systole
- Duroziez's sign: systolic murmur heard over femoral artery with proximal compression and diastolic murmur heard with distal compression
- Hill's sign: defined as popliteal systolic pressure exceeding brachial pressure by 30 mm Hg. Of note is that two studies, with a relatively small number of patients, found that Hill's sign was due to inaccurate noninvasive measurement of pressures in the thigh. Intra-arterial pressure recordings found minimal differences between arm and leg systolic pressures [2,3].

Hemodynamic changes detected by echocardiography

Echocardiography (transthoracic or transesophageal) enables visualization of the valve and identification of congenital abnormalities, rheumatic changes, vegetations, thickening, and/or calcification. Echocardiography also provides information about the size of the LV and aortic root and LV systolic function. Severity of AR may be estimated based on measurement of velocity of regurgitant flow between aorta and left ventricle during diastole by continuous-wave Doppler. The rate of decay of the velocity of flow between aorta and left ventricle during diastole (i.e., pressure half-time) gives an estimate of the gradient between the aorta and left ventricle. A rapid decay indicates equalization of left ventricular and aortic pressures and suggests severe AR. The amount of regurgitant flow can be estimated by several techniques, but a discussion of the relative advantages and disadvantages of these methods is outside the scope of this chapter [4]. Other parameters that can indirectly indicate the hemodynamic severity of AR include (a) measurement of the velocity of tricuspid regurgitation that enables an estimate of pulmonary artery pressures, which in turn may be related to elevated left atrial pressures; and (b) M-mode echocardiography of the mitral valve, which can demonstrate "flutter" of the valve from AR and/or premature closing of the mitral valve during diastole.

The regurgitant fraction tends to decrease in patients with AR as they exercise because (a) the increase in heart rate shortens diastole and (b) peripheral resistance decreases. As the patient exercises more vigorously, further increases in cardiac output are dependent on increased ejection fraction. Thus, some investigators advocate the use of exercise echocardiography in patients with moderate AR. The inability to augment ejection fraction during exercise may be an indication for earlier valve replacement surgery.

Acute aortic regurgitation

Acute AR generally results from endocarditis, aortic dissection, trauma, or failure of a prosthetic valve. The clinical presentation is usually dramatic, with hypotension and pulmonary edema. LV diastolic pressures increase markedly as the LV is suddenly exposed to regurgitant flow from the aorta. In acute AR, the LV does not have time to dilate in response to the regurgitant flow and thus markedly increased diastolic pressures are found.

In acute AR, the "classic" hemodynamic changes associated with chronic AR, for example wide pulse pressure or low diastolic pressure, are absent. There are, however, several characteristic hemodynamic changes that can be observed in these patients:
- Left ventricular and aortic pressures may equalize during diastole. The rate of increase (slope) of the LV pressure during diastole is elevated due to rapid filling from the aorta. This is due to the large volume of blood entering a normal, relatively noncompliant chamber.

- Rapid filling from the aorta can lead to premature closure of the mitral valve. In a heart with a competent aortic valve, LV pressure does not exceed left atrial pressure during diastole and the mitral valve remains open until the left ventricle begins to contract. In acute AR, however, filling of the ventricle from the aorta during diastole leads to a rapid increase in LV pressure. If LV pressure exceeds left atrial pressure, the mitral valve will close before the end of diastole. Premature closure of the mitral valve protects the left atrium and pulmonary circulation from elevated diastolic pressures, but reduces flow of blood from the left atrium to the LV.
- Decreased systemic flow leads to activation of compensatory mechanisms that cause left atrial pressure to rise and can result in elevations of pulmonary capillary wedge pressure and development of pulmonary edema.
- Myocardial ischemia can occur because of inadequate coronary perfusion (even in the absence of coronary artery disease). This occurs as coronary perfusion pressures decrease due to low aortic diastolic pressures and elevated LV diastolic pressure (Figure 11.1).
- Increased LVEDP

Pharmacologic treatment of AR

The preferred treatment of patients with severe AR is valve replacement, but there are patients with less severe disease who will be treated medically. Pharmacologic treatment is based on the principle that the amount of regurgitation is a function of the valve incompetence, length of diastole, and peripheral arterial resistance. Thus in patients with AR, drugs that decrease peripheral resistance (e.g., nifedipine, angiotensin-converting enzyme inhibitors) are beneficial, whereas drugs that lengthen diastole (e.g., beta blockers or rate-slowing calcium channel blockers) are deleterious.

Hemodynamic tracings of a patient with severe AR

These are shown in Figure 11.2 and a further example is given in the case study.

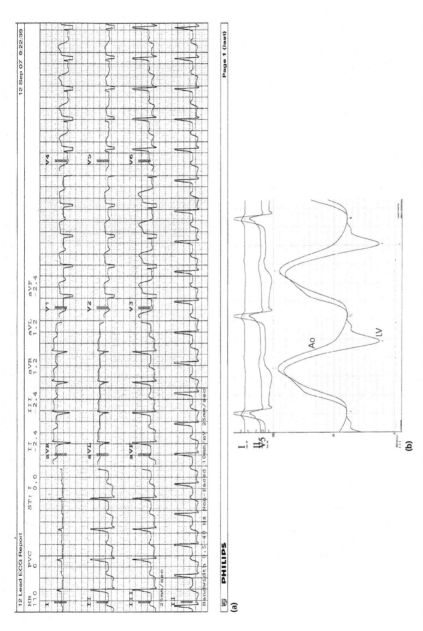

Figure 11.1 Coronary ischemia in a patient with acute on chronic AR. A 31-year-old male with a history of ankylosing spondylitis presented with a one-week history of progressive dyspnea, low-grade fevers (100.5 °F), cough, nausea, and diarrhea. He reported a rapid decline in exercise tolerance over the week and now experiences dyspnea when walking only 10–20 feet. After admission, he developed severe chest pain and an ECG showed anterior ST elevation that was not present on an ECG taken on admission (a). His blood pressure as determined by sphygmomanometry was 90/30 mm Hg. Emergent cardiac catheterization showed no evidence of coronary artery disease, but severe AR with equalization of aortic and left ventricular diastolic pressures (b).

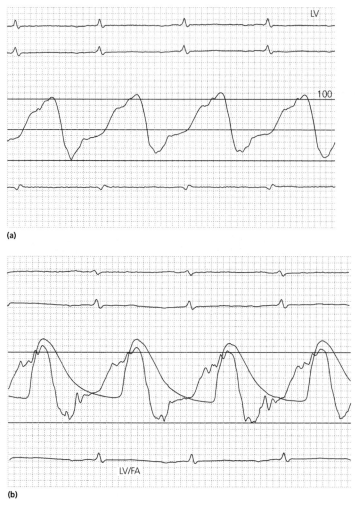

(a)

(b)

Figure 11.2 Left ventricular tracings alone (a), with femoral artery pressure (b), and with PCWP (c) in a patient with severe chronic AR (all tracings are on a 200 mm Hg scale).

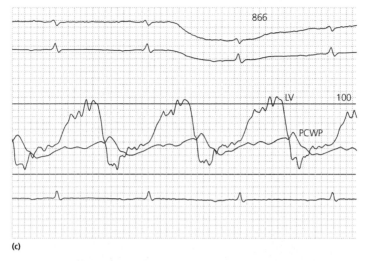

(c)

Figure 11.2 (Continued)

Case study

A 65-year-old male with chronic severe aortic regurgitation was referred for cardiac catheterization prior to valve replacement. He had carried the diagnosis of severe AR for several years and was being treated with enalapril. Annual echocardiograms confirmed the presence of AR but showed no chamber dilation. He had been asymptomatic for years but recently developed dyspnea on exertion.

The hemodynamic tracings are shown in Figure 11.3.

Note that the pulse pressure is 60 mm Hg with an aortic diastolic pressure of 62 mm Hg. A clear dichrotic notch is present on the aortic tracing. While the LV diastolic pressure rises more rapidly than normal, the LVEDP is only 15 mm Hg.

The hemodynamics are not consistent with severe AR. This was confirmed by aortic angiography that revealed 2+ AR. In the absence of elevated filling pressures and with normal LV size, there is no evidence that this patient will improve with valve replacement. Looked at a different way, valve replacement will probably not result in a favorable change in hemodynamics (in AR this usually involves a decrease in LVEDP and an increase in aortic diastolic pressure).

A severe lesion was found in the right coronary artery that was treated by placement of an intracoronary stent. Following the procedure, the patient's symptoms resolved.

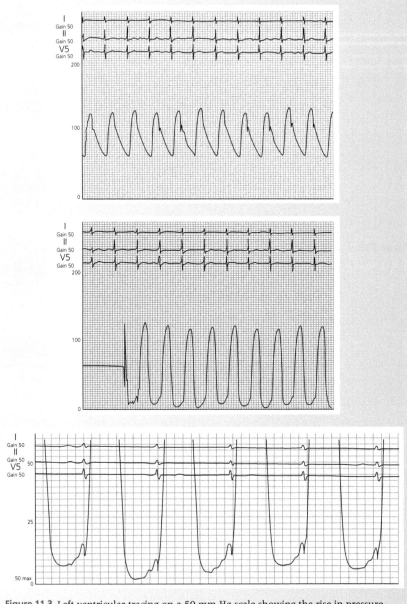

Figure 11.3 Left ventricular tracing on a 50 mm Hg scale showing the rise in pressure during diastole.

Angiographic classification of severity of aortic regurgitation (based on the amount of contrast dye entering the left ventricle during an aortogram)

1+ some dye enters ventricle but clears with every systole
2+ the ventricle becomes completely opacified after several heart beats and remains opacified throughout the cardiac cycle
3+ the ventricle becomes as dark as the aorta after several heart beats
4+ the ventricle becomes darker than the aorta after several heart beats

References

1 Stouffer GA, Uretsky BF. Hemodynamic changes of aortic regurgitation. *Am J Med Sci* 1997;**314**:411–414.
2 Kutryk M, Fitchett D. Hill's sign in aortic regurgitation: enhanced pressure wave transmission or artefact? *Can J Cardiol* 1997;**13**:237–240.
3 HK Kang, GR Andrews, S. Ramamoorthy. A study to evaluate the clinical value of Hill's sign in the assessment of aortic regurgitation. *Nurs Midwifery Res J* 2008;**4**:107–114.
4 Lancellotti P, Tribouilloy C, Hagendorff A, *et al.*; European Association of Echocardiography. European Association of Echocardiography recommendations for the assessment of valvular regurgitation. Part 1: aortic and pulmonary regurgitation (native valve disease). *Eur J Echocardiogr* 2010;**11**:223–244.

CHAPTER 12

Mitral regurgitation

Robert V. Kelly, Mauricio G. Cohen and George A. Stouffer

Patients remain asymptomatic for years with chronic severe mitral regurgitation (MR) before developing exertional dyspnea. In contrast, sudden onset of pulmonary edema is a hallmark of acute MR. The natural history of chronic MR is variable and depends on the regurgitant volume, left ventricular (LV) function, and the underlying cause of MR. Compensatory mechanisms enable the patient to adapt to severe MR (Figure 12.1). The development of symptoms at rest in chronic MR can be an ominous finding, especially if coupled with decrease in LV systolic function.

Pathology

MR can be caused by structural abnormalities of the mitral leaflets, papillary muscles, chordae tendineae, or mitral annulus. A partial list of the causes of MR includes myxomatous changes, congenital abnormalities, chordal rupture, papillary muscle dysfunction or rupture secondary to myocardial ischemia or infarction (MI), endocarditis, trauma, and rheumatic degeneration. In patients with MR due to myocardial ischemia or infarction, the posterior leaflet is most likely to be incompetent, as the posterior papillary muscle is supplied solely by the posterior descending artery, whereas the anterolateral papillary muscle has a dual blood supply, including diagonal branches of the left anterior descending coronary artery and often obtuse marginal branches from the left circumflex artery.

MR can occur in the setting of a normal mitral valve and apparatus when there is pathology of the mitral annulus. In healthy adults, the annulus is about 10 cm in circumference. It is a soft and flexible structure, which contributes to valve closure by enhancing valvular constriction, due to the contraction of the surrounding LV muscle. Dilation of the left ventricle can cause dilatation of the mitral valve annulus and mal-apposition of the mitral leaflets.

Cardiovascular Hemodynamics for the Clinician, Second Edition. Edited by George A. Stouffer.
© 2017 John Wiley & Sons Ltd. Published 2017 by John Wiley & Sons Ltd.

No MR   Severe MR

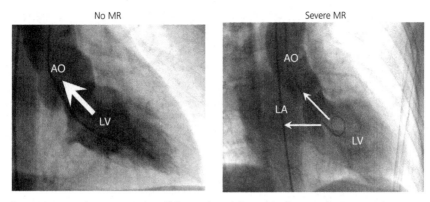

Figure 12.1 Mitral regurgitation. Still frames from left ventriculograms from two patients showing no mitral regurgitation on the left and severe mitral regurgitation on the right. In both cases, dye has been injected into the left ventricle. Note that the left atrium is opacified on the right but not on the left, indicative of mitral regurgitation. The arrow represents blood flow. With a competent mitral valve, all of the blood ejected by the left ventricle goes into the aorta. In patients with mitral regurgitation, a portion of left ventricular stroke volume goes into the left atrium. [Ao = aorta; LA = left atrium; LV = left ventricle.]

Mitral annular calcification (MAC) can also cause regurgitation in severe cases. MAC is associated with hypertension, diabetes, aortic stenosis, Marfan's syndrome, Hurler's syndrome, and chronic renal failure. In severe calcification, a rigid ring of calcium encircles the mitral orifice and calcific spurs may project into the adjacent myocardium. Severe mitral annular calcification may also immobilize the mitral leaflets, resulting in MR.

Acute MR

Acute MR is a rare but potentially life-threatening condition that is generally associated with abrupt onset of dyspnea, heart failure, and shock. Characteristic hemodynamic changes include increased LV preload, increased total stroke volume, compromised forward stroke volume, decreased LV end-systolic diameter, and increased ejection fraction. Causes of acute MR include ruptured papillary muscles (e.g., during acute MI) or rupture chordae (e.g., from myxomatous disease), myocardial ischemia leading to papillary muscle dysfunction, bacterial endocarditis, and trauma. Acute MR is characterized hemodynamically by regurgitation in the absence of any compensatory dilation of a relatively noncompliant left atrium or left ventricle. The lack of time for compensatory mechanisms to develop results in an abrupt rise in left atrial (LA) pressure, which is generally accompanied by large V waves on pulmonary capillary wedge pressure (PCWP) tracing, appearance of large V waves in the PA tracing (so-called Camelback PA tracing, in which V waves are reflected through a compliant pulmonary vasculature; see Figure 12.4) and a rapid Y descent as the distended LA quickly empties.

Hemodynamic concepts in patients with chronic MR

1 The amount of mitral regurgitation is labile and dependent on:
  • Size of regurgitant orifice—the primary determinant of the size of the regurgitant orifice is the underlying pathology. Note, however, that the cross-sectional area of the annulus may be influenced by LV size. LV dilation will result in an increase in the annulus size and the regurgitant orifice, whereas a decrease in LV size (e.g., by diuretics, inotropes, or vasodilators) will cause a reduction in the regurgitant orifice.
  • LA compliance—the left atrium dilates over time in patients with chronic MR so that large regurgitant volumes can be accommodated with minimal increases in pressure.
  • Pressure difference between LV and LA during systole
  • Duration of systole
  • Afterload—systolic blood flow from the left ventricle goes in two directions: into a high-pressure, high-capacitance system (the aorta) and a low-pressure, low-capacitance system (the left atrium). Thus, the amount of regurgitant flow is influenced by the ratio of resistance to flow across the aortic valve to resistance to flow across the mitral valve. Increases in aortic afterload (e.g., blood pressure, aortic stenosis, etc.) will increase mitral regurgitation. Because of blood flow into the left atrium, the effective afterload seen by the LV is reduced regardless of the aortic afterload.
2 In the LV pressure–volume loop there is no true isovolumetric contraction phase, because regurgitant flow across the mitral valve occurs before the aortic valve opens.
3 Left ventricular end-diastolic volume (LVEDV) increases to maintain stroke volume and compensate for the regurgitant volume. Increased diastolic volumes result in increased contractility (via Starling's law). In MR, there is increased stroke volume and stroke work, although effective forward stroke volume may be normal or reduced.
4 The compliance of the left atrium and pulmonary veins is an important determinant of the severity of MR symptoms. In patients with a normal-sized LA and severe MR, marked elevation in LA pressure occurs, with a prominent V wave on the PCWP tracing and significant pulmonary congestion. In patients with acute MR, the left atrium initially operates on the steep portion of the Frank–Starling curve, with a marked rise in pressure for a small increase in volume. In chronic MR, over time the LA dilates and is able to accommodate large regurgitant volumes. This usually occurs over a 6–12-month period. Increased LA compliance is a feature of longstanding MR (i.e., increased LA size with minimal increases in LA pressure). In this situation, longstanding MR shifts the LA Starling curve to the right, minimizing the increases in LA pressures in response to large volume increases.
5 LV loading conditions in MR are favorable for preserved ejection fraction, because LV preload is increased while LV afterload is normal or reduced.

In patients with chronic MR, LV systolic contractility can become progressively impaired, with clinical indexes of LV function (e.g., ejection fraction and fractional shortening) remaining normal. This is why a fall in ejection fraction in patients with severe MR is an ominous finding and why ejection fraction may worsen after mitral valve surgery (as opposed to aortic regurgitation, in which ejection fraction may improve after valve replacement because afterload is decreased).

6 Symptoms commonly occur initially with exercise in patients with MR. There is controversy about whether exertional dyspnea in patients with chronic MR is due to increases in pulmonary artery pressure or to inability to increase cardiac output. Hasuda *et al.* found that exertional dyspnea did not correlate with pulmonary artery pressures, but did correlate with the rise in pulmonary artery pressures per unit of cardiac output in their group of 20 patients with MR or AR [1].

Compensatory mechanisms in chronic MR

The hemodynamic changes of chronic MR can be predicted by understanding the compensatory changes that occur. The heart adapts to chronic MR primarily by LA and LV dilation. The LV adapts to substantial regurgitant volumes by increasing LVEDV to maintain adequate forward cardiac output. According to Laplace's law (wall tension is related to radius × intraventricular pressure), the increased LVEDV increases wall tension to supranormal levels. In chronic MR, LVEDV and LV mass increase, usually in proportion to the degree of LV dilation. The degree of hypertrophy correlates with the amount of chamber dilation so that the ratio of LV mass to end-diastolic volume remains in the normal range (in contrast to the situation in patients with LV pressure overload). At the same time there is a greater volume at a given pressure, resulting in a shift in the pressure–volume relationship (Figure 12.2). In most patients, LV compensation is maintained for years, but eventually LV failure occurs. This results in an increase in preload and LV end-systolic volume (LVESV), and a decrease in LVEF and stroke volume.

LVESV is an important pre-operative prognostic marker, especially in terms of mortality, post-operative heart failure, and post-operative LV systolic function. LVESV index is an important marker of LV function in MR patients and helps with mitral valve surgery decisions. End-systolic diameter (ESD) on echo is also a useful prognostic indicator. An ESD >45 mm is generally used as an indication for surgery, although if mitral valve repair can be accomplished a lower cutoff value has been advocated.

The transition from a compensated state to a decompensated state in chronic MR is not completely understood. LV systolic function begins to decline, LVEDV increases, and filling pressures rise. Thus, chronic decompensated MR results in both systolic and diastolic dysfunction.

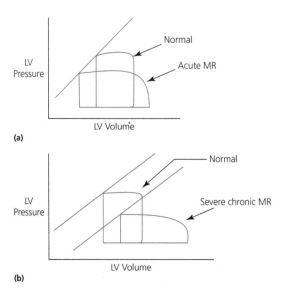

Figure 12.2 Pressure–volume loops in acute MR (a) and chronic MR (b).

Cardiac catheterization and MR hemodynamics

The primary findings at catheterization in chronic MR include:
- Increased LA (or PCWP), pulmonary artery, right ventricular, and right atrial pressures.
- In severe MR, effective cardiac output is usually depressed while stroke volume (i.e., the combination of forward and regurgitant flow) is usually increased. Functional capacity during exercise depends primarily on cardiac output and not the regurgitant volume.
- V waves may or may not be present in the PCWP tracing (Figure 12.3). They occur during ventricular systole and coincide with the T wave on the ECG and descent of pressure (isovolumetric relaxation) on the LV tracing. The V wave represents the rise in LA pressure during ventricular contraction and the height of the V wave is determined by the volume of blood entering the LA, LA compliance, and LA size. Because the size of the V wave is influenced by factors other than regurgitant flow, large V waves are neither sensitive nor specific for MR, and the absence of a significant V wave does not rule out significant MR (for a more detailed discussion of V waves, see Chapter 5).
- There may be a "camelback" appearance to the PA waveform. This tracing is characterized by a bifid appearance in which the systolic peak is followed by a second peak, which is a reflected V wave (Figure 12.4).
- In MR, the A wave is generally not affected. In cases of pure MR, the Y descent in the pulmonary capillary wedge pressure is rapid (pseudoconstriction pattern) as the distended left atrium empties rapidly during early diastole. However, in

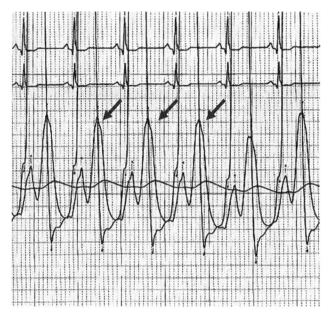

Figure 12.3 Simultaneous LV and PCWP tracing in a patient with severe MR showing a V wave (arrow).

patients with mixed mitral valve disease, the Y descent is gradual. A brief early diastolic pressure gradient between LA and LV may occur in patients with isolated severe MR as a result of increased blood flow across a normal-size mitral orifice early in diastole.

Physical examination

The pulse is sharp in severe chronic MR and the pulse volume is usually normal. The apical impulse is brisk and hyperdynamic. It is often displaced to the left and can be associated with a prominent LV filling thrill. On auscultation, the first heart sound is diminished in severe MR. A wide splitting of S2 is common. It results from the shortening of the LV ejection and an earlier aortic valve closure as a consequence of reduced resistance to LV outflow. If severe pulmonary hypertension develops, P2 can be louder than A2.

There is a pansystolic murmur. In severe MR, it commences immediately after a soft S1. It may extend beyond A2 because of the persisting pressure difference between the LV and LA after aortic closure. The murmur is a blowing high-pitched murmur and is loudest at the apex. It often radiates to the axilla, but it may also radiate to the sternum or aortic valve area if the posterior leaflet is involved, mimicking aortic stenosis. The murmur of MR is usually accentuated by isometric exercise. In papillary dysfunction, the MR murmur may occur later in systole,

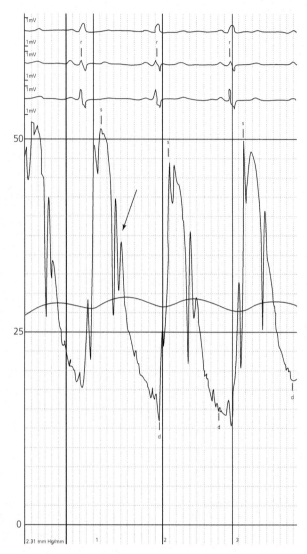

Figure 12.4 Pulmonary artery tracing in a patient with severe MR (the same patient as in Figure 12.3) showing bifid appearance characteristic of a reflected V wave (arrow).

with preservation of a normal S1 because the initial closure of the mitral valve is unaffected. A third heart sound but not a fourth heart sound is typical of chronic MR. In MR caused by mitral valve prolapse and myxomatous degeneration of the valve, the murmur may not be holosystolic, but rather tend to be more early or mid-systolic and have a more musical quality.

In acute severe MR, the patient is almost always symptomatic and often in heart failure. A systolic murmur will be present, although it may not be holosystolic and may disappear in mid or late systole if left atrial pressure is elevated. The murmur of acute MR is generally lower in pitch and softer than the murmur of chronic MR. A S3 and S4 are common, but there may not be a hyperdynamic apical impulse if the ventricle is normal in size.

Echocardiography

The mitral valve, valve apparatus, chordae, and papillary muscles can be visualized on echocardiography. The LA and LV size can be measured. Severity of MR can be defined by several different echo parameters. The intensity of the Doppler signal, the ratio of the regurgitant flow (RF) to the forward flow (FF), the regurgitant jet area, the ratio of regurgitant jet to LA area, and effective regurgitant orifice (ERO) all correlate with the severity of MR. Reversal of Doppler flow in pulmonary veins during systole can also be assessed and is an important indicator of severe MR.

Important points

1 The amount of MR is labile and dependent on
   • Size of regurgitant orifice
   • LA compliance
   • Mean pressure difference between LV and LA
   • Duration of systole
   • LV afterload (i.e., blood pressure)
2 Acute MR is generally associated with abrupt onset of heart failure, normal size LV, hyperdynamic LV, and softer, shorter murmur than chronic MR.
3 Chronic MR is associated with reduced LV afterload. This is why a fall in ejection fraction is ominous and why ejection fraction does not improve after valve replacement
4 LVEDV increases to maintain stroke volume.
5 Pronounced V waves on PCWP tracing are suggestive of MR, but are neither sensitive nor specific

Hemodynamics of mitral regurgitation

Acute
   • Elevated PCWP and PA
   • Prominent V wave
   • Pseudoconstriction (rapid dilation of left atria, RV, and right atria can simulate hemodynamic findings of constrictive pericarditis)
   • Hyperdynamic LV function with increased ejection fraction

- LV is normal in size
- May have hypotension and shock

Chronic compensated
- Normal to mild right heart pressure elevation
- Less prominent V wave
- Mild to moderate LV dilation
- Normal ejection fraction

Chronic decompensated
- Elevated PCWP, PA, and right heart pressures
- Marked LV dilation
- Decreased ejection fraction

Pseudomitral stenosis in a patient with severe mitral regurgitation

The pressure gradient across a stenotic valve is a function of resistance and flow ($P = R \times F$). In patients with mild mitral stenosis (MS) and severe MR, the diastolic gradient across the mitral valve can simulate severe MS because of the excessive flow across the valve. Remember, in MR, flow across the mitral valve is equal to cardiac output + regurgitant volume. Thus in severe MR, flow across the mitral valve may exceed 2 × cardiac output.

Grading severity of mitral regurgitation on LV angiography

1+ Contrast enters LA but clears with each beat and never fills the entire LA
2+ Faint filling of entire LA but the opacification of the LA remains less than that of the LV
3+ Complete opacification of LA with opacification of the LA equal to that of the LV
4+ Complete and dense filling of the LA with the initial beat and opacification of the LA becoming darker than LV; evidence of contrast in the pulmonary veins

---

Reference

1 Hasuda T, Okano Y, Yoshioka T, Nakanishi N, Shimizu M. Pulmonary pressure–flow relation as a determinant factor of exercise capacity and symptoms in patients with regurgitant valvular heart disease. *Int J Cardiol* 2005;**99**:403–407.

CHAPTER 13

The tricuspid valve

David A. Tate and George A. Stouffer

The tricuspid valve separates the right atrium (RA) from the right ventricle (RV). Its three leaflets are unequal in size, with the anterior leaflet usually being the largest. The leaflets are thin and translucent, a design that is adequate to the relatively lower pressures and hemodynamic stresses to which the right-sided valves are subjected under normal circumstances (Figure 13.1). Indeed, although structural tricuspid valvular abnormalities do occur, hemodynamic perturbations involving the tricuspid valve are far more commonly seen in patients with morphologically normal valves subjected to abnormal hemodynamic stresses.

Tricuspid regurgitation

Pathophysiology

Tricuspid regurgitation due to primary structural valvular abnormalities is rare, but will occasionally be seen due to rheumatic heart disease, myxomatous disease (prolapse), infective or marantic endocarditis, carcinoid heart disease, anorectic drugs, trauma, Marfan's syndrome, or Ebstein's anomaly. In addition, the tricuspid valve can be damaged during placement of leads for pacemakers or implantable cardioverter-defibrillators or during right ventricular biopsies in heart transplant recipients.

In contrast, secondary functional tricuspid regurgitation is commonly encountered as a consequence of conditions associated with increased pulmonary arterial pressures, such as left ventricular systolic or diastolic dysfunction, mitral regurgitation, mitral stenosis, primary pulmonary disease, or primary pulmonary hypertension. Dilatation of the tricuspid annulus may also be seen in right ventricular infarction or in dilated cardiomyopathies.

The backward flow of blood from the RV to the RA is often clinically subtle due to the relatively compliant RA and the more conspicuous manifestations

Cardiovascular Hemodynamics for the Clinician, Second Edition. Edited by George A. Stouffer.
© 2017 John Wiley & Sons Ltd. Published 2017 by John Wiley & Sons Ltd.

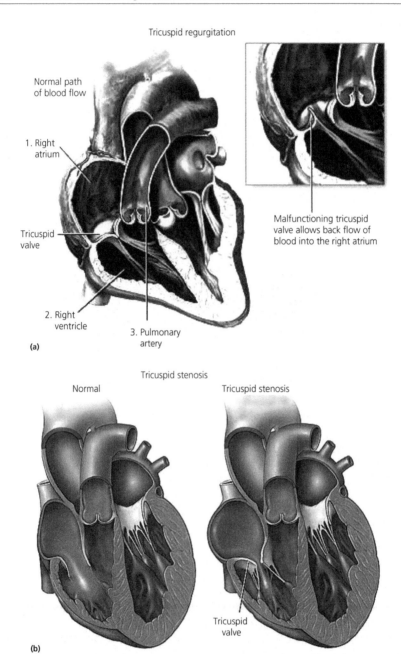

Figure 13.1 Drawing showing tricuspid valve anatomy and pathology.

produced by the underlying primary disease process. Nevertheless, as the regurgitation becomes more severe, the signs and symptoms of elevated systemic venous pressure become evident and, in severe disease, cardiac output is diminished.

Hemodynamic changes detected by physical exam

Symptoms and signs are often due to associated left-sided heart disease or pulmonary disease but, if there is significant tricuspid regurgitation, signs of this are generally evident on the physical exam. As with any cause of right heart failure, there are likely to be congestive findings on physical exam such as pedal edema, ascites, and hepatic enlargement.

Inspection of the jugular veins will generally demonstrate both distention correlating with elevated RA pressure, and a distinct and prominent CV wave reflecting systolic regurgitant flow into the RA. The typical murmur is holosystolic and located at the left sternal edge. Augmentation of the murmur with inspiration helps to distinguish tricuspid from mitral regurgitation.

Hemodynamic changes detected by echocardiography

Two-dimensional (2D) and Doppler echocardiography are invaluable in the evaluation of tricuspid regurgitation [1]. The 2D portion of the study evaluates the structure of the valvular apparatus, but, as already noted, this is normal in the overwhelming majority of cases. RA and RV size, however, give important clues to the duration of the volume and pressure overload.

The Doppler component of the study yields specific hemodynamic information. Color flow and pulse-wave examination reveal the presence, direction, and magnitude of the regurgitant jet. Detection of systolic flow reversal in the inferior vena cava and hepatic veins is generally indicative of severe tricuspid regurgitation. Finally, continuous-wave Doppler and the modified Bernoulli equation can be used to estimate the RV and pulmonary artery systolic pressures. In tricuspid regurgitation, the gradient between the RV and the RA during systole equals four times the square of the velocity. This gradient is then added to the estimated right atrial pressure (the jugular venous pressure) to estimate RV systolic pressure. In the absence of pulmonic stenosis, this also equals pulmonary systolic pressure. It is important to recognize that this calculation estimates the severity of the pulmonary hypertension, not the volumetric severity of the tricuspid regurgitation itself.

Hemodynamic changes evident at catheterization

In the cardiac catheterization laboratory, the findings associated with tricuspid regurgitation are most evident in the RA pressure tracing (Figure 13.2). The normal RA waveform consists of an A wave associated with atrial contraction, a C wave associated with ventricular contraction, and a V wave associated with rising atrial pressure just prior to opening of the tricuspid valve. With volumetrically important tricuspid regurgitation, there is a large systolic wave in the right atrial tracing, reflecting retrograde ejection of blood and consequent transmission of pressure from the RV to the RA. This waveform is variously termed an S wave or

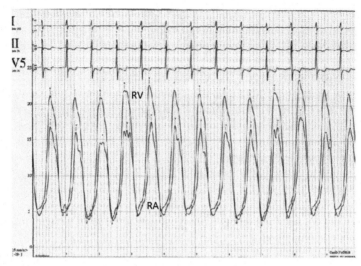

Figure 13.2 Simultaneous RA and RV pressures from a 67-year-old male who had undergone heart transplantation 9 years previously. Source: Rao 2013 [2]. Reproduced with permission of John Wiley and Sons.

a CV wave, as it occurs during systole and subsumes the normally independent C and V waves. The magnitude of the systolic wave is determined by both the severity of the regurgitation and the compliance of the RA [2].

With severe tricuspid regurgitation, the systolic wave in the RA becomes so prominent that the tracing resembles the right ventricular tracing (Figures 13.2 and 13.3). Indeed, in very severe tricuspid regurgitation the RA and RV pressure tracings are virtually identical, reflecting the fact that in the absence of a competent tricuspid valve, the RA and RV become, functionally, a single chamber. While this may be most evident with the simultaneous placement of two fluid-filled catheters in the RA and RV (Figures 13.2 and 13.3), this is procedurally cumbersome and the catheter across the tricuspid valve introduces the possibility of artifactual tricuspid regurgitation. Careful performance and observation of RV to RA "pullback" pressures, paired with Doppler and echocardiographic analysis, can provide compelling evidence for severe tricuspid regurgitation. Similarly, while right ventricular angiography can help assess the severity of tricuspid regurgitation, it is rarely necessary. Moreover, the catheter across the tricuspid valve and the ectopy associated with right ventricular contrast injection often introduce artifactual error. With current echocardiographic and Doppler techniques, angiography generally is of little additional utility.

Catheterization data do not allow definitive distinction between structural and functional tricuspid regurgitation. However, severe tricuspid regurgitation associated with relatively low RV and PA systolic pressures (less than 40 mm Hg) are more likely to be at least partially due to organic valvular disease. On the other

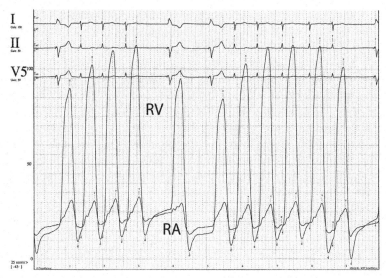

Figure 13.3 Simultaneous RA and RV pressure in a patient with severe tricuspid regurgitation.

hand, tricuspid regurgitation associated with very high RV systolic pressures is much more likely to be functional.

Treatment

In the case of functional tricuspid regurgitation, the mainstay of therapy is treatment of the condition causing pulmonary hypertension. This may be medical therapy as, for example, in the setting of left ventricular failure, or procedural as, for example, in the setting of mitral stenosis. Diuretics may be useful for refractory fluid retention. With structural valve disease, tricuspid valve repair or replacement is appropriate for patients who are either refractory to medical therapy or undergoing surgery for coexistent mitral valve disease. Often a prosthetic ring is used for annuloplasty. If valve replacement is necessary, bioprostheses are favored because the tricuspid valve may be relatively prone to thrombosis.

Tricuspid stenosis

Pathophysiology

Acquired tricuspid stenosis is uncommon. Most cases are due to rheumatic heart disease, carcinoid heart disease, or stenosis of a prosthetic valve initially placed for tricuspid regurgitation. When rheumatic tricuspid stenosis is present, it is generally associated with mitral stenosis, which accounts for most of the presenting signs and symptoms. The signs and symptoms of tricuspid stenosis may be mimicked by tumors (myxoma or metastasis) or vegetations that obstruct RV inflow.

Hemodynamic changes detected by physical exam

The signs and symptoms of tricuspid stenosis are primarily due to increased systemic venous pressure. Peripheral edema, ascites, hepatic enlargement, and right upper quadrant discomfort may develop with chronic tricuspid stenosis or regurgitation. Decreased cardiac output may cause pronounced fatigue. Jugular venous pressure is increased and, if the patient is in sinus rhythm, there is a prominent A wave due to impaired RV filling during atrial systole. However, due to the increased right atrial pressure, these patients are often in atrial fibrillation. Though clinically subtle, the finding of a blunted or absent Y descent supports the diagnosis. The murmur of tricuspid stenosis is a low-pitched diastolic murmur at the lower left sternal edge, although this is often obscured by or difficult to differentiate from the usually associated mitral stenosis murmur. Accentuation of the murmur during inspiration may help to identify a component of tricuspid stenosis, even if there is concurrent mitral stenosis.

Hemodynamic changes detected by echocardiography

Echocardiography typically reveals thickened tricuspid leaflets, decreased mobility, scarred chordae, and sometimes doming of the leaflets if they remain pliable. Carcinoid heart disease is associated with a distinctive morphology of a thickened tricuspid valve that is narrowed and fixed in the open position. The pandiastolic gradient of tricuspid stenosis is reflected in both the slow E to A slope of the M-mode echocardiogram and in the slowly falling velocity of the turbulent flow on Doppler assessment. Doppler evaluation also allows estimation of the diastolic pressure gradient by the modified Bernoulli equation.

Hemodynamic changes evident at catheterization

With modern echocardiographic and Doppler techniques, cardiac catheterization is generally not necessary for the diagnosis of tricuspid stenosis. When the diagnosis is in doubt, however, careful invasive determination of the transvalvular gradient is necessary. In most cases, a careful RV to RA pullback will reveal the gradient. However, the gradients are generally small, in the range of 4–8 mm Hg. If the cardiac output is low, tricuspid gradients are particularly likely to be low and may not be adequately evaluated with a catheter pullback. In this case, separate simultaneous catheters should be placed in the RA and RV. Clinically, significant tricuspid stenosis is usually associated with a valve area of 1.5 cm^2 or less.

Treatment

Treatment of tricuspid stenosis includes diuretics and occasionally nitrates to relieve venous congestion. Refractory patients can undergo tricuspid valve replacement, but in most cases the concomitant mitral valve disease primarily determines the indication and timing of surgery. A surgical approach may also be indicated for debulking of obstructive tumors or myxoma. The early experience with percutaneous balloon valvuloplasty for tricuspid stenosis is encouraging.

Case study of a patient with tricuspid stenosis

A 49-year-old male is referred for catheterization due to atypical chest pain, mild pedal edema, and an echocardiogram suggesting recurrent tricuspid stenosis with a mean gradient of 6 mm Hg (Figure 13.4a). Ten years previously, he had undergone tricuspid valve replacement with a Hancock porcine bioprosthetic valve for tricuspid stenosis due to carcinoid tumor. Coronary angiography revealed no hemodynamically significant stenoses. To evaluate the gradient across the tricuspid valve, separate catheters were placed in the RA and RV.

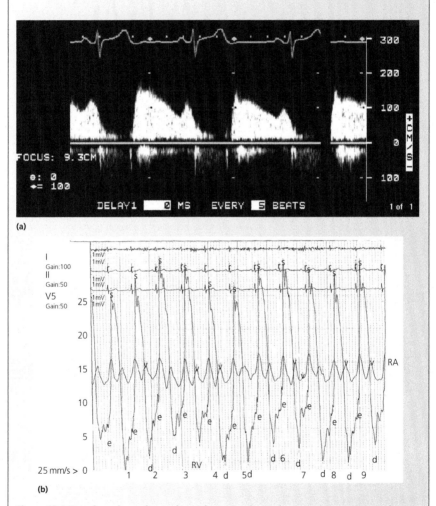

(a)

(b)

Figure 13.4 Doppler echocardiography and invasive hemodynamics in a patient with severe tricuspid stenosis. Doppler recording across the tricuspid valve (a) and simultaneous RA and RV pressures (b) were recorded in a patient with severe tricuspid stenosis. Panel (c) highlights the transvalvular gradient during diastole.

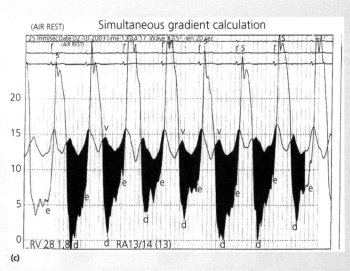

Figure 13.4 (Continued)

Hemodynamic tracings showed a pandiastolic gradient between the RA and RV (Figure 13.4). The mean RA pressure was 13 mm Hg, and the RV end-diastolic pressure was 8 mm Hg. The mean gradient was 7.3 mm Hg, and the calculated valve area was 1 cm².

Because of the relatively mild symptoms and the morbidity of a repeat operation, the patient was managed conservatively with diuretic therapy.

References

1 Lancellotti P, Moura L, Pierard LA, *et al.* European Association of Echocardiography recommendations for the assessment of valvular regurgitation. Part 2: mitral and tricuspid regurgitation (native valve disease). *Eur J Echocardiogr* 2010;**11**(4):307–332.
2 Rao S, Tate DA, Stouffer GA. Hemodynamic findings in severe tricuspid regurgitation. *Catheter Cardiovasc Interv* 2013;**81**(1):162–169.

CHAPTER 14

Hemodynamic findings in pulmonic valve disease

Cynthia Zhou, Anand Shah and George A. Stouffer

Hemodynamically significant pulmonic valve disease is rare and usually diagnosed at birth or in childhood. Pulmonary stenosis (PS) is commonly due to isolated valvular obstruction, but may also be due to either subvalvular or supravalvular obstruction. PS is typically first diagnosed in childhood, and it accounts for approximately 8% of all congenital heart defects [1]. The clinical presentation of PS varies from critical stenosis in newborns to asymptomatic mild stenosis without the need for therapy.

Severe pulmonary regurgitation (PR) most commonly occurs as a sequelae of treatment of PS or Tetralogy of Fallot, with fewer cases of primary pulmonic valvular regurgitation [2]. The amount of PR is influenced by valvular integrity, right ventricular (RV) size, and RV diastolic pressures. In chronic severe PR, the RV remodels to accommodate the regurgitant flow and RV stroke volume increases to maintain effective forward blood flow. Hemodynamic changes include a widened pulmonary artery (PA) pulse pressure and low PA diastolic pressures. As the amount of regurgitation increases, RV end-diastolic pressure becomes elevated and systemic cardiac output is reduced, especially with exercise. "Ventricularization" of the PA pressure tracing, in which the contour of the PA pressure is similar to the contour of the RV pressure, is a specific but not sensitive finding in severe PR.

Pulmonic valve stenosis

The stenotic area in PS can be either valvular, subvalvular, or supravalvular (Figure 14.1) [3]. PS is often seen in conjunction with other congenital heart abnormalities. Most adults with mild to moderate PS are asymptomatic and it will be discovered when a murmur is found during routine physical examination. Patients with more severe PS may experience exertional dyspnea and fatigue.

Mild, moderate, and severe PS as determined by echocardiography are defined as peak pressure gradients of <36 mm Hg, 36–64 mm Hg, and >64 mm Hg, respectively [4].

Cardiovascular Hemodynamics for the Clinician, Second Edition. Edited by George A. Stouffer.
© 2017 John Wiley & Sons Ltd. Published 2017 by John Wiley & Sons Ltd.

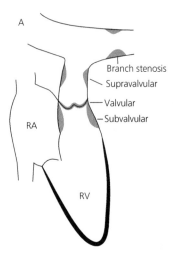

Figure 14.1 Schematic showing various locations of stenotic areas in patients with PS.

Long-term outcomes of patients with PS are dependent on pressure gradient across the valve, with patients with invasively measured peak-to-peak gradient of ≤25 mm Hg having normal survival and no progression of their stenosis in 25 years of follow-up, and patients with a gradient between 25 and 49 mm Hg having a 20% chance of needing an intervention [5].

Valvular pulmonary stenosis
In valvular PS, the pulmonary valve is generally shaped like a dome and has a narrow central opening. Alternatively, the valve may be dysplastic with myxomatous thickened leaflets, which is seen in Noonan syndrome. There can be a stenotic bicuspid or unicuspid pulmonary valve in Tetralogy of Fallot. Valvular PS can also be associated with other congenital heart defects such as atrial septal defect (ASD), Ebstein's anomaly, double outlet right ventricle, and transposition of the great arteries.

Subvalvular pulmonary stenosis
Subvalvular PS can be infundibular or subinfundibular. Primary infundibular PS is generally seen as part of Tetralogy of Fallot, while secondary infundibular hypertrophy may occur in valvular PS and result in dynamic RVOT obstruction. Subinfundibular PS is very rare and referred to as double chambered right ventricle (DCRV).

Supravalvular pulmonary stenosis
Supravalvular PS can occur as a result of congenital rubella syndrome or can be found in association with other congenital abnormalities, such as in Williams–Beuren, Noonan, Allagile, DiGeorge, and Leopard syndromes. The stenosis can be found in the common pulmonary trunk, the bifurcation, or the pulmonary branches (Figure 14.1).

Non-invasive imaging

The clinical standard to diagnose PS and quantify its severity is transthoracic 2D echocardiography with Doppler imaging. The valve morphology can be assessed and peak and mean gradients can be measured by Doppler imaging. Computed tomography (CT) can be used to image the anatomy of the right ventricular outflow tract (RVOT) and the pulmonary arterial tree, but lacks the ability to analyze function.

Magnetic resonance imaging (MRI) is beneficial for analyzing the anatomy of the RVOT, the pulmonary artery, and its branches. The exact location of the stenosis can be identified, which enables a distinction between valvular, subvalvular, and supravalvular stenosis. MRI is considered the standard for assessment and quantification of right ventricular volume, mass and function.

Cardiac catheterization and invasive hemodynamics

Right heart catheterization has been the traditional way of measuring the severity of PS and is still used prior to treatment, but has largely been supplanted by echocardiography for establishing the diagnosis of PS. Pressure gradients can be measured directly (Figures 14.2 and 14.3) and angiography (Figure 14.4) provides information on the anatomy. Cardiac catheterization also provides the opportunity for treatment via balloon valvuloplasty.

Hemodynamic findings associated with PS include fixed outflow tract obstruction (Figures 14.2a and 14.3a) and diastolic dysfunction (Figures 14.2b and 14.3b). Over time, the RV will hypertrophy in patients with PS in response to the pressure overload. Increased wall thickness causes the RV to become stiffer and less compliant and higher end-diastolic pressures are required to maintain RV filling. This, in turn, leads to higher RA pressures (Figures 14.2b and 14.3b), which will further increase if RV systolic function starts to fail.

Unlike mitral and aortic stenosis in which severity is estimated by calculated valve area, this is rarely used in PS. Rather, severity and need for treatment are generally determined based on peak-to-peak gradient across the pulmonic valve (Table 14.1). The success of treatment is also determined by measuring pressure gradients, with treatment considered a success when the invasive gradient is <30 mm Hg.

Treatment of PS

The preferred treatment is balloon pulmonary valvuloplasty (BPV), as long-term outcomes are generally good with consistent reductions in pressure gradients. Analysis of multiple studies showed that 8–10% of patients have restenosis at <2 year follow-up, where restenosis is defined as an invasive gradient >50 mm Hg [3]. The three studies with intervention in adults showed a drop from 107±29 mm Hg to 37±25 mm Hg, 91±46 mm Hg to 38±32 mm Hg, and 105±39 mm Hg to 34±26 mm Hg [3].

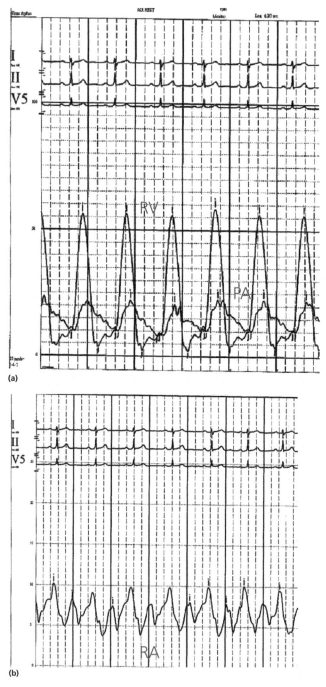

(a)

(b)

Figure 14.2 Simultaneous RV and PA tracings (a) and RA tracing (b) in a 28-year-old female with moderate PS.

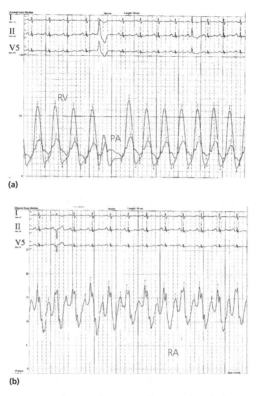

(a)

(b)

Figure 14.3 Simultaneous RV and PA tracings (a) and RA tracing (b) in a 42-year-old female with moderate PS.

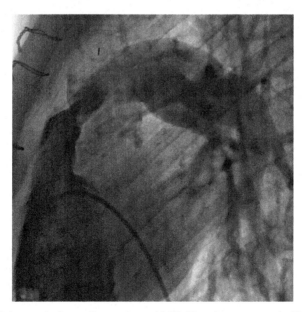

Figure 14.4 Right ventriculogram in a patient with PS. Note the post-stenotic dilation.

Table 14.1 Severity grading of pulmonary stenosis [4].

	Mild	Moderate	Severe
Peak Doppler velocity (m/s)	<3	3–4	>4
Peak Doppler gradient (mm Hg)	<36	36–64	>64
Mean Doppler gradient (mm Hg)			>40

Different thresholds for treatment have been proposed. Class 1 indications for BPV in the AHA/ACCF guidelines are RV to pulmonary artery peak-to-peak gradient greater than 40 mm Hg at catheterization or symptoms (exertional dyspnea, angina, syncope, or presyncope) plus an RV to pulmonary artery peak-to-peak gradient >30 mm Hg at catheterization. Class IIb indication is lack of symptoms with RV to pulmonary artery peak-to-peak gradient 30–39 mm Hg at catheterization [6,7]. Others have proposed treatment (either surgery or BPV) for any obstruction in the RVOT and/or pulmonary valve with a Doppler-derived peak instantaneous gradient >64 mm Hg (peak velocity >4 m/s) or PS with symptoms, decreased RV function, right-to-left shunting via an ASD, or significant arrhythmias [3].

Pulmonic regurgitation

Although many adults have modest amounts of pulmonic valve regurgitation on echocardiography, severe PR is rarely seen. The most common cause of severe PR is as sequelae of treatment of a congenital disorder involving stenosis of the pulmonic valve and/or RVOT, most frequently Tetralogy of Fallot or PS [8,9]. Treatment with either surgical valvotomy or balloon valvuloplasty can eventually result in significant PR due to dilation of the annulus and/or damage to the pulmonic valve leaflets [10]. Severe PR in the absence of prior treatment of RVOT obstruction or PS is rare and usually due to (a) a dilated pulmonary annulus, which can be congenital or acquired (e.g., pulmonary hypertension, Marfan's syndrome, idiopathic pulmonary artery dilation, or connective tissue disorders); (b) congenitally abnormal pulmonic valve (e.g., absent valves, absent leaflets, bicuspid valve, malformed tricuspid valve, or quadricuspid valve); or (c) acquired abnormalities of the pulmonic valve (e.g., infective endocarditis, carcinoid, syphilis, rheumatic heart disease, rheumatoid arthritis, or trauma from PA catheters) [2,10].

Hemodynamic changes in chronic PR

Hemodynamic changes associated with chronic PR result from pulmonary artery to RV blood flow during diastole and compensatory responses of the RV to increased diastolic filling. In mild PR, increased RV stroke volume and/or heart

Table 14.2 Hemodynamic findings in severe PR.

- Wide pulmonary artery pulse pressure
- Low pulmonary artery diastolic pressure
- A rapid dicrotic collapse that leads to early equilibration of the PA and RV diastolic pressures
- RV and PA pressures that may equalize during diastole ("ventricularization" of PA pressure)
- A rate of increase (slope) of RV diastolic pressures that is elevated due to rapid filling from the PA
- Rapid filling from the PA, which can lead to premature closure of the tricuspid valve

rate leads to an increase in RV output across the pulmonic valve, thus maintaining systemic cardiac output. As the severity of PR increases, the RV begins to remodel and dilate. This remodeling allows the maintenance of RV output with relatively normal filling pressures. In patients with severe PR, chronic volume overload can result in increased RV end-diastolic volume and increased RV diastolic pressures. If the degree of regurgitation exceeds the ability of the RV to remodel, this can result in increased RV systolic volume, RV systolic dysfunction, and impaired systemic cardiac output.

Common hemodynamic manifestations of severe PR are shown in Table 14.2. PA pressure manifestations associated with chronic PR are a wide pulse pressure and a low diastolic pressure (similar to aortic pressures in aortic valve insufficiency). Other hemodynamic changes result from an increased RV stroke volume coupled with low afterload (due to regurgitant flow across the pulmonic valve and decreased pulmonary vascular resistance). These include:
- A rapid dicrotic collapse that leads to early equilibration of the PA and RV diastolic pressures (Figures 14.5 and 14.6)
- RV and PA pressures that may equalize during diastole ("ventricularization" of PA pressure; Figure 14.6)
- A rate of increase (slope) of RV diastolic pressures that is elevated due to rapid filling from the PA (Figure 14.7)
- Rapid filling from the PA, which can lead to premature closure of the tricuspid valve (Figure 14.7)

In chronic severe PR, RV stiffness can play an important role in the hemodynamic response, since increased stiffness will raise RV diastolic pressure and therefore decrease the pressure gradient for PR. In a series of repaired tetralogy patients, RV stiffness was seen to prevent dilation despite the increased preload associated with chronic PR. The clinical benefit of this was demonstrated by better exercise tolerance [11].

A few additional factors influence the hemodynamics in patients with severe PR. Increased airway or intrathoracic pressure can increase the resistance in the pulmonary microvasculature, increasing RV afterload and therefore the amount of PR. For example, small incremental changes in airway pressures in mechanically ventilated patients can influence the degree of PR. Chronic PR can be associated with branch pulmonary stenosis, which can mimic findings of PS and result in a gradient between RV and PA systolic pressures. RA contraction can contribute to

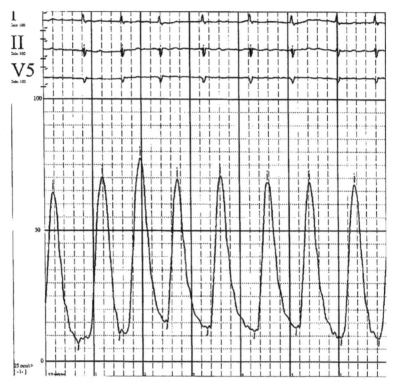

Figure 14.5 PA tracing in a female with severe PR. Note the wide pulse pressure and low pulmonary artery diastolic pressure.

forward flow in patients with severe PR and RV systolic failure, leading to late diastolic forward flow in the PA. Lastly, PR is exacerbated by conditions that lead to elevated arteriolar resistance to pulmonary artery outflow, such as bronchopulmonary disease, left ventricular dysfunction, or pulmonary vascular disease [2].

Right ventricular function in chronic PR

The ability of the RV to maintain system cardiac output in the presence of significant PR is facilitated by the relatively low resistance of the pulmonary microvasculature. However, over time, the increased volume results in increased diastolic pressures and RV remodeling, with hemodynamic findings depending on the degree of regurgitation and extent of RV remodeling. In mild to moderate PR, filling from the PA enables the RV to increase stroke volume by increasing RV end-diastolic volume (i.e., Starling's Law). As PR becomes more severe, the RV dilates in order to handle increased volumes with minimal changes in RV diastolic pressures. In some patients with PR and dilated right ventricles, RV myocardial contractile function declines.

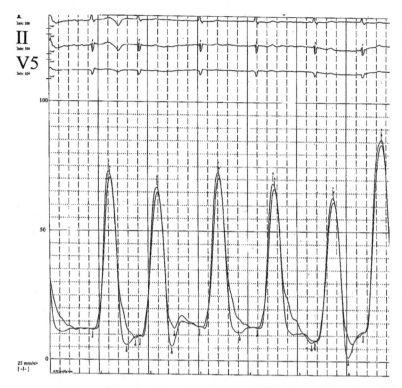

Figure 14.6 Simultaneous RV and PA tracings in a 75-year-old female with severe PR.

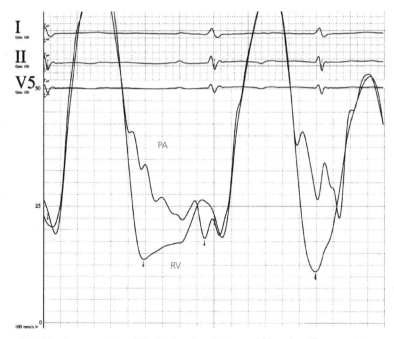

Figure 14.7 Simultaneous RV and PA tracings in a 69-year-old female with severe PR.

The development of RV dysfunction leads to further increases in RV diastolic pressures and eventually to development of fluid overload, signs of right heart failure, and decreased cardiac output. With progressive RV and tricuspid annular dilation, tricuspid regurgitation ensues, which in turn can lead to further RV and RA dilation.

The remodeling process can be reversed in some patients with PR by valve replacement [12]. In a study of 170 patients with severe chronic PR, there were significant reductions in RV volumes and improvement in RV systolic function following pulmonary valve replacement. Changes in RV function tended to be irreversible when RV end-diastolic volume index exceeded 163 mL/m^2 or end-systolic volume index exceeded 80 mL/m^2 [13].

Hemodynamic changes detected by non-invasive imaging in chronic PR

Echocardiography enables visualization of the pulmonic valve and identification of congenital abnormalities, vegetations, thickening, and/or calcification [14]. The rate of decay of the velocity of flow between the pulmonary artery and RV during diastole (i.e., pressure half-time) gives an estimate of the gradient between the pulmonary artery and RV. A rapid decay indicates equalization of RV and PA pressures and suggests severe PR. Other echocardiographic measurements of the hemodynamic effects of PR include RV size, RV systolic function, evidence of elevated RA pressures, amount of tricuspid regurgitation, and estimation of PA systolic pressure by measurement of the velocity of tricuspid regurgitation.

Cardiovascular magnetic resonance (CMR) imaging provides quantitative assessment of RV volume and systolic function, valvular insufficiency, and regurgitant volume and fraction. CMR is unique in that it directly quantifies valvular regurgitation in mL/min rather than providing an estimate based on a surrogate measure. In patients who cannot have a CMR, CT scanning can be used to measure RV volume and systolic function. Rarely, the severity of PR is assessed angiographically by injecting a large volume of contrast into the proximal PA and observing retrograde filling of the RV. The severity is estimated using the four-point scale utilized to measure regurgitant flow across other cardiac valves.

Natural history of chronic PR

In general, even severe PR is well tolerated for many years, with symptoms developing only when RV failure occurs. One study examining severe PR found that 6% of patients developed symptoms within 20 years and that 29% developed symptoms by 40 years [15]. Late complications of severe PR include RV dilation, RV dysfunction, secondary tricuspid regurgitation, development of atrial or ventricular arrhythmias, and/or deteriorating exercise capacity. Percutaneous pulmonary valve implantation has been associated with hemodynamic improvement in patients with severe PR following Tetralogy of Fallot repair [12,16].

Pregnancy

Early in pregnancy, stroke volume increases, heart rate increases 15–20%, and left ventricular end-diastolic volume increases; the total effect is a 30–50% increase in cardiac output by the end of the first trimester, with peak cardiac output occurring between the second and third trimesters [17]. Additionally, vascular resistance decreases by 30–50% by the end of the second trimester, and then rises toward the end of the third trimester. Significant hemodynamic changes occur during delivery, including catecholamine-induced increases in heart rate, stroke volume, and cardiac output. Arterial blood pressure increases during each contraction by up to 15–20 mm Hg.

Pregnancy is well tolerated in women with mild to moderate PS, but the increased cardiac output of pregnancy can lead to right-sided heart failure in severe PS. Uncorrected severe PS has been linked to an increased risk of pre-term birth and fetal mortality of 4.8%. Severe PR has been associated with a progressive RV dilatation that may persist after pregnancy. In one study, severe PR was found to be an independent predictor of maternal complications, particularly in patients with impaired right ventricular function [17–19].

Ideally, intervention should take place in severe PS or severe PR prior to pregnancy.

References

1 van der Linde D, Konings EEM, Slager MA, *et al*. Birth prevalence of congenital heart disease worldwide: a systematic review and meta-analysis. *J Am Coll Cardiol* 2011;**58**(21):2241–2247.
2 Rommel JJ, Yadav PK, Stouffer GA. Causes and hemodynamic findings in chronic severe pulmonary regurgitation. *Catheter Cardiovasc Interv* 2015. Online first, doi:10.1002/ccd.26073
3 Cuypers JAAE, Witsenburg M, van der Linde D, Roos-Hesselink JW. Pulmonary stenosis: update on diagnosis and therapeutic options. *Heart* 2013;**99**(5):339–347.
4 Baumgartner HJ, Hung J, Bermejo JB, *et al*. Echocardiographic assessment of valve stenosis: EAE/ASE recommendations for clinical practice. *Eur J Echocardiogr* 2009;**10**:1–25.
5 Hayes CJ, Gersony WM, Driscoll DJ, *et al*. Second natural history study of congenital heart defects. Results of treatment of patients with pulmonary valvar stenosis. *Circulation* 1993;87 (2 suppl):I28–I37.
6 Bonow RO, Carabello BA, Chatterjee K, *et al*. ACC/AHA 2006 guidelines for the management of patients with valvular heart disease: a report of the American College of Cardiology/American Heart Association Task Force on Practice Guidelines (Writing Committee to Revise the 1998 Guidelines for the Management of Patients with Valvular Heart Disease). *J Am Coll Cardiol* 2006;**48**(3):e1–e148.
7 Nishimura RA, Otto CM, Bonow RO, *et al*. 2014 AHA/ACC guideline for the management of patients with valvular heart disease: a report of the American College of Cardiology/American Heart Association Task Force on Practice Guidelines. *J Am Coll Cardiol* 2014;**63**(22):e57–e185.

8 Waller BF, Howard J, Fess S. Pathology of pulmonic valve stenosis and pure regurgitation. *Clin Cardiol* 1995;**18**(1):45–50.

9 Shah PM. Tricuspid and pulmonary valve disease evaluation and management. *Rev Esp Cardiol* 2010;**63**(11):1349–1365.

10 Fitzgerald KP, Lim MJ. The pulmonary valve. *Cardiol Clin* 2011;**29**(2):223–227. doi:10.1016/j. ccl.2011.01.006

11 Gatzoulis MA, Clark AL, Cullen S, Newman CG, Redington AN. Right ventricular diastolic function 15 to 35 years after repair of tetralogy of Fallot. Restrictive physiology predicts superior exercise performance. *Circulation* 1995;**91**(6):1775–1781.

12 Weinberg CR, McElhinney DB. Pulmonary valve replacement in Tetralogy of Fallot. *Circulation* 2014;**130**(9):795–798.

13 Lee C, Kim YM, Lee CH, *et al*. Outcomes of pulmonary valve replacement in 170 patients with chronic pulmonary regurgitation after relief of right ventricular outflow tract obstruction: implications for optimal timing of pulmonary valve replacement. *J Am Coll Cardiol* 2012;**60**(11):1005–1014.

14 Lancellotti P, Tribouilloy C, Hagendorff A, *et al*. European Association of Echocardiography recommendations for the assessment of valvular regurgitation. Part 1: aortic and pulmonary regurgitation (native valve disease). *Eur J Echocardiogr* 2010;**11**(3):223–244. doi:10.1093/ ejechocard/jeq030

15 Shimazaki Y, Blackstone EH, Kirklin JW. The natural history of isolated congenital pulmonary valve incompetence: surgical implications. *Thorac Cardiovasc Surg* 1984;**32**(4):257–259.

16 Armstrong AK, Balzer DT, Cabalka AK, *et al*. One-year follow-up of the Melody transcatheter pulmonary valve multicenter post-approval study. *JACC Cardiovasc Interv* 2014;**7**(11):1254–1262.

17 Nanna M, Stergiopoulos K. Pregnancy complicated by valvular heart disease: an update. *J Am Heart Assoc* 2014;**3**(3):e000712.

18 Drenthen W, Pieper PG, Roos-Hesselink JW, *et al*. Outcome of pregnancy in women with congenital heart disease: a literature review. *J Am Coll Cardiol* 2007;**49**(24):2303–2311.

19 Khairy P, Ouyang DW, Fernandes SM, Lee-Parritz A, Economy KE, Landzberg MJ. Pregnancy outcomes in women with congenital heart disease. *Circulation* 2006;**113**(4): 517–524.

PART III
Cardiomyopathies

CHAPTER 15

Hypertrophic cardiomyopathy

Jayadeep S. Varanasi and George A. Stouffer

Hypertrophic cardiomyopathy (HCM) is the name given to a heterogeneous family of disorders characterized by genetic defects involving myocyte sarcomeric proteins. More than 1400 mutations in 11 genes encoding proteins have been described, with the most common defect being a mutation in the gene that encodes beta-myosin heavy chain, but defects in other genes encoding for sarcomeric proteins including troponin T, troponin I, myosin light chains, alpha tropomyosin, and myosin-binding protein C have been implicated in causing HCM. Inheritance is usually autosomal dominant with variable penetrance. Classically, HCM was defined by excessive septal hypertrophy (usually the width of the septum on echocardiography exceeding 1.5 cm) with or without the presence of outflow tract obstruction, and even today most studies of HCM use echocardiographic, rather than genetic, criteria to determine eligibility.

Various microscopic features of HCM distinguish it from other diseases that cause left ventricular hypertrophy (LVH). The principal aspect of HCM is myocyte disarray in which cells lose their normal parallel arrangement. Individual myocytes often show variability in size and may form circular patterns around areas of fibrous tissue. Myocyte disarray can be seen in other illnesses; however, it tends to affect less of the left ventricle when caused by hypertension or aortic stenosis. In HCM, intramyocardial arteries are often obliterated, creating small areas of fibrosis within the ventricular wall, especially within the interventricular septum.

On gross examination in patients with HCM, there is increased myocardial mass with a normal or small left ventricular chamber size. The disease usually affects the left ventricle more than the right ventricle, with the interventricular septum and anterolateral free wall being the most common segments involved. The hypertrophy is often asymmetric, with differing wall thicknesses noted in contiguous segments. Left atrial enlargement is common because of both

Cardiovascular Hemodynamics for the Clinician, Second Edition. Edited by George A. Stouffer.
© 2017 John Wiley & Sons Ltd. Published 2017 by John Wiley & Sons Ltd.

impaired ventricular relaxation and mitral regurgitation. Along with fibrosis in the ventricular wall, a fibrotic plaque is sometimes seen on the interventricular septum and is thought to be the result of repetitive contact between the anterior mitral leaflet and the septum. "Burned-out" HCM, in which there is LV wall thinning, chamber enlargement, and systolic dysfunction resembling dilated cardiomyopathy, develops in 5–10% of patients.

Several anatomic variants of HCM have been described. The most well-known phenotype from a hemodynamic standpoint is hypertrophic obstructive cardiomyopathy (HOCM; also known as idiopathic hypertrophic subaortic stenosis). It was formally described as a distinct clinical entity in 1958, and consists of narrowing of the left ventricular outflow tract (LVOT) with ventricular contraction causing a dynamic pressure gradient (Figure 15.1). This anatomic pattern occurs in 25–50% of cases of HCM and will be the type of HCM that we concentrate on in this chapter. Other anatomic forms of HCM that have been described include apical HCM [1], concentric hypertrophy, localized hypertrophy (e.g., posterior portion of septum, posterobasal free wall of the LV, or at the mid-ventricular level), and HCM of the elderly, characterized by severe concentric LVH, a small LV cavity, and hypertension [2]. The vast majority of intraventricular pressure gradients are localized to the LVOT, although mid-cavity obstruction has also been reported. Note that in the rest of this chapter HCM will refer to all types of hypertrophic cardiomyopathy, while HOCM will refer only to hypertrophic cardiomyopathy in which there is a pressure gradient in the left ventricle at rest or with provocation.

The most feared complication of HCM is sudden cardiac death. HCM is one of the most common causes of sudden death in individuals between the ages of 12 and 35 and is also a common cause of death in young athletes. Not all patients with HCM are symptomatic, but in those who are, dyspnea, angina, and palpitations are common.

Physical exam

Signs of LVH, such as an S4 and laterally displaced precordial impulse, may be present. Most patients with intraventricular gradients have a double or triple apical impulse. Atrial contraction may be noted as a presystolic apical impulse, as well as a prominent A wave in the jugular venous pulsation. The carotid pulse may display a "spike and dome" configuration. In patients with an LVOT obstruction, there is a harsh mid-systolic murmur that commences well after the first heart sound and becomes louder with maneuvers that decrease LV size and filling pressures (e.g., standing from squatting, Valsalva, or dehydration). The murmur often decreases with handgrip exercise. A murmur of mitral regurgitation may be present as well.

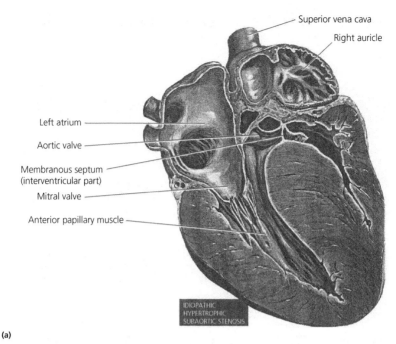

- Superior vena cava
- Right auricle
- Left atrium
- Aortic valve
- Membranous septum (interventricular part)
- Mitral valve
- Anterior papillary muscle

IDIOPATHIC HYPERTROPHIC SUBAORTIC STENOSIS

(a)

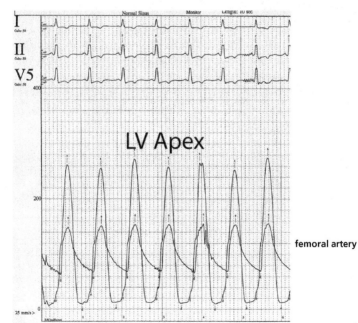

(b)

Figure 15.1 Eccentric hypertrophy and LV outflow tract gradient in HOCM. HOCM is characterized by asymmetric septal hypertrophy (a) which causes an obstruction to LV outflow and a pressure drop in the LV outflow tract (b).

Hemodynamics

An understanding of the hemodynamic manifestations of HOCM can be facilitated by considering causative factors separately, while realizing that in a given patient there will be significant interactions between these factors. The four factors that will be discussed here are diastolic dysfunction, LVOT obstruction, mitral regurgitation, and abnormal coronary flow reserve (Table 15.1).

Diastolic dysfunction is present, to some degree, in almost all patients with HCM. Diastolic dysfunction progresses as the ventricle hypertrophies and becomes less compliant. Higher pressures are required to fill the ventricle, leading to increased left atrial, pulmonary artery (PA), right ventricular (RV), and right atrial pressures. Progressive diastolic dysfunction results in clinical manifestations of congestive heart failure in some patients with HOCM.

Outflow tract obstruction in patients with HOCM is "dynamic," which means that the resistance to flow changes depending on filling pressures, afterload (e.g., aortic pressure), and force of contractility. LVOT obstruction changes in severity depending on the force of systolic contraction and the dimensions of the LV (in contrast to aortic stenosis, which is a fixed obstruction since it is valvular and not muscular). Thus, patients with HOCM may not have any obstruction while at rest, but may develop significant pressure gradients during any activity that increases the force of cardiac contraction (e.g., exercise, emotional stress) or at times when their LV is smaller because of incomplete filling (e.g., dehydration). This obstruction can cause pressure gradients of greater than 100 mm Hg and is thought to be one etiology of exercise-induced syncope in these patients (another potential etiology is arrhythmias).

LVOT gradients can be provoked using methods that decrease filling pressures and stroke volume (e.g., Valsalva maneuver or nitroglycerin) or methods that increase the force of contraction (post-PVC or isoproterenol infusion). Dobutamine should be avoided, as it can cause subaortic pressure gradients in normal hearts due to catecholamine stimulant effects.

Mitral regurgitation is thought to be caused by systolic anterior motion (SAM) of the mitral valve during mid-systole, which interferes with normal valve closure.

Table 15.1 Hemodynamic findings in HOCM.

Spike and dome configuration of arterial pulse	On aortic pressure tracing, there is a rapid rise during systole, which is followed by a mild drop in pressure and then a secondary peak
Systolic intraventricular pressure gradient	Simultaneous intraventricular and aortic pressure tracings will show a difference in maximum systolic pressure at rest and/or with provocation
Diastolic dysfunction	LV end-diastolic pressure will be elevated, the rapid phase of LV filling will be prolonged, and atrial contribution to LV filling will be accentuated
Brockenbrough sign	Aortic pulse pressure fails to widen during a post-extrasystolic beat

Mitral regurgitation is usually mild, but can become significant, especially in association with large subaortic pressure gradients. The magnitude of pressure gradients measured at cardiac catheterization correlates well with Doppler velocities and with the duration of SAM. Prolonged mitral valve septal coaptation (>30% of systole) is invariably associated with high LVOT gradients and mild to severe mitral regurgitation. Although the role of SAM in producing the gradient is controversial, there is a close relationship between the degree of SAM and the size of the LVOT gradient in patients with subaortic obstruction (as opposed to mid-cavity obstruction) [3,4].

Coronary flow reserve, the ratio of the maximal to the resting coronary blood flow and thus an index of the ability to increase coronary flow under physiologic stress, is abnormal in most patients with HOCM. A study of 20 patients with HCM found higher resting coronary blood flow and lower coronary resistance in comparison to 28 controls. Most patients with HCM achieved maximum coronary vasodilation and flow at modest increases in heart rate. Higher heart rates resulted in severe myocardial ischemia, elevation in LV end-diastolic pressure (LVEDP), and a decline in coronary flow [5]. The same group of investigators, in a subsequent study of 50 patients with HCM, found that patients with LVOT obstruction at rest had higher coronary flow and regional myocardial oxygen consumption at rest and with pacing compared to patients with HCM but without obstruction. In patients with obstruction, transmural coronary flow reserve was exhausted at a heart rate of 130 bpm. Interestingly, in patients without obstruction, myocardial ischemia occurred at a lower coronary flow than in patients with obstruction [6]. A more recent study comparing coronary blood flow in eight patients with symptomatic HCM to eight matched controls found that patients with HCM had higher resting coronary blood flow, lower coronary resistance, and lower coronary flow reserve. Patients with HCM also had abnormal phasic coronary flow characteristics. These results are consistent with the reduction of coronary flow reserve in patients with HCM being caused by near maximal vasodilation of the microcirculation in the basal state [7].

Findings at cardiac catheterization

Cardiac catheterization is usually not needed to confirm the diagnosis, but occasionally patients with HCM will undergo catheterization for evaluation of chest pain or congestive heart failure.

Left atrium or pulmonary capillary wedge pressure

Pulmonary capillary wedge pressure (PCWP) is generally elevated in patients with HCM, even more so when there is significant mitral regurgitation. The A wave may be accentuated due to a stiff ventricle and the V wave can be increased, either from mitral regurgitation or reduced LA compliance. RV systolic and PA pressures are generally only mildly elevated, and cardiac output is preserved, until LV failure occurs.

As an example of filling pressures in patients with HCM, a study of 20 patients with HCM (9 with significant outflow tract gradients) compared to 28 controls found higher LVEDP (16 ± 6 versus 11 ± 3 mm Hg) and mean PCWP (13 ± 5 versus 7 ± 3 mm Hg) [5].

LV pressure

LVEDP is generally elevated, but there are no pathognomonic findings for HCM in the LV pressure tracing. The rapid filling phase of LV may be significantly prolonged and a prominent atrial contraction wave may be present (Figure 15.2). The upstroke of the LV pressure tracing may have a notch that corresponds with the anterior leaflet of the mitral valve coming into contact with the septum because of SAM.

Aortic pressure

A variable finding in HOCM is that the dynamic nature of the outflow tract obstruction causes a "spike and dome" configuration of the aortic or peripheral pulse (Figure 15.3). This is known as a bisferiens pulse, a name derived from Latin *bis* (= two) + *feriere* (= to beat). The bisferiens pulse is characterized by an initial rapid rise in aortic pressure (spike), followed by a slight drop in pressure (dip), and then a secondary peak (dome), and is most prominent in central aortic pressure, but can also be transmitted to the carotids. It is enhanced by maneuvers that increase intraventricular pressure gradients (e.g., following a PVC or by the Valsalva maneuver), and in patients with obstruction only during provocation, a normal-appearing pressure tracing will often be replaced by the spike and dome during provocative maneuvers. A bisferiens pulse should be not confused with the dicrotic pulse, a pulse with an exaggerated dicrotic wave. A bisferiens pulse is most commonly associated with HOCM, but can also be seen in severe aortic regurgitation.

Outflow tract gradient

A gradient can be demonstrated by comparing pressure in the LV apex (using an end-hole catheter) to aortic pressure or by a slow pullback of the catheter through the LV (Figure 15.4). In the cardiac catheterization laboratory, dynamic outflow tract obstruction can be provoked by a variety of maneuvers, including methods that decrease preload and/or afterload (e.g., Valsalva maneuver, administration of amyl nitrate; Figure 15.5) or methods that increase the force

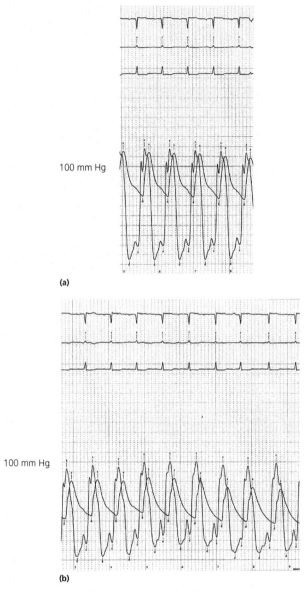

(a)

(b)

Figure 15.2 LV tracings in a patient with HOCM. In panel (a), pressures are obtained at baseline. Note the elevated LVEDP, prominent A wave in LV tracing, and lack of an outflow tract gradient. Panel (b) was obtained after inhalation of amyl nitrate. LVEDP is increased and an A wave is prominent. Aortic pressure is decreased compared to basal conditions and a small outflow tract gradient is present.

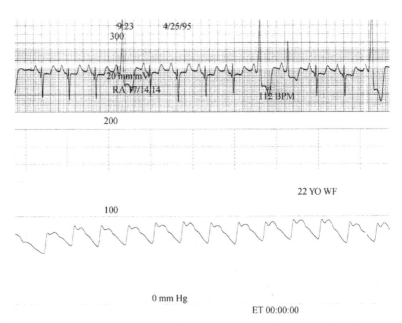

Figure 15.3 Aortic pressure in a patient with HOCM demonstrating the "spike and dome" configuration.

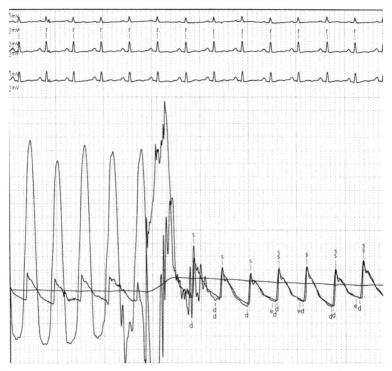

Figure 15.4 LV to aortic pullback using a dual lumen end-hole catheter during amyl nitrate administration in a patient with HOCM. Aortic pressure is measured continuously through the second lumen.

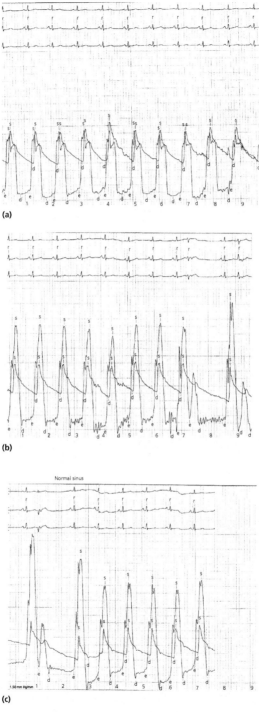

Figure 15.5 Demonstration of a provocable gradient with inhalation of amyl nitrate. There is no left ventricular outflow tract gradient under basal conditions (a). Following inhalation of amyl nitrate, aortic pressure falls, and a gradient is apparent (b). Over time, aortic pressure continues to fall and the gradient increases (c). All tracings are recorded on a 200 mm Hg scale.

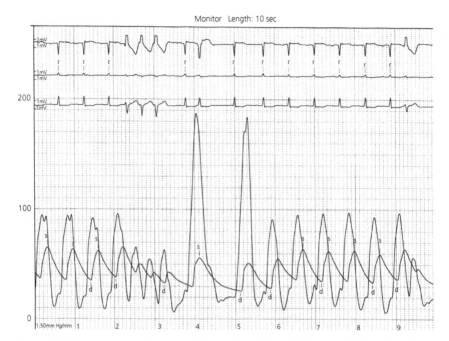

Figure 15.6 Demonstration of a provocable gradient with PVCs during administration of amyl nitrate.

of contraction (e.g., isoproterenol infusion or PVC; Figure 15.6). LV outflow obstruction can be reduced or eliminated by maneuvers that increase chamber size (e.g., hydration).

The Brockenbrough–Braunwald–Morrow sign was originally described in 1961. This sign is present if the aortic pulse pressure falls in the first normal beat post PVC in HOCM (Figure 15.7). While originally thought to be specific for HOCM, it has since been described in some cases of aortic stenosis.

RV intraventricular gradient is common in infants and children with HOCM, but is rarely seen in adults. Maron [8] reported that RV obstruction was observed in 60% of infants with HOCM and that RV outflow tract obstruction was frequently greater than LV outflow tract obstruction.

Echocardiography

Since the initial development of ultrasonic evaluation of the heart, echocardiography has been the gold standard for diagnosing HOCM. The cardinal echocardiographic features of HOCM are LVH, an intraventricular pressure gradient, and

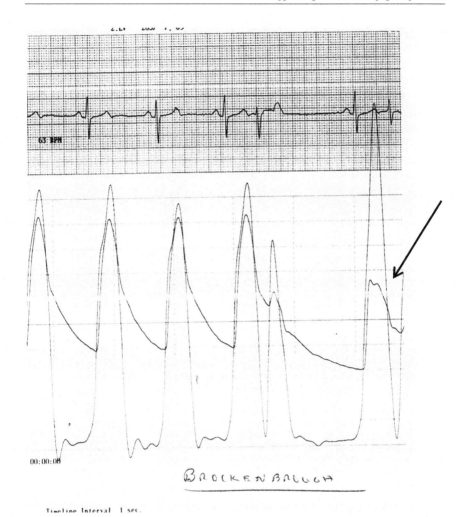

Figure 15.7 Brockenbrough–Braunwald–Morrow sign. Pulse pressure falls in the first normal beat post-PVC (arrows) in HOCM (a) but not in aortic stenosis (b).

SAM of the mitral valve. There is considerable variability in the degree and pattern of hypertrophy and in some patients there is variation in the extent of LVH from region to region. The finding of a thickened septum that is at least 1.3–1.5 times the thickness of the posterior wall when measured in diastole just prior to atrial systole has been a commonly used criterion for the diagnosis of asymmetric septal hypertrophy.

An intraventricular pressure gradient as measured by continuous-wave Doppler interrogation in the aortic outflow tract is present in some patients.

Provocative maneuvers (e.g., inhalation of amyl nitrate, Valsalva maneuver) can be performed in the echocardiography laboratory. Some investigators have criticized these maneuvers as being nonphysiologic and advocated using echocardiography in conjunction with treadmill or bicycle exercise testing to determine provocable gradients.

The American College of Cardiology/European Society of Cardiology Clinical Expert Consensus [9] has recommended classifying patients with HCM into one of three groups based on the representative peak instantaneous gradient as assessed with continuous-wave Doppler: (a) resting obstruction—gradient under basal (resting) conditions equal to or greater than 30 mm Hg (2.7 m/s by Doppler); (b) provocable obstruction—gradient less than 30 mm Hg under basal conditions and equal to or greater than 30 mm Hg with provocation; and (c) nonobstruction—gradient less than 30 mm Hg at rest and with provocation. A resting outflow tract gradient of ≥30 mm Hg (measured by continuous-wave Doppler) is an independent determinant of symptoms of progressive heart failure and death.

Other common echocardiographic findings in HCM include normal systolic function, diastolic dysfunction with reduced LV compliance, and a mitral valve E/A ratio less than 1.0 (usually <0.8) and an enlarged left atrium [10].

Septal reduction for refractory symptoms

Invasive treatments are reserved for patients who have severe refractory symptoms (class III or IV) despite medical treatment and intraventricular gradients of more than 50 mm Hg. The classic Morrow myectomy is performed through an aortotomy and involves resection of a relatively small amount of tissue from the proximal septum. Surgical resection of the hypertrophied septum has an initial success rate of 90% in decreasing symptoms and LV outflow obstruction. In a study of 64 patients who underwent transaortic myectomy, there was a sustained improvement in symptoms and a decrease in LVOT resting gradient from 73.2 ± 14.8 mm Hg to 13.6 ± 2.7 mm Hg at an average follow-up of 4.6 years (4 months to 12 years) [11]. Another study of 20 patients who underwent either myectomy or mitral valve replacement as treatment for an outflow tract gradient found a sustained reduction in gradient, a decrease in basal coronary blood flow, and a decrease in coronary blood flow and myocardial oxygen consumption during rapid atrial pacing [12].

Alcohol septal ablation has been developed as a treatment for LV outflow obstruction due to septal hypertrophy. In this procedure, alcohol is injected into a septal branch of the left anterior descending artery, causing localized infarction of the septum. Alcohol septal ablation appears to elicit a sustained reduction in outflow tract gradient. In a study of 50 patients, septal ablation (mean creatine kinase value 413 ± 193 U/L) reduced LVOT gradients from 80 ± 33 to 18 ± 17 mm Hg after 4–6 months and to 17 ± 15 mm Hg after 12–18 months [13].

There is considerable controversy about proper patient selection for alcohol septal ablation and surgical myectomy. Current guidelines emphasize several important points: (a) both ASA and myectomy are effective at reducing LVOT gradient; (b) myectomy produces more complete gradient relief, particularly in patients <65 years of age; (c) residual gradients are more common after alcohol septal ablation [9,14].

Dual-chamber pacing has largely been abandoned as a treatment option in HOCM because data from randomised, double-blind, crossover trials failed to show any benefit. RV pacing causes the interventricular septum to move paradoxically, and in theory this should increase LVOT dimensions and thus reduce LVOT blood velocities, which results in less SAM of the mitral valve and less mitral regurgitation. While initially proposed in 1975, interest in AV sequential pacing for HCM was revived by a study of DDD devices in 84 patients with obstructive HCM and severe symptoms refractory to medical therapy [15]. Symptoms were abolished in 33.3% of the patients, reduced in 56%, and unchanged in 8%. At a mean follow-up of 2.3 ± 0.8 years only four patients had to undergo a surgical procedure. In this study there was significant improvement in NYHA class, in exercise capacity, and in resting LVOT gradient.

Subsequent studies produced less enthusiastic results and dual-chamber pacing is rarely utilized as a treatment for HOCM. In a multicenter, randomized, double-blind, crossover study of permanent DDD pacing in 48 patients with drug-refractory HOCM, Maron *et al.* found an average reduction of outflow gradient of 40%, but no change in exercise capacity, peak oxygen consumption, or LV wall thickness in the overall group [16].

Case study

A 75-year-old male with a history of atrial fibrillation reported increasing dyspnea on exertion and lower-extremity edema. A nuclear stress test was suggestive of ischemia and he was referred for cardiac catheterization. Simultaneous measurement of LV apex and femoral artery pressures revealed no gradient under basal conditions. Initiation of a PVC elicited a Brockenbrough sign (Figure 15.8a) and Valsalva maneuver precipitated a marked, transient increase in LVOT gradient (Figures 15.8b, 15.8c). These findings are consistent with HOCM.

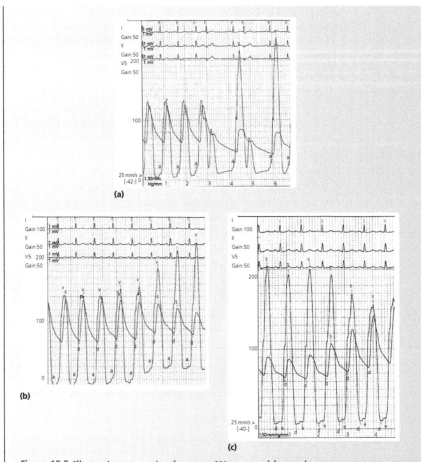

Figure 15.8 Illustrative case—simultaneous LV apex and femoral artery pressures demonstrating a Brockenbrough sign (a) and precipitation of an intraventricular gradient during Valsalva maneuver, onset in (b) and offset in (c).

References

1 Louie EK, Maron BJ. Apical hypertrophic cardiomyopathy: clinical and two-dimensional echocardiographic assessment. *Ann Intern Med* 1987;**106**:663–670.

2 Topol EJ, Traill TA, Fortuin NJ. Hypertensive hypertrophic cardiomyopathy of the elderly. *N Engl J Med* 1985;**312**:277–283.

3 Maron BJ, Bonow RO, Cannon IRO, Leon MB, Epstein SE. Hypertrophic cardiomyopathy: interrelations of clinical manifestations, pathophysiology, and therapy. *N Engl J Med* 1987; **316**:780–789; 844–852.

4 Panza JA, Petrone RK, Fananapazir L, Maron BJ. Utility of continuous wave Doppler echocardiography in the noninvasive assessment of left ventricular outflow tract pressure gradient in patients with hypertrophic cardiomyopathy. *J Am Coll Cardiol* 1992;**19**:91–99.

5 Cannon RO III, Rosing DR, Maron BJ, *et al*. Myocardial ischemia in patients with hypertrophic cardiomyopathy: contribution of inadequate vasodilator reserve and elevated left ventricular filling pressures. *Circulation* 1985;**71**:234–243.

6 Cannon RO III, Schenke WH, Maron BJ, *et al*. Differences in coronary flow and myocardial metabolism at rest and during pacing between patients with obstructive and patients with nonobstructive hypertrophic cardiomyopathy. *J Am Coll Cardiol* 1987;**10**:53–62.

7 Yang EH, Yeo TC, Higano ST, Nishimura RA, Lerman A. Coronary hemodynamics in patients with symptomatic hypertrophic cardiomyopathy. *Am J Cardiol* 2004;**94**:685–687.

8 Maron BJ. Hypertrophic cardiomyopathy. *Curr Probl Cardiol* 1993;**18**:637–704.

9 Maron BJ, McKenna WJ, Danielson GK, *et al*. American College of Cardiology/European Society of Cardiology clinical expert consensus document on hypertrophic cardiomyopathy. A report of the American College of Cardiology Foundation Task Force on Clinical Expert Consensus Documents and the European Society of Cardiology Committee for Practice Guidelines. *J Am Coll Cardiol* 2003;**42**:1687–1713.

10 Maron BJ, Maron MS. Hypertrophic cardiomyopathy. *Lancet* 2013;**381**:242–255.

11 Minami K, Woltersdorf H, Kleikamp G, Bothig D, Koertke H, Koerfer R. Long-term results after myectomy in 64 patients with hypertrophic obstructive cardiomyopathy (HOCM). Morphological and hemodynamic aspects. *J Cardiovasc Surg (Torino)* 2000;**41**:801–806.

12 Cannon RO III, McIntosh CL, Schenke WH, Maron BJ, Bonow RO, Epstein SE. Effect of surgical reduction of left ventricular outflow obstruction on hemodynamics, coronary flow, and myocardial metabolism in hypertrophic cardiomyopathy. *Circulation* 1989;**79**:766–775.

13 Boekstegers P, Steinbigler P, Molnar A, *et al*. Pressure-guided nonsurgical myocardial reduction induced by small septal infarctions in hypertrophic obstructive cardiomyopathy. *J Am Coll Cardiol* 2001;**38**:846–853.

14 Gersh BJ, Maron BJ, Bonow RO, *et al*. 2011 ACCF/AHA guideline for the diagnosis and treatment of hypertrophic cardiomyopathy: a report of the American College of Cardiology Foundation/American Heart Association Task Force on practice guidelines. *J Am Coll Cardiol* 2011;**58**(25):e212–e260.

15 Fananapazir L, Epstein ND, Curiel RV, Panza JA, Tripodi D, McAreavey D. Long-term results of dual-chamber (DDD) pacing in obstructive hypertrophic cardiomyopathy. *Circulation* 1994;**90**:2731–2742.

16 Maron BJ, Nishimura RA, McKenna WJ, Rakowski H, Josephson ME, Kieval RS. Assessment of permanent dual-chamber pacing as a treatment for drug-refractory symptomatic patients with obstructive hypertrophic cardiomyopathy. A randomized, double-blind, crossover study (M-PATHY). *Circulation* 1999;**99**:2927–2933.

CHAPTER 16

Heart failure

Geoffrey T. Jao, Steven Filby and Patricia P. Chang

Heart failure (HF) is a clinical syndrome caused by failure of the heart to meet the demands of the body, with symptoms due to elevated intracardiac filling pressures and/or decreased effective cardiac output. The most common classification of HF is based on the left ventricular ejection fraction (LVEF), as determined by some form of cardiac imaging (most commonly an echocardiogram). The LVEF cutoff for HF with reduced ejection fraction (HFrEF, also known as systolic heart failure) is <50%, or more strictly <40%. Patients with LVEF >50% are considered to have HF with preserved ejection fraction (HFpEF, previously known as diastolic heart failure). While these two entities are indistinguishable based on clinical signs and symptoms alone, they differ in all other aspects: gross anatomy, histology, radiographic and hemodynamic findings, and, not surprisingly, treatment effects. The etiology of HF is due to some form of myocardial insult (Table 16.1), with HFrEF better understood than HFpEF.

The pressure–volume loops best illustrate the hemodynamic differences between HFrEF and HFpEF (Figure 16.1). Since patients with HFrEF have reduced myocardial contractility, the left ventricle dilates to accommodate a higher preload necessary to maintain an effective cardiac output. In hemodynamic terms, a patient with HFrEF has higher left ventricular end-diastolic volume (LVEDV) and pressure (LVEDP), as well as lower stroke volume, pulse pressure, and effective cardiac output, which then translate to higher left ventricular end-systolic volume (LVESV) and pressure (LVESP). As the degree of systolic dysfunction worsens, the pressure–volume loop further shifts toward the right. Likewise, in the presence of significant mitral regurgitation, the stroke volume and effective cardiac output are further reduced due to the absence of isovolumetric contraction.

The exact mechanism causing HFpEF is still unknown. An autopsy series of patients with HFpEF showed more cardiac hypertrophy, epicardial coronary artery disease, coronary microvascular rarefaction, and myocardial fibrosis compared to

Cardiovascular Hemodynamics for the Clinician, Second Edition. Edited by George A. Stouffer.
© 2017 John Wiley & Sons Ltd. Published 2017 by John Wiley & Sons Ltd.

Table 16.1 Common etiologies of heart failure.

Coronary artery disease

Hypertension

Primary valvular disease

Tachycardia-mediated cardiomyopathy

Toxins (ethanol, anthracyclines, her2-neu receptor antagonist, and tyrosine kinase inhibitors)

Stress-induced cardiomyopathy (aka Takotsubo cardiomyopathy)

Congenital heart disease

Infectious (HIV, Chagas' disease, coxsackie, echovirus, Lyme disease)

Infiltrative disease (hemochromatosis, amyloidosis, sarcoidosis)

Peripartum cardiomyopathy

Myocarditis (giant cell myocarditis, lymphocytic myocarditis, eosinophilic myocarditis/hypersensitivity)

Connective tissue disease (systemic lupus erythematosis)

Nutritional deficiencies (selenium, copper)

Metabolic (thyroid disease)

Hereditary (neuromuscular disorders [Duchenne's muscular dystrophy], X-linked, mitochondrial [MELAS syndrome], storage disease)

High-output states (arteriovenous fistula, hyperthyroidism, beriberi)

Hypertrophic cardiomyopathy

Restrictive cardiomyopathy

Idiopathic

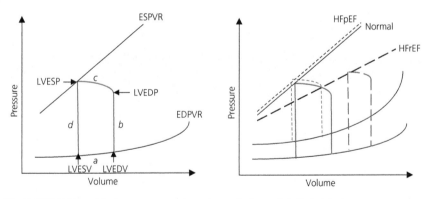

Figure 16.1 Left ventricular pressure–volume loops. Left panel: left ventricular pressure–volume loop demonstrates pressure and volume changes during the cardiac cycle: (a) the left ventricle fills during diastole, followed by (b) isovolumetric contraction at end-diastole, which ends when the aortic valve opens (at the highest LVEDV and LVEDP), followed by (c) left ventricular ejection (systole), followed by (d) isovolumetric relaxation (beginning with the aortic valve closing). The slope of the end-systolic pressure–volume relationship (ESPVR) represents end-systolic elastance (Ees), which provides an index of contractility. The end-diastolic pressure–volume relationship (EDPVR) represents the passive filling (compliance) for the LV, and the slope of this curve is ventricular stiffness (the reciprocal of ventricular compliance). Stroke volume is the difference of LVEDV and LVESV (SV = EDV − ESV). Pulse pressure is represented as the difference of LVESP and LVEDP. Right panel: pressure–volume loops for normal (solid line), HFpEF (thin dash line), and HFrEF (bold dash line).

age-matched control subjects [1]. In contrast to HFrEF, the resulting "stiffer" left ventricle develops higher filling pressures given the same incremental changes in volume (Figure 16.1). Thus, a much lower LVEDV is needed to overcome the aortic pressure, resulting in reduced stroke volume, effective cardiac output, and LVESV. LVEF, defined as the ratio of stroke volume to LVEDV, is preserved because both the numerator and denominator are reduced.

History, physical examination, cardiac biomarkers, chest X-ray, and occasionally cardiac imaging are central in the medical management of acute on chronic heart failure. In some cases it may be difficult to estimate accurately the true hemodynamic status of the chronic HF patient using these tools alone. Physical examination findings of HF can be absent in as many as 40% of patients with elevated pulmonary capillary wedge pressures (PCWP) [2, 3]. Additionally, the chest X-ray often does not show evidence of pulmonary congestion in advanced HF patients due to increased pulmonary lymphatic drainage [4]. In this light, judicious utilization of right heart catheterization can be very helpful in some clinical scenarios.

It is noteworthy that *routine* pulmonary artery catheter (PAC) use has never been shown to improve mortality or long-term clinical outcomes in patients with HF [5–12]. In the randomized, multicenter Evaluation Study of Congestive Heart Failure and Pulmonary Artery Catheterization Effectiveness (ESCAPE) trial, the addition of routine PAC to clinical assessment, compared to clinical assessment alone, did not improve clinical outcomes in patients with severe symptomatic and recurrent systolic heart failure [12]. Clinical status significantly and continuously improved in both groups, but there was a consistent trend suggesting greater clinical improvement in the PAC group (especially at the 1-month but not at the 6-month follow-up). Not surprisingly, inpatient mortality and survival at 6 months were similar in both groups and adverse in-hospital events (driven by PAC infection) were higher in the PAC group. As is true for most advanced HF patients, improvements in functionality and quality of life are more meaningful than prolongation of life. Thus, PAC can be useful for optimizing hemodynamic management of the decompensated HF patient when clinically indicated. Table 16.2 lists some of the indications for right heart catheterization.

The hemodynamic findings of HFrEF and HFpEF are often similar in terms of elevated intracardiac filling pressures, but decreased effective cardiac output is usually seen only in advanced HFpEF, whereas it is seen earlier in HFrEF. Patients with chronic HF usually have higher baseline intracardiac pressures than those with acute HF, because chronic HF patients typically require higher filling pressures to maintain optimal cardiac output (as illustrated by the Frank–Starling relationship, Figure 16.2). Thus the "normal" parameters are slightly higher for chronic HFrEF patients than the "ideal" normal range for patients with normal cardiac function. Specific conditions such as restrictive cardiomyopathy, constrictive pericarditis, and hypertrophic cardiomyopathy will be discussed elsewhere in this book.

Table 16.2 Indications for right heart catheterization in patients with heart failure.

Determination of true hemodynamic/intravascular status when noninvasive clinical evaluation alone is insufficient

Initiation of and dose optimization of inotropes and/or vasodilators

Perioperative monitoring and management of the high-risk patient undergoing cardiothoracic surgery

Gold standard for diagnosis and management of pulmonary hypertension

Hemodynamic monitoring, including evaluation of pulmonary vascular resistance, of end-stage HF patients awaiting cardiac transplantation

Differentiation of constrictive pericarditis from restrictive cardiomyopathy (together with left heart catheterization)

Determination of valvular heart disease severity when other diagnostics (e.g., echocardiography) are equivocal

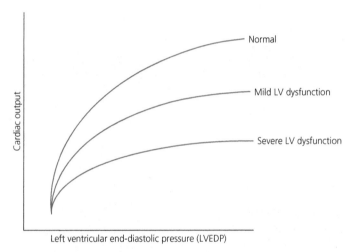

Figure 16.2 Frank-Starling curve of cardiac output as a function of LVEDP. Idealized Frank–Starling curves with varying degrees of left ventricular contractile dysfunction. In the normal heart, an increase in preload results in a steep increase in cardiac output. With left ventricular systolic dysfunction, the curves are displaced down and rightward, such that higher filling pressures are needed to maintain the same amount of cardiac output.

Directly measured intracardiac pressures

The best measurement of LV preload is left atrial (LA) pressure. In practice, LA pressure is difficult to obtain and thus two surrogate measurements are commonly used (Figure 16.3): left ventricular end diastolic pressure (LVEDP) and pulmonary capillary wedge pressure (PCWP).

Left ventricular end-diastolic pressure

Since LVEDP is measured at the end of diastole, the major contribution is from atrial contraction for patients in sinus rhythm. While it is noteworthy that the end-diastolic pressure–volume relationship (EDPVR) is curvilinear (Figure 16.1),

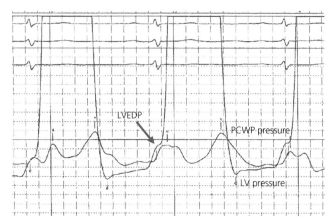

Figure 16.3 Simultaneous left ventricular and pulmonary capillary wedge pressures in a 59-year-old female. [LVEDP = left ventricular end diastolic pressure.]

the more severe the degree of systolic and diastolic dysfunction, the less likely this generalization is to hold. In HFrEF where the left ventricular chamber size is dilated, increased LVEDV is needed to produce a proportionate increase in LVEDP, which in turn is needed to optimize cardiac output. In contrast, the abnormal left ventricular relaxation or ventricular stiffness in HFpEF creates a stiff and poorly compliant LV, thus a relatively small change in LVEDV leads to elevation in LVEDP.

Direct measurement of the LVEDP is achieved by placing a catheter into the left ventricle via arterial access (Figure 16.3).

Pulmonary capillary wedge pressure

The PCWP profile is different in acute and chronic HF patients. For the patient who sustained an acute myocardial injury, for example secondary to sudden complete occlusion of the proximal left anterior descending artery with resultant myocardial dysfunction, a sudden rise in PCWP to 17–20 mm Hg could be sufficient to cause acute pulmonary edema. In contrast, a patient with chronic HF often needs a mean PCWP of 17–20 mm Hg to optimize cardiac output, as explained by the Frank-Starling mechanism (Figure 16.2).

The PCWP waveform in HF patients is often characterized by a prominent V wave (Figure 16.4). This V wave morphology may be due to a noncompliant LV or LA, and/or due to moderate to severe functional mitral regurgitation (from left ventricular dilatation), often seen in HFrEF. The calculated mean PCWP will be elevated and not accurately reflective of LV preload, as the increased pressure in the V waves is transmitted to the pulmonary vessels.

Pulmonary artery pressure

Pulmonary hypertension (PH) is defined as mean pulmonary artery pressure (mPAP) >25 mm Hg. World Health Organization Group 2 refers to PH due to left heart disease (i.e., pulmonary venous hypertension or post-capillary PH) [13],

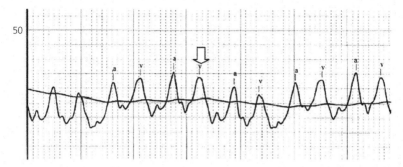

Figure 16.4 Pulmonary capillary wedge pressure tracing in a patient with dilated cardiomyopathy and severe mitral regurgitation. The mean PCWP is elevated at approximately 25 mm Hg and prominent V waves are also noted (arrow).

and is by far the most common cause of PH and right-sided HF. Up to 60% of patients with severe systolic dysfunction and up to 70% of patients with isolated LV diastolic dysfunction may present with PH [14]. PH carries a poor prognosis for patients with chronic heart failure [15]. PH is further discussed in Chapter 26.

The PA diastolic pressure should correlate well with the PCWP in the absence of significant pulmonary vasculature remodeling. It is important to mention that the mPAP is used to calculate the transpulmonary gradient, pulmonary vascular resistance, and the right ventricular stroke work index, all of which are important parameters in deciding eligibility for ventricular assist device implantation or heart transplantation.

Right ventricular pressures

In the absence of pulmonic stenosis, the RV systolic pressure should correlate well with the PA systolic pressure. The RV diastolic pressure should also correlate well with the mean right atrial pressure in the absence of pathologic tricuspid regurgitation. An elevated RV systolic pressure usually indicates preserved RV myocardial contractility. One needs to consider RV failure if the RV systolic pressure is low in the setting of elevated right atrial pressure (>15 mm Hg) and depressed cardiac index (<2.0 mL/min/m2) [13].

Right atrial pressure (normal 2–8 mm Hg)

Examination of the jugular venous pulse and sonographic assessment of the jugular vein and inferior vena cava are noninvasive estimates of right atrial pressure (RAP). Typically, the mean PCWP is greater than the mean RAP in chronic HF and in normal hearts. Tricuspid regurgitation can raise the mean RAP above the mean PCWP and show a prominent V wave on the RA waveform. In patients with predominantly right-sided HF, the mean RAP can dominate the right atrial waveform with a prominent V wave and steep Y descent.

Derived parameters from measured intracardiac pressures

Mixed venous oxygen saturation (normal ~75%)

The mixed venous oxygen saturation (SvO_2) is a marker of adequacy of tissue perfusion and decreases when oxygen delivery falls or tissue oxygen demand increases. It is directly measured in a blood sample obtained from the pulmonary artery. SvO_2 in HF patients is usually decreased, often less than 60%, and may be as low as 30% in severely decompensated patients. Measurement of SvO_2 is useful to monitor progression of disease in HF patients and has been proposed as an easy alternative to the more conventional hemodynamic parameters (i.e., cardiac output) to estimate hypoperfusion, as SvO_2 is a critical component of the Fick equation for derivation of cardiac output.

SvO_2 is directly related to cardiac output, hemoglobin, and arterial saturation and inversely related to the metabolic rate. By using the derivation of the Fick equation, the mixed venous saturation can be determined by:

$$SvO_2 = SaO_2 - \left[\left(VO_2\right)/\left(Hb \times 1.36 \times Q\right)\right]$$

where:
SvO_2 = mixed venous saturation
SaO_2 = arterial oxygen saturation
VO_2 = oxygen consumption
Hg = hemoglobin
Q = cardiac output

Cardiac output and cardiac index

Cardiac output (CO) and cardiac index (CI) in HFrEF and severe HFpEF are low. In new acute HF, a cardiac index <2.2 L/min/m² characterizes cardiogenic shock. However, patients with chronic HF adapt to a low cardiac index by increasing oxygen extraction in tissue (which results in a decrease in mixed venous oxygen saturation). As such, chronic HFrEF patients may have cardiac indices as low as 1.0–1.5 L/min/min² without demonstrating clinical signs of shock. CO is derived from either the thermodilution method or by the Fick principle, as discussed in Chapter 6. Each CO derivation method has strengths and limitations depending on certain conditions. The Fick method is based on a calculation of oxygen consumption (VO_2) divided by the arteriovenous oxygen difference ($C_a - C_v$):

$$CO = \left[VO_2 \times BSA\right]/\left[hemoglobin \times 1.36 \times 10\left(SaO_2 - SvO_2\right)\right]$$

While hemoglobin, arterial oxygen saturation, and mixed venous oxygen saturation are directly measured, the patient's VO_2 rarely is, and thus an average value (e.g., 130 cc/min/m²) is used for every patient. However, every patient is unlikely to have the same VO_2; thus a patient with end-stage HF may have falsely elevated Fick-derived CO and CI. While the cardiac output is often important for decision making, understanding the potential limitations and observing the trend of CO during PAC-guided therapy remains vital for optimal clinical management.

Transpulmonary gradient (TPG) and pulmonary vascular resistance (PVR)

The transpulmonary gradient (TPG) is the difference between PCWP and mPAP. PVR is TPG divided by the cardiac output:

$$PVR = (mPAP - mPCWP) / CO$$

A TPG that exceeds 15 mm Hg or a PVR >3 Woods units suggests pulmonary vascular remodeling secondary to longstanding pulmonary venous hypertension. A PVR >5 Woods units is an absolute contraindication to heart transplantation, as it increases the risk for right heart failure of the cardiac allograft. Implantation of an LVAD can decrease the TPG and PVR, but persistent elevation is concerning for development or progression of post-LVAD RV dysfunction [16].

Right ventricular stroke work index (normal 5–10 g-m^2/beat)

Right ventricular stroke work (RVSW) and right ventricular stroke work index (RVSWI) are hemodynamic surrogates of right ventricular function. They are calculated based on direct measurements from a PAC as well as derived parameters to derive stroke volume (SV) and stroke volume index (SVI). The calculations are as follows:

$$RVSW = (mPAP - RAP) \times SV \times 0.0136 = (mPAP - RAP) \times CO/HR \times 0.0136$$
$$RVSWI = (mPAP - RAP) \times SVI \times 0.0136 = (mPAP - RAP) \times CO/HR/BSA \times 0.0136$$

A RVSWI <5 g-m^2/beat (together with MELD-A score >14, PCWP >20 mm Hg, and VO_2 <14 mL/kg/min) among ambulatory NYHA stage III HF patients was associated with death, need for ventricular assist device implantation, and heart transplantation at 1 year [17]. Low RVSWI and low PAP may also predict right heart failure and need for right ventricular assist device after left ventricular assist device implantation [18].

Aortic pressure and pulsus alternans

In contrast to acute HF, aortic pressure in chronic HF may be normal or even elevated. Changes in aortic pulse pressure correlate with changes in cardiac index. Pulsus alternans may also be seen on the aortic pressure tracing (Figure 16.5), noted by the beat-to-beat variation in the peak systolic pressure amplitude. While the precise mechanism of pulsus alternans is not known, it is a sign of severe left ventricular dysfunction. Proposed mechanisms include changes in preload and contractility leading to alterations in stroke volume [19, 20]. Post-ectopic potentiation and increased preload may play a role in the initiation of pulsus alternans. Pulsus alternans is more common during tachycardia and occurs more frequently with inotropic therapy. It should be noted that the absence of pulsus alternans

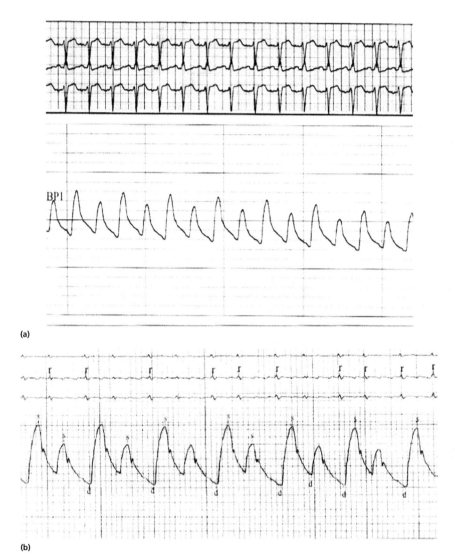

(a)

(b)

Figure 16.5 Aortic pressure tracing showing pulsus alternans (a). The beat-to-beat variation in aortic pressure amplitude is evident. The pressure tracing in panel (b) represents "pseudo-pulsus alternans." In this example, the beat-to-beat variation in aortic pressure amplitude is due to atrial flutter.

does not exclude severe left ventricular dysfunction. In one study, only 19.1% of patients with moderate to severe left ventricular dysfunction (mean LVEF 35%) had pulsus alternans at rest [20]. Pulsus alternans as a result of severe right-sided HF may also be seen on pulmonary artery pressure tracings.

Ambulatory monitoring of pulmonary artery pressures (CardioMEMS)

The goal of ambulatory monitoring of PA pressures is to assess fluid status in heart failure patients remotely and intervene before the patient worsens to the point of requiring hospital admission. The first such system, CardioMEMS, was FDA (Food and Drug Administration) approved in 2014 and consists of a battery-free capacitive pressure sensor permanently implanted in the PA, and a station that acquires and processes signals from the implantable device and transmits PA pressure measurements to a remote database that is monitored by the treating physician (Figure 16.6). The CardioMEMS device was evaluated in the prospective, multicentered, randomized, single-blinded CHAMPION (CardioMEMS Heart Sensor Allows Monitoring of Pressure to Improve Outcomes in NYHA Class III Heart Failure Patients) trial. In this study of 550 HYHA class III heart failure patients with at least one hospitalization in the prior year, there was a statistically significant reduction in heart failure–related hospitalizations/patient/6 months from 0.44 to 0.32 [21].

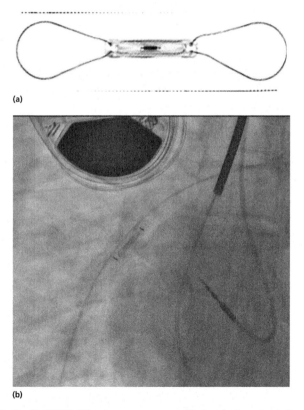

(a)

(b)

Figure 16.6 The CardioMEMS HF system pressure-monitoring device prior to implantation (a) and after implantation in a branch of the right pulmonary artery (b).

Important points: Hemodynamics in HF

- Chronic HF patients typically have higher baseline intracardiac filling pressures
- Mixed venous saturation (SvO_2) is a useful surrogate measurement for the assessment of cardiac output
- Both the Fick and thermodilution methods for assessment of cardiac output have limitations
- Low right ventricular stroke work index can predict right ventricular failure
- Pulmonary vascular remodeling (TPG >15 mm Hg and PVR >3 Woods units) can increase the risk of right ventricular failure
- Pulsus alternans is a sign of a failing ventricle
- Invasive hemodynamic monitoring, mostly commonly with a pulmonary artery catheter, can be useful in the assessment and management of HF patients

References

1 Mohammed SF, Hussain S, Mirzoyev SA, *et al.* Coronary microvascular rarefaction and myocardial fibrosis in heart failure with preserved ejection fraction. *Circulation* 2015;**131**: 550–559.
2 Stevenson LW, Perloff JK. The limited reliability of physical signs for estimating hemodynamics in chronic heart failure. *JAMA* 1989;**261**:884–888.
3 Butman SM, Ewy Ga, Standen JR, Kern KB, Hahn E. Bedside cardiovascular examination in patients with severe chronic heart failure: importance of rest or inducible jugular venous distention. *J Am Coll Cardiol* 1993;**22**:968–974.
4 Chakko S, Woska D, Martinez H, *et al.* Clinical, radiographic, and hemodynamic correlations in chronic congestive heart failure: conflicting results may lead to inappropriate care. *Am J Med* 1991;**90**:353–359.
5 Matthay MA, Chatterjee K. Bedside catheterization of the pulmonary artery: risks compared with benefits. *Ann Intern Med* 1988;**109**(10):826–834.
6 Fein AM, Goldberg SK, Walkenstein MD, Dershaw B, Braitman L, Lippman ML. Is pulmonary artery catheterization necessary for the diagnosis of pulmonary edema? *Am Rev Resp Dis* 1984;**129**(6):1006–1009.
7 Harvey S, Harrison DA, Singer M, *et al.* Assessment of clinical effectiveness of pulmonary artery catheters in the management of patients in intensive care units (PAC-Man): a randomized controlled trial. *Lancet* 2005;**366**:472–477.
8 Bernard GR, Sopko G, Cerra F, *et al.* Pulmonary artery catheterization and clinical outcomes: National Heart, Lung, and Blood Institute and Food and Drug Administration Workshop Report. *Consensus Statement. JAMA* 2000;**283**(19):2568–2572.
9 Connors AF Jr, McCaffree DR, Gray BA. Evaluation of right-heart catheterization in the critically ill patient without acute myocardial infarction. *N Engl J Med* 1983; **308**(5):263–267.
10 Connors AF Jr, Speroff T, Dawson NV, *et al.*, for SUPPORT Investigators. The effectiveness of right heart catheterization in the initial care of critically ill patients. *JAMA* 1996; **276**(11):889–897.
11 Eisenberg P, Jaffe AS, Schuster DP. Clinical evaluation compared to pulmonary artery catheterization in the hemodynamic assessment of critically ill patients. *Crit Care Med* 1984;**12**(7):549–553.

12 Binanay C, Califf RM, Hasselblad V, *et al.* Evaluation study of congestive heart failure and pulmonary artery catheterization effectiveness: the ESCAPE trial. *JAMA* 2005;**294**(13):1625–1633.

13 Galie N, Hoeper MM, Humbert M, *et al.* Guidelines for the diagnosis and treatment of pulmonary hypertension. *Eur Heart J* 2009;**30**:2493–2537.

14 Ghio S, Gavazzi A, Campana C, *et al.* Independent and additive prognostic value of right ventricular systolic function and pulmonary artery pressure in patients with chronic heart failure. *J Am Coll Cardiol* 2001;**37**:183–188.

15 Grigioni F, Potena L, Galie N, *et al.* Prognostic implication of serial assessments of pulmonary hypertension in severe chronic heart failure. *J Heart Lung Transplant* 2006;**25**:1241–1246.

16 Neragi-Miandoab S, Goldstein D, Bello R, Michler R, D'Allesandro D. Right ventricular dysfunction following continuous flow left ventricular assist device placement in 51 patients: predictors and outcomes. *J Cardiothorac Surg* 2012;**7**:60.

17 Kato TS, Stevens GR, Jiang J, *et al.* Risk stratification of ambulatory patients with advanced heart failure undergoing evaluation for heart transplantation. *J Heart Lung Transplant* 2013;**32**(3):333–340.

18 Ochai Y, McCarthy PM, Smidera NG, *et al.* Predictors of severe RV failure after implantable LVAD insertion: analysis of 245 patients. *Circulation* 2002;**106**(suppl I):I198–I202.

19 Gleason WL, Braunwald E. Studies on Starling's law of the heart. VI. Relationships between left ventricular end diastolic volume and stroke volume in man with observations on the mechanism of pulsus alternans. *Circulation* 1962;**25**:841–848.

20 Kodama M, Kato K, Hirono S, *et al.* Linkage between mechanical and electrical alternans in patients with chronic heart failure. *J Cardiovasc Electrophysiol* 2004;**15**(3):295–299.

21 Abraham WT, Adamson PB, Bourge RC, *et al.* and CHAMPION Trial Study Group. Wireless pulmonary artery haemodynamic monitoring in chronic heart failure: a randomised controlled trial. *Lancet* 2011;**377**(9766):658–666.

CHAPTER 17

Restrictive cardiomyopathy

David P. McLaughlin and George A. Stouffer

Restrictive cardiomyopathy is a disease of the myocardium characterized by impaired relaxation and diastolic dysfunction of either or both ventricles. The disease is progressive and as the ventricles become less distensible, diastolic filling and cardiac output are impaired and filling pressures increase. A reduction in systolic function may also occur as the disease progresses. Initial symptoms are usually low output–type complaints (e.g., exertional dyspnea or exercise intolerance) because of inability to augment stroke volume. As right atrial (RA) pressure increases, symptoms of systemic venous congestion may predominate. Further increases in RA and pulmonary capillary wedge (PCW) pressures will be accompanied by symptoms of orthopnea and paroxysmal nocturnal dyspnea. The clinical presentation of restrictive cardiomyopathy can be similar to constrictive pericarditis and differentiation of these processes can be difficult. Additionally, some disease processes (e.g., amyloid) can involve both myocardium and pericardium, leading to a mixed hemodynamic profile.

Causes of restrictive cardiomyopathy include amyloidosis, hemochromocytosis, metabolic storage diseases, hypereosinophilic syndrome, metastatic malignancies, sarcoid, carcinoid, idiopathic, endomyocardial fibrosis, and mediastinal radiation.

Hemodynamic principles

The hemodynamic findings of restrictive cardiomyopathy and constrictive pericarditis are similar. Chapter 18 contains a more detailed description of the findings in constrictive pericarditis.

1 Diastolic filling is impaired and determined by the degree of restriction.
- Pressures during diastole are elevated and similar in all cardiac chambers. Right and left ventricular diastolic pressures are elevated and equal in early diastole, but generally end-diastolic pressures differ by more than 5 mm Hg;

Cardiovascular Hemodynamics for the Clinician, Second Edition. Edited by George A. Stouffer.
© 2017 John Wiley & Sons Ltd. Published 2017 by John Wiley & Sons Ltd.

in contrast to constrictive pericarditis, where left ventricular end-diastolic pressure (LVEDP) and right ventricular end-diastolic pressure (RVEDP) will be similar.
* The difference between LVEDP and RVEDP is accentuated by exercise.
* Stroke volume is decreased. Cardiac output will fall in the absence of tachycardia.
* Severe pulmonary hypertension is more common than in constrictive pericarditis. RV and pulmonary systolic pressures may exceed 50 mm Hg.
* Pulsus paradoxus is not found in restrictive cardiomyopathy because of a stiff, noncompliant septum.
2 Almost all ventricular filling occurs in early diastole.
* Exaggerated Y descent in atrial tracings (Figure 17.1).
* Usual respiratory variation of atrial pressures is reduced, but the Y descent may become deeper during inspiration.
* RA tracing may have a classic M or W configuration.
* Dip and plateau configuration in RV and LV tracings.

Differentiating restrictive cardiomyopathy from constrictive pericarditis

The hemodynamic effects of restrictive cardiomyopathy are similar to those of constrictive pericarditis, and it is generally difficult to make a correct diagnosis based on hemodynamics alone. Hemodynamic criteria that favor restrictive cardiomyopathy include:
* Equalization of left and right ventricular filling pressures, but with a difference of more than 5 mm Hg between LVEDP and RVEDP. Remember that the studies from which the 5 mm Hg cutoff was determined were generally performed with high-fidelity manometric catheters.
* RVEDP does not exceed one-third of the level of the right ventricular systolic pressure.
* RV systolic pressure may be greater than 50 mm Hg.
* Concordance, defined as an inspiratory decrease in both RV and LV systolic pressures during normal respiration (Figure 17.1). This is in contrast to discordance, which is an increase in RV systolic pressure simultaneous with a decrease in LV systolic pressure (seen in constrictive pericarditis). The difference in ventricular interdependence is due to the effects of respiration on ventricular filling. It is imperative to record RV and LV simultaneously on a 200 mm Hg scale on slow sweep speed and to assess several respiratory cycles.

A review of 82 cases of constrictive pericarditis and 37 cases of restrictive cardiomyopathy found that the predictive accuracy of a difference between RVEDP and LVEDP >5 mm Hg was 85%, the predictive accuracy of RV systolic pressure >50 mm Hg was 70%, and the predictive accuracy of a ratio of RVEDP to RV systolic pressure of less than 0.33 was 76%. If all three criteria were

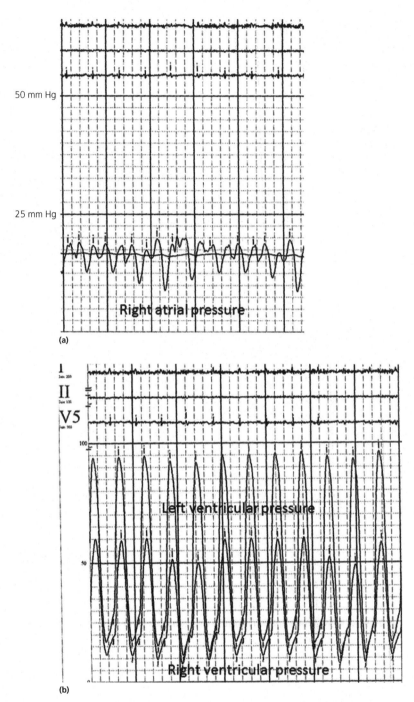

50 mm Hg

25 mm Hg

Right atrial pressure

(a)

I

II

V5

100

Left ventricular pressure

50

Right ventricular pressure

(b)

Figure 17.1 Pressure tracings from a patient with amyloidosis. Note the elevated RA pressures with an exaggerated Y descent (a). Simultaneous RV and LV pressures shows equalization during diastole (most notable during expiration) and concordance in which RV and LV systolic pressures both decrease with inspiration (b).

concordant, the probability of having classified the patient correctly was greater than 90%. However, one-fourth of patients could not be classified by hemodynamic criteria [1].

A more detailed description of hemodynamic findings that can be used to differentiate restrictive cardiomyopathy from constrictive pericarditis can be found in Chapter 18.

Echocardiography

The ventricles are usually normal in size. LV hypertrophy is frequently present (of note is that decreased R wave amplitude on ECG coupled with LV hypertrophy on echo is frequently a clue to restrictive cardiomyopathies). Mitral inflow velocity in restrictive cardiomyopathy is typically one of a prominent E wave, decreased A wave, an increased ratio of early diastolic filling to atrial filling (>2), decreased deceleration time (<150 ms), and a decreased isovolumic relaxation time (<70 ms). Cardiac valves may be involved in restrictive cardiomyopathy, leading to regurgitation.

Respiratory variation in mitral valve inflow is less in restrictive cardiomyopathy compared to constrictive pericarditis. An echocardiographic study of 30 patients (19 with constrictive pericarditis and 11 with restrictive cardiomyopathy) found that significant respiratory variation in the ventricular inflow peak velocity ≥10% predicted constrictive pericarditis with a sensitivity and specificity of 84% and 91%, respectively [2]. Remember that mitral valve inflow velocity is dependent on preload and that marked elevation in LA pressure may mask respiratory variation [3]. Reducing preload (e.g., by head-up tilting) may accentuate respiratory variation in inflow velocity.

Doppler findings in Constrictive Pericarditis and Restrictive Cardiomyopathy

- RV and LV inflow show prominent E wave due to rapid early diastolic filling
- Short deceleration time of E wave as filling abruptly stops
- Small A wave as little filling occurs in late diastole following atrial contraction

---

Case study

A 49-year-old female with pulmonary sarcoidosis reported increasing dyspnea associated with chest tightness. Echocardiogram showed normal LV chamber size, wall thickness, and function. Initial hemodynamic evaluation in the cardiac catheterization laboratory showed a mean RA pressure of 8 mm Hg. The waveform had a "W" configuration with accentuation of the Y descent during inspiration (Figure 17.2a). RA and LV pressures during diastole were similar (Figure 17.2b). The RV pressure tracing showed a "dip and plateau" configuration

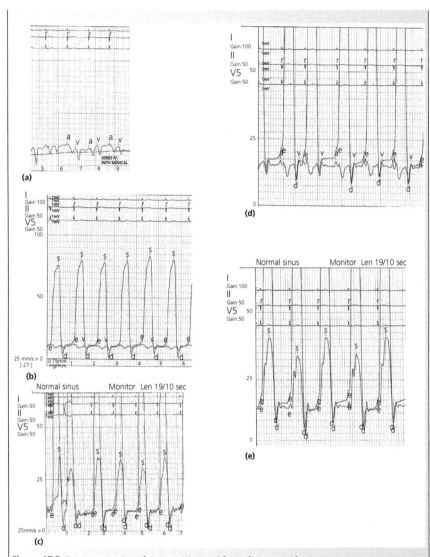

Figure 17.2 Pressure tracings from a patient with cardiac sarcoidosis.

and RV diastolic pressures approximated LV diastolic pressures (Figure 17.2c). Following rapid infusion of 500 mL of saline, RA, RVEDP, and LVEDP increased markedly. RA, RV, and LV pressures were similar during diastole, but some separation of RA and LV at the end of diastole (Figure 17.2d) and RVEDP from LVEDP (Figure 17.2e) were evident. These findings are consistent with restrictive cardiomyopathy from sarcoid.

References

1 Vaitkus PT, Kussmaul WG. Constrictive pericarditis versus restrictive cardiomyopathy: a reappraisal and update of diagnostic criteria. *Am Heart J* 1991;**122**:1431–1441.
2 Rajagopalan N, Garcia MJ, Rodriguez L, *et al.* Comparison of new Doppler echocardiographic methods to differentiate constrictive pericardial heart disease and restrictive cardiomyopathy. *Am J Cardiol* 2001;**87**:86–94.
3 Ha JW, Oh JK, Ling LH, Nishimura RA, Seward JB, Tajik AJ. Annulus paradoxus: transmitral flow velocity to mitral annular velocity ratio is inversely proportional to pulmonary capillary wedge pressure in patients with constrictive pericarditis. *Circulation* 2001;**104**:976–978.

PART IV

Pericardial disease

CHAPTER 18

Constrictive pericarditis

David P. McLaughlin and George A. Stouffer

The pericardium is a two-layered sac that encircles the heart. The visceral pericardium is a mesothelial monolayer that is adherent to the epicardium, which is reflected back on itself at the level of the great vessels. The cardiac chambers are covered by the pericardium, with the exception of the left atrium and pulmonary veins, which are mostly outside of the pericardium. The parietal layer is a tough, fibrous outer layer. In the potential space that exists between these two layers there is normally 5–50 mL of serous fluid. The normal pericardium serves three primary functions: fixing the heart within the mediastinum, limiting the spread of adjacent infections, and limiting acute cardiac distention during sudden increases in intracardiac volumes.

Constrictive pericarditis is a condition characterized by a dense, fibrous thickening of the pericardium that adheres to and encases the myocardium, resulting in impaired diastolic ventricular filling. The general paradigm is that constrictive pericarditis occurs over a period of years, due either to an acute insult (e.g., an infection) that elicits a chronic fibrosing reaction or to a chronic insult that stimulates a persistent reaction (e.g., renal failure). In the past the most common etiology was tuberculosis, but currently idiopathic pericardial constriction is the most frequent offender.

Clinically, constrictive pericarditis is generally a chronic disease with symptom progression over a period of years. The clinical presentation is that of right-sided heart failure and may resemble restrictive cardiomyopathy, cirrhosis, or cor pulmonale, among other conditions. Occasionally patients will go for years without the correct diagnosis being made. Recently, the advent of newer diagnostic technologies and a change in the predominant etiologies of constriction have led to increasing recognition of subacute presentations occurring over a period of months [1].

Pericardial constriction occurring after acute pericarditis of any cause is rare, but can occur early or later after the insult. Constrictive physiology can occur in the weeks following cardiac surgery or acute pericarditis. This often resolves and

Cardiovascular Hemodynamics for the Clinician, Second Edition. Edited by George A. Stouffer.
© 2017 John Wiley & Sons Ltd. Published 2017 by John Wiley & Sons Ltd.

the possible transient nature must be carefully considered when planning treatment. In patients with permanent constrictive pericarditis, the presentation is usually years after the initial insult. Constriction following radiation therapy for malignancy can be a difficult diagnostic dilemma, as it can coexist with radiation-induced restrictive myocardial disease.

A study of 500 patients with acute pericarditis found that the risk of developing chronic constrictive pericarditis was low, but varied depending on the etiology. The incidence rate of constrictive pericarditis per 1000 person-years was 0.8 cases for idiopathic/viral pericarditis, 4.4 cases for connective tissue disease/pericardial injury syndrome, 6.3 cases for neoplastic pericarditis, 31.7 cases for tuberculous pericarditis, and 52.7 cases for bacterial pericarditis [2].

Hemodynamics of constrictive pericarditis

Elevation of and equalization of diastolic pressures are the hallmarks of constriction (Table 18.1). Right atrial (RA), left atrial (LA), right ventricular (RV), and left ventricular (LV) diastolic pressures are elevated and nearly identical. In contrast to the normal heart, where pressures in the cardiac chambers are independent (i.e., unrelated) during diastole, in constrictive pericarditis the stiff pericardium limits expansion of the cardiac chambers. The chambers can fill beyond a certain limited point only by compressing other chambers and thus the diastolic pressures equalize. The ventricular waveform has a characteristic square root sign due to the rapid rise in early diastolic pressure prior to reaching the constraining effects of the rigid pericardium (Figure 18.1).

Hemodynamic principles

1 Diastolic filling is impaired and determined by degree of constriction.
   • Pressures during diastole are elevated and equal in all cardiac chambers. Right and left ventricular end-diastolic pressures (RVEDP and LVEDP) are elevated and within 5 mm Hg of each other.

Table 18.1 Hemodynamic findings in constrictive pericarditis.

• Almost all ventricular filling occurs in early to mid-diastole
• Elevation of atrial pressures
• Equalization of early and mid-diastolic pressures (e.g., RV and LV or RA and LV)
• Increase in RA pressure during inspiration (Kussmaul's sign)
• Exaggerated X and Y descents
• Intrathoracic pressure is not transmitted to the cardiac chambers
• Ventricular systolic discordance—defined as inspiratory augmentation of RV systolic pressure simultaneous with a decrease in LV systolic pressure. Occurs due to the effects of respiration on ventricular filling

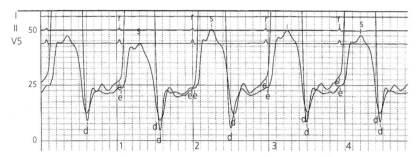

Figure 18.1 Ventricular pressure tracings in constrictive pericarditis. Simultaneous LV and RV tracings in a patient with constrictive pericarditis. Note the "dip and plateau" configuration and the near equalization during mid and late diastole. Operative findings in this patient included a dense, adherent pericardium. Central venous pressure dropped by approximately 15 mm Hg in the operating room with removal of the pericardium from the anterior RV and the RA.

- Stroke volume is decreased. Cardiac output will fall in the absence of tachycardia.
- Hypovolemia may mask constriction because diastolic filling pressures do not appear elevated (especially in patients who are over-diuresed). Fluid challenge may help in diagnosis.
- Severe pulmonary hypertension is rare. Usually RV and pulmonary artery (PA) systolic pressures are <50 mm Hg.

2 Almost all ventricular filling occurs in early diastole (Figure 18.2).
- Exaggerated Y descent.
- RA tracing may have classic M or W configuration (Figure 18.3).
- Dip and plateau configuration in RV and LV tracings.

3 In severe constrictive pericarditis, intrathoracic pressure is not communicated to the intrapericardial space (Figure 18.4).
- Central venous pressure (CVP) and RA pressure do not decrease, and may actually increase, with inspiration. Classically this is described as Kussmaul's sign, which is defined as a reversal of the normal pattern of decreasing jugular venous pressures during inspiration [3]. Venous flow to RA does not accelerate with inspiration.
- Pulsus paradoxus is minimal or absent in rigid constrictive pericarditis because ventricular filling is not affected by intrathoracic pressure. In some cases the pericardium retains some elasticity as it thickens and pulsus paradoxus may be present.
- Interdependence of ventricular filling—on inspiration, intrathoracic pressure and pulmonary venous pressure decrease, but LA pressure does not. A reduced pulmonary vein to LA pressure gradient results in decreased flow into the LA and LV. Decreased LV filling during diastole allows for increased RV filling, which leads to an increase in flow across the tricuspid valve. Thus on inspiration, RV systolic pressure increases while LV systolic pressure decreases. On expiration, increased LV filling occurs at the expense of RV filling and the opposite effect occurs on mitral valve and tricuspid valve flow.

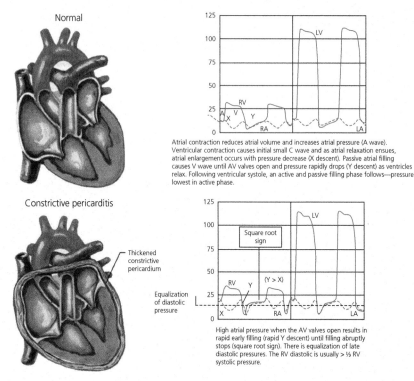

Atrial contraction reduces atrial volume and increases atrial pressure (A wave). Ventricular contraction causes initial small C wave and as atrial relaxation ensues, atrial enlargement occurs with pressure decrease (X descent). Passive atrial filling causes V wave until AV valves open and pressure rapidly drops (Y descent) as ventricles relax. Following ventricular systole, an active and passive filling phase follows—pressure lowest in active phase.

High atrial pressure when the AV valves open results in rapid early filling (rapid Y descent) until filling abruptly stops (square root sign). There is equalization of late diastolic pressures. The RV diastolic is usually > ⅓ RV systolic pressure.

Figure 18.2 Comparison of intracardiac pressures in the normal heart and in constrictive pericarditis.

4 Constrictive physiology can be mimicked by restrictive cardiomyopathy and acute volume overload of the heart.

The differentiation of constrictive pericarditis from restrictive cardiomyopathy based solely on hemodynamics is difficult and will be discussed in more detail later in this chapter. Pseudoconstriction occurs when LV or RV volume overload happens rapidly, such that the pericardium does not have time to expand to accommodate the increased size. It is defined as constrictive-appearing physiology in the absence of pericardial pathology, and as such is a diagnosis of exclusion. The following list gives the most common causes of pseudoconstrictive physiology. Bradycardia is listed but does not cause compressive physiology per se. It is mentioned here only in that the ventricular waveform can manifest a square root appearance in patients with heart rates in the 40s.

• Large RV infarcts
• Acute RV volume overload (e.g., pulmonary embolus)
• Acute severe mitral regurgitation
• Acute severe tricuspid regurgitation

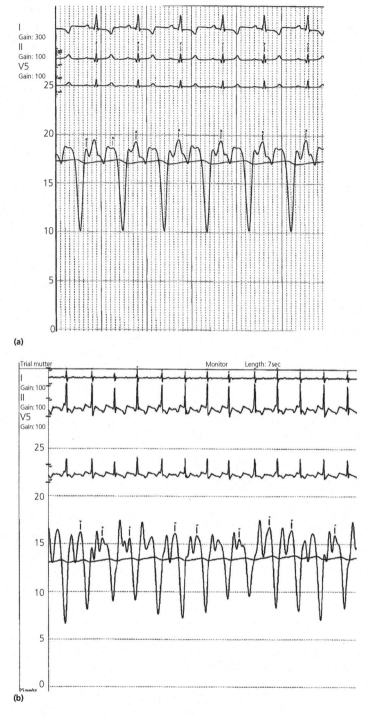

Figure 18.3 RA tracings from two patients with constrictive pericarditis. Note the elevated RA pressure, prominent Y descent, and lack of respiratory variation (both patients were breathing normally during these recordings).

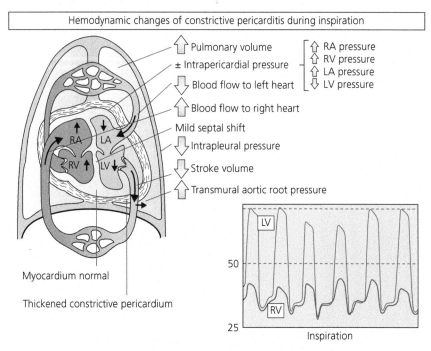

Figure 18.4 Effect of respiration on blood flow in mild constrictive pericarditis.

- Acute severe aortic regurgitation
- Severe bradycardia
- Aneurysms

Physical exam

The most obvious findings are related to elevated right heart pressures and include elevated CVP, hepatomegaly, ascites, and peripheral edema. The general physical examination in patients with constrictive pericarditis is not unlike that for those with right heart failure of any cause. There are, however, a few fairly specific physical findings that are important to recognize.

Careful examination of CVP will invariably reveal elevation. Normally, inspiration leads to a fall in CVP, as the negative thoracic pressure generated in the thorax is transmitted to the right-sided cardiac chambers. Kussmaul described a paradoxical rise in CVP with inspiration in patients with pericardial constriction that is rare in restrictive myocardial disease. Occasionally, prominent X and Y descents can be seen on examination of the neck veins. Friedreich's sign, the sudden collapse of previously distended neck veins during early diastole, is found in patients with constrictive pericarditis. A high-pitched early diastolic sound or pericardial knock occurring before a typical S3 is often heard.

Pericardial imaging techniques

Plain chest X-ray has some value in chronic pericardial constriction, as calcification of the pericardium can be seen in up to 25% of cases. Pericardial thickening can be seen on echocardiography, but must be distinguished from gain artifact or harmonics. Pericardial effusion is occasionally present and typically small. CT scanning and cardiac MRI are now the gold standard of cardiac imaging modalities used in diagnosing constriction. A pericardial thickness of >3 mm is suggestive of pericardial constriction, but it is important to note that pericardial thickening on imaging is absent in up to 20% of cases. Similarly, not all patients with thickened pericardium will have constrictive pericarditis, although a thickness of >6 mm adds considerable specificity to the diagnosis.

Findings at cardiac catheterization

1 Diastolic pressures are elevated. Equalization of diastolic pressures can be observed in the normal heart when filling pressures are low and paradoxically constrictive pericarditis can be masked with hypovolemia. Thus, it is essential that IV fluids be given in sufficient quantifies to increase diastolic pressures before the diagnosis of constrictive pericarditis can be considered.
2 Prominent Y descent on RA tracing. X descent is usually preserved.
3 Right and left ventricular diastolic pressures are elevated and similar. In a study of 15 patients with surgically proven constrictive pericarditis, LVEDP minus RVEDP (determined using high-fidelity manometric catheters) at end-expiration was 4±4 mm Hg [4]. While comparison of LVEDP and RVEDP is the time-honored way to evaluate for constrictive pericarditis, a comparison of mean pressures in the RA and the LA (or PCWP) may be more useful, as such recordings are less subject to artifacts.
4 LV diastolic pressures and RA pressures are similar.
5 Characteristic dip and plateau configuration to LV and RV pressure tracings.
6 RA pressure does not decrease with inspiration (i.e., Kussmaul's sign). The Y descent may become more prominent with inspiration in patients with some remaining elasticity in their pericardium.
7 Ventricular systolic discordance is thought by some to be the most specific hemodynamic sign of constrictive pericarditis. This is defined as inspiratory augmentation of RV systolic pressure simultaneous with a decrease in LV systolic pressure and occurs due to the effects of respiration on ventricular filling (Figure 18.5). Inspiration augments right heart filling at the expense of left heart filling. This is reflected as a drop in LV systolic pressure on particular cycles when the RV is rising. It is imperative to record RV and LV simultaneously on a 200 mm Hg scale on slow sweep speed and to assess several respiratory cycles.

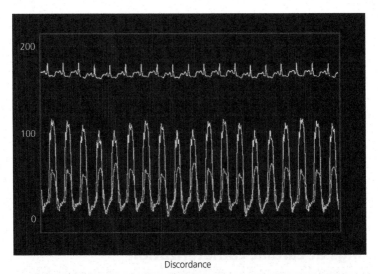

Discordance

Concordance

Figure 18.5 Examples of concordance and discordance. Source: Courtesy of Cardiovillage.com.

8 The RVEDP is usually greater than one-third the RV systolic pressure. In a study of 15 patients with surgically proven constrictive pericarditis, the ratio of RVEDP to RVSP was 0.57 ± 0.14 [4].

9 Pulmonary artery diastolic pressure (and occasionally PCWP) can be less than LVEDP during inspiration. The pulmonary artery, but not the LA, is subject to intrathoracic pressure changes in patients with constrictive pericarditis and thus will fall with inspiration.

Sensitivity and specificity of various hemodynamic findings in constrictive pericarditis

A study from the Mayo Clinic of 15 patients with constrictive pericarditis and 7 patients with restrictive cardiomyopathy provides some useful information [4]. Note, however, that this study was performed with high-fidelity manometric catheters. The small, soft fluid-filled catheters that are commonly used in cardiac catheterization laboratories can distort waveforms to a significant extent.

- Sensitivity and specificity of an LVEDP–RVEDP ≤5 mm Hg for the diagnosis of constrictive pericarditis were 60% and 71%, respectively.
- Sensitivity and specificity of an RVEDP/RV systolic pressure >1/3 for the diagnosis of constrictive pericarditis were 93% and 57%, respectively.
- Ventricular concordance/discordance was 100% sensitive and specific.
- Respiratory change in RA pressure <3 mm Hg was 93% sensitive and 48% specific.

Another study found that Kussmaul's sign was neither sensitive nor specific for constrictive pericarditis. In a study of 135 patients, Kussmaul's sign was present in only 21% of patients with surgically proven constrictive pericarditis [1]. Kussmaul's sign may also occur in right-sided heart failure, right ventricular infarction, and tricuspid stenosis.

Findings on echocardiography

The two-dimensional and Doppler echocardiographic features of constriction include a thickened pericardium, abnormal ventricular septal motion, flattening of the left ventricular posterior wall during diastole, respiratory variation in ventricular size, dilated inferior vena cava (IVC), impaired diastolic filling, and dissociation of intracardiac and intrathoracic pressures [5,6]. In constrictive pericarditis, there is a decrease in the mitral inflow velocity of greater than 25% with respiration. Also with respiration, variation in ventricular filling can sometimes be seen. During inspiration, a decrease in LV filling makes more room for RV filling, as the interventricular septum moves to the left and hepatic diastolic flow velocities increase during inspiration. During expiration, left ventricular filling increases, which decreases right heart filling and therefore hepatic diastolic forward flow velocity is decreased. In constriction, diastolic forward flow is usually greater than systolic forward flow. Additionally, hepatic diastolic flow reversal is increased, as the inflow across the tricuspid valve is interrupted by the pericardium and movement of the septum toward the right ventricle with expiration. Plethora of the IVC is common and failure of the IVC to decrease in diameter by 50% during the respiratory cycle is the echo equivalent of Kussmaul's sign. M-mode imaging can demonstrate an early diastolic notch of the interventricular septum corresponding to rapid cessation of filling, the pericardial knock, and the onset of the plateau phase of the ventricular diastolic waveform.

Differentiation of constrictive pericarditis and restrictive cardiomyopathy

Constrictive pericarditis and restrictive cardiomyopathy are very different diseases sharing a similar hemodynamic profile. Both have as the primary hemodynamic abnormality altered mid to late diastolic filling of the ventricles, leading to a syndrome of congestive heart failure. Often the heart failure is insidious in onset and predominantly right sided. These syndromes may mimic many other disease entities and it is common for both conditions to go undiagnosed for years.

In the case of constrictive pericarditis, the impediment to filling is caused by the thickened unyielding pericardium. In restrictive cardiomyopathy, the abnormality is a result of a poorly compliant myocardium that limits the ability of the ventricles to expand and accept the filling volume of the atria. Rarely there is overlap and both entities can coexist (e.g., radiation-induced myopericardial disease). The possibility of constriction or restriction should be entertained in any patient presenting with heart failure and normal systolic function (although systolic function will decline as restrictive cardiomyopathy progresses), particularly when other causes of this entity are not present.

Although the differentiation of these two entities can be quite challenging to the clinician, a thorough understanding of both the similarities and differences is imperative to arriving at the correct diagnosis. Hemodynamic factors that are helpful in differentiating constrictive pericarditis from restrictive cardiomyopathy are listed in Table 18.2, and some generalities regarding the effects of respiration on hemodynamic findings in restrictive cardiomyopathy, constrictive pericarditis, and cardiac tamponade are shown in Table 18.3. Experience teaches that it is rare to arrive at a firm diagnosis of either restrictive cardiomyopathy or constrictive pericarditis based on hemodynamics alone.

Table 18.2 Hemodynamic findings in constrictive pericarditis and restrictive cardiomyopathy.

	Constrictive pericarditis	Restrictive cardiomyopathy
LV systolic function	Usually normal	May be reduced
PA systolic pressure	Usually <50 mm Hg	May be >50 mm Hg
RV/LV systolic pressure	Discordant	Concordant
RVEDP/LVEDP separation	<5 mm Hg	>5 mm Hg
RVEDP/RV systolic pressure	>1/3	<1/3
Kussmaul's sign	Present	Absent

Table 18.3 Effects of respiration on hemodynamic findings in restrictive cardiomyopathy, constrictive pericarditis, and cardiac tamponade.

	Restrictive cardiomyopathy	Constrictive pericarditis	Cardiac tamponade
Intrathoracic pressure	Transmitted to intracardiac chambers and pulmonary venous circulation	Not transmitted to intracardiac chambers but to pulmonary venous circulation	Right-sided chambers have increased filling during inspiration whereas left-sided chambers have increased filling during expiration The inferior vena cava shows little or no change on respiration
RA pressure	Decreases with inspiration	Increases or does not change with inspiration (Kussmaul's sign)	Decreases with inspiration
Mitral inflow on echocardiography	No significant change in mitral E wave, deceleration time, or isovolumic relaxation time (IVRT) with phases of respiration	Marked respiratory variation in biventricular inflow Decrease of >25% in mitral E wave velocity and prolonged IVRT on inspiration	Mitral valve E wave velocity decreases and IVRT increases by more than 30% on inspiration compared with expiration Tricuspid valve E wave velocity increases with respiration
LV systolic pressure	Decreases with inspiration	Decreases with inspiration	Exaggerated decrease in LV systolic pressure with inspiration (pulsus paradoxus)
RV systolic pressure	Decreases with inspiration	Increases with inspiration	Increases with inspiration
Ventricular interdependence	Concordant	Discordant	

Case study

A 54-year-old male with end-stage renal failure was admitted to the hospital with signs and symptoms of right heart failure. He had been admitted 10 times during the previous 2-year period. Past medical history was remarkable for an episode of uremic pericarditis 8 years previously requiring pericardiocentesis. The pericardium was calcified on fluoroscopy (Figure 18.6a). Hemodynamics revealed elevated RA pressure with prominent Y descent and minimal variation with respiration (Figure 18.6b). Simultaneous recording of RV and LV pressures (Figure 18.6c) showed end-diastolic equalization and systolic discordance. LV and RA pressures were equal during diastole (Figure 18.6d). These findings are all consistent with constrictive pericarditis.

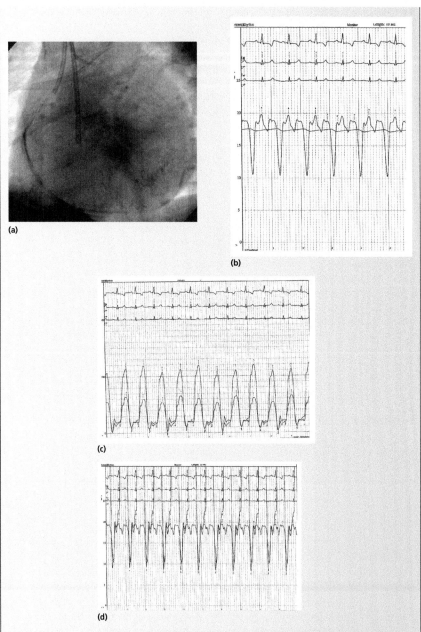

Figure 18.6 Case of constrictive pericarditis. Note the calcification of the pericardium on fluoroscopy of the heart (a, LAO projection). RA pressure is elevated with prominent Y descent and minimal variation with respiration (b). Simultaneous recording of RV and LV pressures (c) showed diastolic equalization and systolic discordance. LV and RA pressures were equal during diastole (d). These findings are all consistent with constrictive pericarditis.

References

1 Ling LH, Oh JK, Schaff HV, *et al.* Constrictive pericarditis in the modern era: evolving clinical spectrum and impact on outcome after pericardiectomy. *Circulation* 1999;**100**:1380–1386.

2 Imazio M, Brucato A, Maestroni S, *et al.* Risk of constrictive pericarditis after acute pericarditis. *Circulation* 2011;**124**:1270–1275.

3 Bilchick KC, Wise RA. Paradoxical physical findings described by Kussmaul: pulsus paradoxus and Kussmaul's sign. *Lancet* 2002;**359**:1940–1942.

4 Hurrell DG, Nishimura RA, Higano ST, *et al.* Value of dynamic respiratory changes in left and right ventricular pressures for the diagnosis of constrictive pericarditis. *Circulation* 1996;**93**:2007–2013.

5 Hatle LK, Appleton CP, Popp RL. Differentiation of constrictive pericarditis and restrictive cardiomyopathy by Doppler echocardiography. *Circulation* 1989;**79**:357–370.

6 Welch TD, Ling LH, Espinosa RE, *et al.* Echocardiographic diagnosis of constrictive pericarditis Mayo Clinic criteria. *Circ Cardiovasc Imaging* 2014;**7**:526–534.

CHAPTER 19

Cardiac tamponade

Siva B. Mohan and George A. Stouffer

The pericardium is a fibroserous sac consisting of two parts: (a) a strong external layer composed of tough fibrous tissue, called the fibrous pericardium; and (b) an internal double-layered sac (visceral and parietal pericardium) composed of a transparent membrane called the serous pericardium. The parietal pericardium is fused to the internal surface of the fibrous pericardium. The visceral pericardium is reflected onto the heart, where it forms the epicardium, the external layer of the heart wall. The potential space between the parietal and visceral layers of the serous pericardium is called the pericardial cavity. It normally contains a thin film of serous fluid that enables the heart to move and beat in a frictionless environment. The pericardium stabilizes the heart within the thoracic cavity by virtue of its ligamentous attachments, and also prevents extreme dilatation in the setting of a sudden rise of intracardiac volume.

The normal pericardial space contains 15–40 mL of pericardial fluid. A myriad of conditions produce pathologic accumulation of fluid in the pericardial cavity. Fluid that accumulates in the pericardial space can be serous, sero-sanguineous, hemorrhagic, chylous, or a combination of the above. Once a critical threshold of pericardial fluid is reached, the pericardial pressure rises in a nonlinear fashion, resulting in hemodynamic compromise or cardiac tamponade (Figure 19.1).

Hemodynamic pathophysiology

The primary hemodynamic pathophysiologic process in the development of tamponade is increased pericardial pressure that impairs diastolic filling [1–6]. Normal pericardial pressure is zero; any increase can have hemodynamic consequences. One way of looking at tamponade is that the effusion competes with the cardiac chambers to occupy the limited volume within and surrounded by the pericardium. Another way to think of tamponade is as a rubber band around

Cardiovascular Hemodynamics for the Clinician, Second Edition. Edited by George A. Stouffer.
© 2017 John Wiley & Sons Ltd. Published 2017 by John Wiley & Sons Ltd.

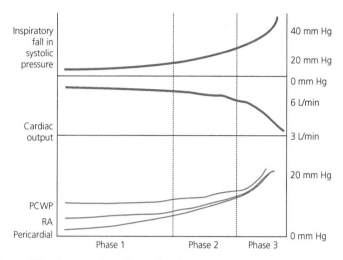

Figure 19.1 Schematic of the phases of cardiac tamponade. Source: Courtesy of Cardiovillage.com.

the cardiac chambers, exerting a constrictive force and preventing adequate expansion. Resultant elevations in intracardiac diastolic pressures impair systemic and pulmonary venous return, leading to venous congestion and reduced cardiac output (Figure 19.2). As pericardial pressures increase, a variety of compensatory mechanisms are elicited, including sympathetic nervous system activation, which leads to tachycardia, increased ejection fraction, peripheral vasoconstriction, and sodium and fluid retention.

The pericardium is a relatively noncompliant structure and thus the relationship between pericardial pressure and volume is nonlinear. Pericardial pressure rises exponentially as pericardial fluid volume increases after a certain threshold is reached. Factors that influence the development of hemodynamic compromise in the setting of a pericardial effusion include the rate at which the fluid accumulates, the amount of pericardial fluid, the compliance of the pericardium, the size of the pericardial space, and ventricular compliance. The pericardium expands only minimally in the acute setting, but can greatly increase in size over prolonged periods of time. Thus, patients with a slowly developing effusion may be asymptomatic even with a large-volume effusion. In contrast, if the rate of accumulation is rapid, even a small volume of effusion may trigger hemodynamic compromise (e.g., in the setting of cardiac trauma). The inherent compliance of the pericardium also plays a role in determining the hemodynamic significance of an effusion. Several disease processes may render the pericardium more stiff or noncompliant, allowing for a smaller effusion to cause cardiac tamponade. Left and right ventricular hypertrophy renders the heart most resistant to elevated pericardial pressures.

The hemodynamic effects of increased pericardial pressure occur on a spectrum and cardiac tamponade can be divided into three phases [5,7]. As the pericardial

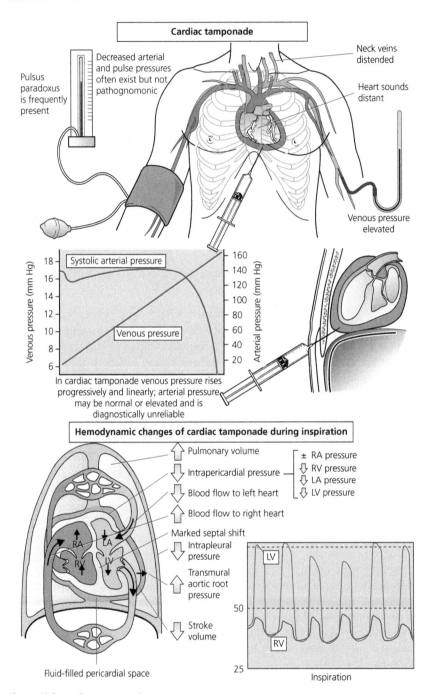

Figure 19.2 Cardiac tamponade.

fluid accumulates, the pericardial pressure rises. Increasing pericardial pressure leads to increasing right atrial (RA) pressure. At this point, clinical signs of tamponade may be absent as the right heart, including right ventricular (RV) stroke volume, but not the left heart is compromised (phase 1). As pericardial fluid continues to accumulate and pericardial pressure rises, pulmonary capillary wedge pressure (PCWP) begins to rise and external compression of both left and right ventricles is present (phase 2). End-diastolic pressures (EDP) throughout the cardiac chambers are elevated and within 5 mm Hg of each other, including RA, RVEDP, pulmonary artery, PCWP, and LVEDP. At this stage, classic signs and symptoms of cardiac tamponade are usually seen. In this phase, compensatory tachycardia maintains cardiac output in the presence of diminished stroke volume. Eventually, if pericardial pressures continue to rise and approximate RA and RV diastolic pressures, cardiac output falls, and cardiac tamponade progresses to shock with impaired tissue perfusion (phase 3).

Hemodynamic findings

See Table 19.1.
1 Elevated pericardial pressure (Figure 19.2).
2 Elevated and near equalization of end-diastolic pressures (RA, RVEDP, pulmonary artery, PCWP, and LVEDP). Since cardiac filling pressure is intracardiac minus pericardial pressure, intracardiac pressures must increase as pericardial pressure increases to maintain a pressure gradient between the atria and ventricles (remember that blood flow through the heart is determined by pressure gradients).
3 Elevated RA pressures with a prominent X descent and blunted Y descent. In the setting of a hemodynamically significant pericardial effusion, diastolic filling is impaired and affected by pericardial pressure. A unique feature of cardiac tamponade is the continuous compression of the heart throughout the cardiac cycle. This limits the fall in ventricular pressure during early diastole and thus causes a decrease in the normal atrium to ventricular pressure gradient in early diastole. This, in turn, restricts the amount of early diastolic filling of the ventricles and blunts the Y descent seen in the atrial pressure tracings (Figure 19.3).

Table 19.1 Findings on catheterization.

Elevated diastolic pressures and equalization of end-diastolic pressures
X descent is preserved, but Y descent is small or absent on RA pressure tracing
Pericardial pressure is elevated
RV pressure does not fall in early diastole (i.e., there is no dip and plateau configuration)
Pulsus paradoxus

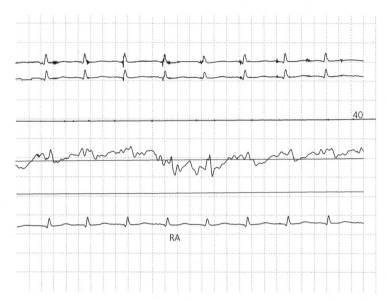

Figure 19.3 RA pressure tracing in a patient with tamponade. Note the increased RA pressures, preserved respiratory variation, and blunted Y descent.

In patients with tamponade, a relatively larger amount of atrial filling occurs following ventricular contraction, since as blood is ejected to the great vessels during ventricular systole, ventricular volume transiently falls, enabling atrial expansion and filling. RA pressure drops immediately following ventricular contraction as atrial volume increases; this large swing in RA pressure gradient in the setting of cardiac tamponade elicits an exaggerated RA X descent. The X descent may be exaggerated during inspiration since a decrease in pericardial pressure leads to augmentation of blood flow to the RV during inspiration (Figure 19.2). Conversely, the Y descent corresponds to passive ventricular filling and is blunted.

Following removal of pericardial fluid with a resulting reduction in pericardial pressure, the Y descent in the RA tracing will become more apparent (Figure 19.4).

4 RV pressure tracing lacks the "dip and plateau" of constrictive pericarditis. Unlike constrictive pericarditis, cardiac tamponade is not characterized by rapid ventricular filling in early diastole, nor does RV pressure fall below pericardial pressure in early diastole. Therefore, there is no "dip and plateau" configuration in the RV tracing. RV hypertrophy is one exception to the rule. Because of the thickness of the RV free wall, early passive diastolic filling may still occur, and therein the Y descent is preserved.

5 Pulsus paradoxus, an exaggerated decrease in arterial systolic pressure during inspiration. It is because of compromised LV diastolic filling during inspiration. This is due to a chain of events: (a) pericardial and RA pressures decrease due to negative intrathoracic pressure; (b) this results in augmented systemic

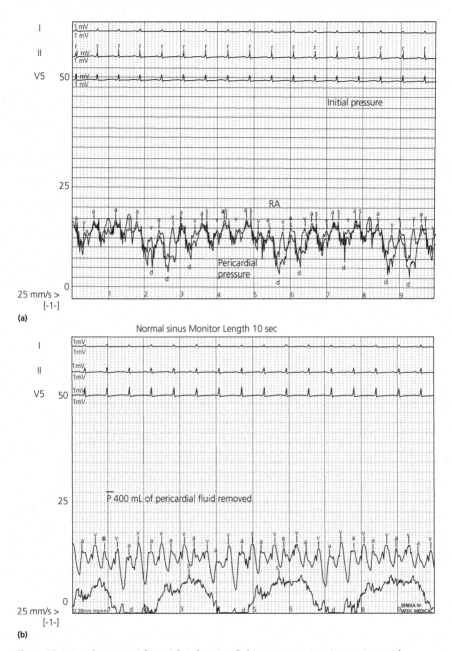

Figure 19.4 Simultaneous right atrial and pericardial pressure tracings in a patient with tamponade before and after the removal of 400 mL of pericardial fluid.

venous return to right-sided chambers and a marked increase in RV volume; (c) this results in an increase in RV filling during inspiration that, in the setting of cardiac tamponade, compromises LV filling. Note that it is normal to have a drop in systolic blood pressure with inspiration and that pulsus paradoxus is defined by the magnitude of the decrease (an "exaggerated" drop). Pulsus paradoxus is variously defined as a drop of >12 mm Hg, a drop of ≥10 mm Hg, or a drop of ≥9% during normal inspiration (Figure 19.5). Note that pulsus paradoxus may not be present in patients with tamponade and

- acute aortic regurgitation (i.e., acute aortic dissection)
- elevated LVEDP
- atrial septal defect
- pulmonary hypertension
- right ventricular hypertrophy

6 Respiratory variation in atrial pressures. Negative thoracic pressure is transmitted to the fluid-filled pericardial space, unlike the situation in constrictive pericarditis, and influences atrial pressures.

7 Inspiratory traction. Described by Boltwood *et al.*, this is the diastolic equalization of PCWP and RA pressures, predominantly during inspiration [8]. It is due to inspiratory traction of the taut pericardium by the diaphragm.

8 Stroke volume is decreased. Cardiac output will fall in absence of tachycardia.

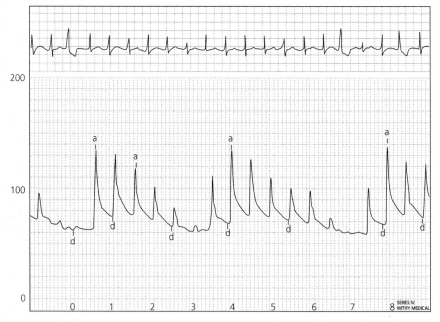

Figure 19.5 Aortic pressure tracing in a patient with tamponade showing pulsus paradoxus. Source: Courtesy of Cardiovillage.com.

Several clinical scenarios can mask the clinical diagnosis of tamponade. In the setting of hypovolemia and suspected tamponade, the typical hemodynamic findings may be masked. Low-pressure effusions equilibrate only with right-sided diastolic pressures and at first only during inspiration. A fluid bolus may elicit classic findings. Severe left ventricular dysfunction may also mask tamponade. In this setting, LV diastolic pressures are higher than RV diastolic pressures and the diagnosis of cardiac tamponade should be dependent on demonstrating elevated pericardial pressures equal to RA pressures. Regional cardiac tamponade can occur when some, but not all, cardiac chambers are compressed by loculated effusions. Typical hemodynamic abnormalities maybe found only in the compressed chambers or zones. In some cases, loculation may also produce classic tamponade, presumably by "stretching" the pericardium.

Tremendous efforts are expended in determining whether a patient is "in tamponade" and, thus, qualifies for emergent therapy. It is important to note that increased pericardial pressure is a clinical spectrum rather than an all-or-none phenomenon. The important questions are "What is the approximate pericardial pressure?" and "What effect is the pericardial fluid having on cardiac output, arterial blood pressure, and intracardiac pressures?" The determination of the need for pericardiocentesis must weigh the risk of the procedure versus these questions and other important considerations, including the rate of accumulation and the potential diagnostic value of obtaining pericardial fluid. The European Society of Cardiology Working Group on Myocardial and Pericardial Diseases has proposed a stepwise scoring system to be used in patients with suspect tamponade. A score ≥6 warrants immediate pericardiocentesis in the absence of contraindications [9].

Physical exam findings

The physical examination can provide clues to cardiac tamponade. Sinus tachy-cardia and hypotension with narrow pulse pressure are hallmarks. The clinician must remain aware that blood pressure may remain normal or even elevated until cardiovascular collapse is imminent.

Pulsus paradoxus, as already described, is an "exaggerated" drop in systolic blood pressure during normal inspiration (not forced inspiration). This is a common finding in moderate to severe tamponade. To measure pulsus paradoxus, the sphygmomanometer should be inflated to suprasystolic pressure, deflating until Korotkoff sounds are initially heard in expiration only. Then, the cuff should be deflated until Korotkoff sounds are heard throughout the respiratory cycle. The difference of these two pressures is the "paradox" (normal pulsus paradox is <10–12 mm Hg). This finding is neither specific nor sensitive and may be seen in other conditions, including constrictive pericarditis, severe obstructive pulmonary disease, restrictive cardiomyopathy, pulmonary embolus, obesity, and right ventricular infarction (Figure 19.6).

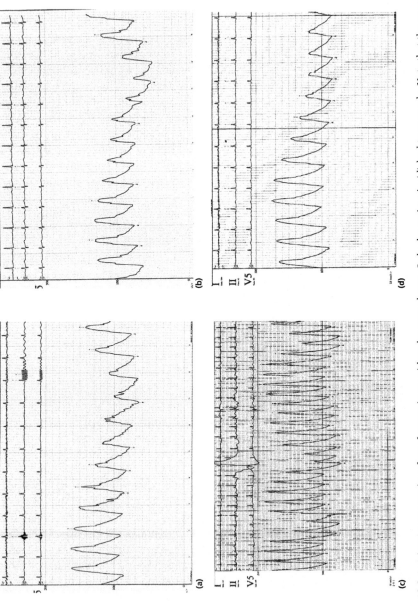

Figure 19.6 Aortic pressure tracings from four patients with pulsus paradoxus. Only the patient in (d) had tamponade. Note that the recording in (c) is made at a speed slower than normal to show several respiratory cycles.

Jugular venous distension is usually present with a preserved X descent. In tamponade, venous waves in the neck are not outward pulsations, but rather X descents are apparent as a collapse from a high standing pressure level. The Y descent is typically not seen.

Kussmaul's sign, which was originally described as an increase in the jugular venous pressure with inspiration but is now commonly used to describe the lack of a decrease in JVP with inspiration, is not classically seen in tamponade without a component of constrictive disease (i.e., effusive–constrictive disease) [10].

Beck's Triad, described in 1935, is a cluster of findings in cardiac tamponade characterized by hypotension, muffled heart sounds, and jugular venous distension.

Pericardial friction rub may be heard in the setting of pericarditis.

Hemodynamics of cardiac tamponade as measured with echocardiography

The echocardiogram is a useful tool in the diagnosis of cardiac tamponade; however, it is important to note that cardiac tamponade is a clinical diagnosis. The echocardiogram is a relatively quick, noninvasive test, which may aid the clinician in delineating the size, morphology, hemodynamic impact, and location of the effusion. Important findings on echocardiography include the following:

- The presence of an effusion is the only sensitive sign in tamponade. The absolute size of the effusion is not as useful in predicting tamponade, with the caveat that larger effusions confer greater risk of tamponade.
- RV diastolic collapse occurring in early diastole is believed to occur only with higher pericardial pressures. However, the lack of RV diastolic collapse does not indicate a nonhemodynamically significant effusion.
- RA collapse occurring in late diastole or early systole is a relatively early sign of increased pericardial pressure.
- Small chamber sizes.
- Inferior vena cava plethora with attenuated respiratory variation.
- Significant changes in inflow across both mitral and tricuspid valves during inspiration. Doppler transmitral flow velocity paradoxus, a reciprocal respiratory variation in transvalvular right- and left-sided flow velocities, has been thought to be a sensitive sign of tamponade. Normally there is no substantial variation in early diastolic filling velocities throughout the respiratory cycle. With cardiac tamponade, there are exaggerated increases in right-sided flow velocities and exaggerated decreases in left-sided flow velocities during inspiration (Figure 19.7). A substantial decrease in Doppler transmitral flow

Note the respiratory variation
in mitral valve flow

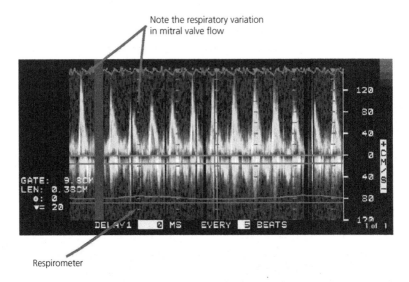

Respirometer

Figure 19.7 Doppler recording of LV inflow with a superimposed respirometer in a patient with tamponade. Note the decrease in mitral valve flow during inspiration.

velocity with inspiration (>25%) may serve as an indicator of flow velocity paradoxus and tamponade physiology.
• Abnormal septal motion. On inspiration the ventricular septum moves toward the left heart, whereas the septum moves toward the right heart on expiration. The filling of the different ventricles is dependent on the position in the respiratory cycle; an echocardiographic demonstration of pulsus paradoxus.

Case study

A 42-year-old female with metastatic lung cancer presented with fatigue and dyspnea on minimal exertion. She was found to have a large pericardial effusion with tamponade physiology on echocardiography (Figure 19.8). On examination, she had muffled heart sounds, JVP at 16 cm, and a blood pressure of 92/68 mm Hg with a heart rate of 112 bpm. Her pulsus paradoxus was 15–18 mm Hg. She was referred for right heart catheterization and pericardiocentesis. The initial RA waveform showed exaggerated X descent with blunted Y descent (Figure 19.9a). The RV waveform showed elevated RV diastolic pressures with minimal change from early diastole to late diastole (Figure 19.9b). Pericardial pressure was elevated and equalized with RA pressure during inspiration (Figure 19.9c). Pericardiocentesis was performed and 600 mL of fluid was removed. The final pericardial pressure was 0 mm Hg. Following pericardiocentesis, Y descents were apparent on RA tracing and evidence of early diastolic filling was also apparent on RV tracing.

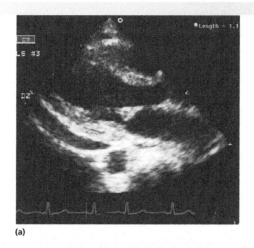

(a)

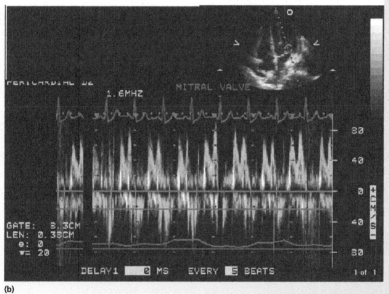

(b)

Figure 19.8 Echocardiographic findings from the patient described in the case study. Panel (a) is a still 2D frame from the parasternal long axis showing a 1.1 cm pericardial effusion. Panel (b) is a Doppler image with the probe at the level of the mitral valve.

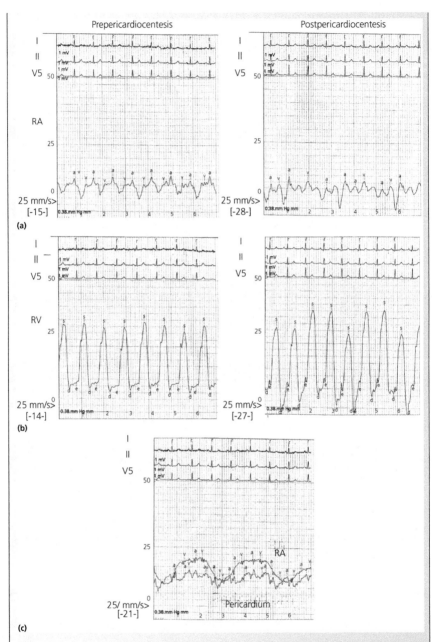

(a)

(b)

(c)

Figure 19.9 Pressure tracings from the patient described in the case study. RA (a) and RV (b) tracings before and after pericardiocentesis. Simultaneous RA and pericardial pressures after the removal of several hundred milliliters of pericardial fluid (c). Note that the scale is not accurate in (c) because the patient is no longer completely supine, but rather the thorax is partially inclined in order to facilitate pericardiocentesis.

References

1 Kern MJ, Aguirre FV. Interpretation of cardiac pathophysiology from pressure waveform analysis: pericardial compressive hemodynamics. Part I. *Cathet Cardiovasc Diagn* 1992;**25**:336–342.
2 Kern MJ, Aguirre FV. Interpretation of cardiac pathophysiology from pressure waveform analysis: pericardial compressive hemodynamics. Part II. *Cathet Cardiovasc Diagn* 1992;**26**:34–40.
3 Kern MJ, Aguirre FV. Interpretation of cardiac pathophysiology from pressure waveform analysis: pericardial compressive hemodynamics. Part III. *Cathet Cardiovasc Diagn* 1992;**26**:152–158.
4 Spodick DH. Acute cardiac tamponade. *N Engl J Med* 2003;**349**:684–690.
5 Reddy PS, Curtiss EI, Uretsky BF. Spectrum of hemodynamic changes in cardiac tamponade. *Am J Cardiol* 1990;**66**:1487–1491.
6 Reddy PS, Curtiss EI, O'Toole JD, Shaver JA. Cardiac tamponade: hemodynamic observations in man. *Circulation* 1978;**58**:265–272.
7 Spodick DH. Pathophysiology of cardiac tamponade. *Chest* 1998;**113**:1372–1378.
8 Boltwood C, Rieders D, Gregory KW. Inspiratory tracking sign in pericardial disease. *Circulation* 1984;**70**(suppl II):103.
9 Ristić AD, Imazio M, Adler Y, *et al.* Triage strategy for urgent management of cardiac tamponade: a position statement of the European Society of Cardiology Working Group on Myocardial and Pericardial Diseases. *Eur Heart J* 2014. Online first, doi: 10.1093/eurheartj/ehu217
10 Bilchick KC, Wise RA. Paradoxical physical findings described by Kussmaul: pulsus paradoxus and Kussmaul's sign. *Lancet* 2002;**359**:1940–1942.

CHAPTER 20

Effusive–constrictive pericarditis

Eric M. Crespo, Sidney C. Smith and George A. Stouffer

Effusive–constrictive pericarditis is an uncommon syndrome characterized by constriction of the heart by the visceral pericardium in the presence of a tense pericardial effusion. In these patients, pericardiocentesis converts the hemodynamics from those typical of tamponade to those of constriction. It is diagnosed when elevated right atrial pressures persist despite reduction of intrapericardial pressures to normal levels by pericardiocentesis. Although first observed in the 1960s [1], it was not well described until the publication of a 13-patient case series by Hancock in 1971 [2]. Since that time there has been a paucity of medical literature on the topic, and it was not until the recent publication of a case series by Sagrista-Sauleda that more complete information about the etiology, incidence, and prognosis of effusive–constrictive pericarditis became known [3].

In their series, Sagrista-Sauleda and colleagues prospectively evaluated 1184 patients presenting to their institution with pericarditis of any type over a 15-year period. Based on their data, the authors estimate that the prevalence of effusive–constrictive pericarditis is approximately 1.3% of all patients with pericarditis and 6.8% of patients with clinical tamponade. Additionally, they found that although effusive–constrictive pericarditis can occur with all types of pericarditis, it is relatively more frequent with radiation-related pericardial disease and less often associated with postsurgical pericarditis. Other studies have shown a relatively higher frequency with tuberculous pericarditis [4]. The etiology and incidence, however, will likely vary between institutions and between different parts of the world based on the most common causes of pericarditis in each location. The majority of patients diagnosed with effusive–constrictive pericarditis will progress to chronic constriction, but a proportion of those with idiopathic disease may have only temporary cardiac constriction and then go on to eventual full resolution [3,5].

Patients tend to have a subacute presentation and are often initially believed to have cardiac tamponade. The true diagnosis can only be made after constrictive physiology persists despite normal pericardial pressures. Thus, continuous monitoring of intracardiac filling pressures during pericardiocentesis is required to arrive at the correct diagnosis.

Hemodynamics of effusive–constrictive pericarditis

The hallmark of effusive–constrictive pericarditis is the persistence of elevated right atrial pressure after intrapericardial pressure has been reduced to normal levels by pericardiocentesis. As in both constrictive pericarditis and cardiac tamponade, the expansion of the cardiac chambers during diastole is limited and there are elevation and equalization of diastolic pressures in the atria and ventricles. Prior to drainage of the effusion, the predominant hemodynamic findings are those of cardiac tamponade with a preserved X descent and an absent or attenuated Y descent on the right atrial pressure tracing. Once the effusion has been drained, constrictive physiology predominates, with return and exaggeration of the Y descent leading to a classic M- or W-shaped configuration of the right atrial pressure waveform. The ventricular pressure tracings demonstrate the square root sign due to rapid ventricular filling in early diastole.

In a study of 68 patients with tuberculous pericarditis, Ntsekhe *et al.* found that 36 patients (53%) had effusive–constrictive physiology as defined by these hemodynamic findings during combined pericardiocentesis and cardiac catheterization: (a) mean pericardial pressure of >8 mm Hg prior to fluid removal; (b) difference between right atrial pressure and intrapericardial pressure of ≤4 mm Hg; (c) mean pericardial pressure of 0 ± 4 mm Hg after pericardiocentesis; and (d) mean right atrial pressure of ≥11 mm Hg or failure to decrease by 50% or more of the pre-pericardiocentesis level [4]. They found that patients with effusive-constrictive pericarditis were younger, had a higher pre-pericardiocentesis right atrial pressure, and higher serum and pericardial fluid levels of interleukin-10.

For detailed descriptions of the hemodynamic principles and findings of constrictive pericarditis and cardiac tamponade, refer to Chapters 18 and 19.

Physical examination

The findings on initial physical examination are similar to those for a patient presenting with cardiac tamponade. Patients will have elevated jugular venous pressure (JVP), and careful examination of the neck veins may reveal a prominent X descent and an absent Y descent. Kussmaul's sign, an increase in central venous pressure with inspiration, may be present and manifest as either increased or unchanged (i.e., failure to decrease) JVP during inspiration. Other sequelae of elevated right heart pressures may be noted, including hepatomegaly, ascites, and peripheral edema. Arterial pulsus paradoxus (inspiratory decrease in systolic pressure by ≥10 mm Hg) may also be noted. Additionally, a pericardial friction rub or pericardial knock may sometimes be auscultated. It should be kept in mind, however, that the sensitivity and specificity of different physical examination findings are not well defined.

Pericardial imaging techniques

A discussion of pericardial imaging can be found in Chapter 18. It is possible that pericardial calcification may be less common among patients with effusive–constrictive pericarditis than it is among those with strictly constrictive disease. In the series by Sagrista-Sauleda and colleagues, none of the patients with effusive–constrictive pericarditis was noted to have pericardial calcification on radiographic examination [3].

Findings on echocardiography

As with the hemodynamic findings during catheterization, the echocardiographic findings will fall somewhere on a spectrum between the findings of cardiac tamponade and those of constriction, depending on whether the effusion has been drained and intrapericardial pressure has normalized. Refer to Chapters 18 and 19 for further discussion of the echocardiographic findings in constrictive pericarditis and cardiac tamponade.

Case study

A 53-year-old previously healthy man presented to the hospital with a complaint of progressive dyspnea on exertion, mild pretibial edema, and pleuritic central chest pain. His symptoms had been progressing over the course of two weeks, and had only become prominent over the last few days. One week prior to the onset of symptoms he had suffered a fall of approximately 8 feet in which he landed directly on his left chest and shoulder. Chest X-ray revealed cardiomegaly, but no pericardial calcification or pulmonary edema. Echocardiogram revealed a large (>2 cm) circumferential pericardial effusion with mild early diastolic collapse of the right ventricle and exaggerated respiratory variation in mitral inflow velocity. Right heart catheterization revealed the findings in Table 20.1.

The persistent elevation in right atrial pressure despite normalization of intrapericardial pressure is consistent with the diagnosis of effusive–constrictive pericarditis. In this case the etiology was felt to be the patient's recent trauma, with bleeding into the pericardium leading to pericardial irritation and inflammation. Despite continued elevation of cardiac filling pressures, the patient's symptoms resolved completely. He was prescribed high-dose ibuprofen and scheduled for outpatient follow-up.

Table 20.1 Findings on right heart catheterization.

	Before pericardiocentesis (mm Hg)	After pericardiocentesis (230 mL of serosanguinous fluid, mm Hg)
Right atrium	17	14
Right ventricular end-diastolic pressure	16	16
Pulmonary capillary wedge pressure	17	14
Pericardial pressure	13	0

References

1 Spodick DH, Kumar S. Subacute constrictive pericarditis with cardiac tamponade. *Dis Chest* 1968;**54**(1):62–66.

2 Hancock EW. Subacute effusive–constrictive pericarditis. *Circulation* 1971;**43**(2):183–192.

3 Sagrista-Sauleda J, Angel J, Sanchez A, Permanyer-Miralda G, Soler-Soler J. Effusive–constrictive pericarditis. *N Engl J Med* 2004;**350**(5):469–475.

4 Ntsekhe M, Matthews K, Syed FF, *et al.* Prevalence, hemodynamics, and cytokine profile of effusive-constrictive pericarditis in patients with tuberculous pericardial effusion. *PloS One* 2013;**8**(10):e77532.

5 Sagrista-Sauleda J, Permanyer-Miralda G, Candell-Riera J, Angel J, Soler-Soler J. Transient cardiac constriction: an unrecognized pattern of evolution in effusive acute idiopathic pericarditis. *Am J Cardiol* 1987;**59**(9):961–966.

PART V
Hemodynamic support

CHAPTER 21

Hemodynamics of intra-aortic balloon counterpulsation

Richard A. Santa-Cruz and George A. Stouffer

History and uses

The idea of using diastolic augmentation to treat left ventricular failure was first proposed in the 1950s. The earliest method involved removing blood from the femoral artery during systole and replacing this volume rapidly during diastole. In the early 1960s an experimental prototype of the intra-aortic balloon pump (IABP) was developed, in which inflation and deflation were triggered by the electrocardiogram (ECG). The initial use of IABP in clinical practice was in 1968. The early devices were 15 French in size and required surgical insertion and removal. Subsequent improvements included a dramatic reduction in size, enabling percutaneous insertion.

Current indications for IABP include cardiogenic shock or left ventricular failure, unstable ischemic syndromes, mechanical complications of acute myocardial infarction, ischemic ventricular arrhythmias, severe mitral regurgitation, stabilization of patients undergoing coronary artery bypass grafting with high-risk anatomy (e.g., severe left main disease), failure to separate a patient from cardiopulmonary bypass, high-risk coronary intervention, or as a bridge to a left ventricular assist device (LVAD) or heart transplantation (Table 21.1). Relative contraindications to IABP usage are listed in Table 21.2.

Description

The IABP consists of a polyurethane balloon placed in the patient's descending aorta and a console that rapidly shuttles a gas, either helium or carbon dioxide, into and out of the balloon. Helium is most commonly used and has the advantage of a lower density and therefore a better rapid diffusion coefficient. Carbon dioxide, on the

Cardiovascular Hemodynamics for the Clinician, Second Edition. Edited by George A. Stouffer.
© 2017 John Wiley & Sons Ltd. Published 2017 by John Wiley & Sons Ltd.

Table 21.1 Indications for IABP.

Complicated acute myocardial infarction
Refractory unstable angina
Cardiogenic shock (including right ventricular failure)
Mechanical complications of acute myocardial infarction or trauma
Severe coronary artery disease with hemodynamic compromise
Left main disease
Support of high-risk coronary interventions
Induction and weaning of cardiopulmonary bypass
Bridge to cardiac transplantation
Refractory ventricular arrhythmias
Noncardiac surgery for high-risk cardiovascular patients
Severe mitral regurgitation

Table 21.2 Relative contraindications for IABP.

Severe peripheral vascular disease
Active hemorrhage
Severe thrombocytopenia
Contraindication to anticoagulation
Moderate to severe aortic insufficiency

other hand, has an increased solubility in blood and thereby reduces the potential consequences of gas embolization following a balloon rupture.

The IABP is placed with one tip below the origin of the left subclavian artery (a useful angiographic marker is the left main stem bronchus). The other tip should be positioned above the renal arteries. It is important to match the appropriate balloon size to patient size, since mismatches can cause either ineffective counterpulsation or possible mechanical trauma to the aorta. In general, a 40 cc balloon size is used, although sizes from 25–50 cc are available.

Hemodynamic effects

An IABP produces hemodynamic effects through the cardiac cycle. During diastole, the IABP inflates, thereby displacing blood from the descending aorta. The balloon deflates immediately before systole, resulting in decreased aortic

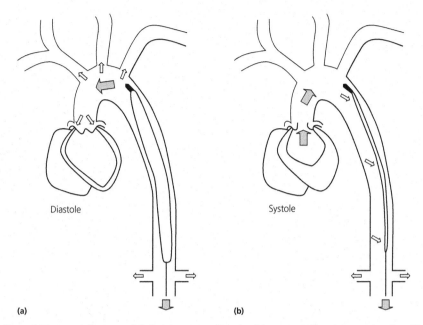

Figure 21.1 IABP inflation and deflation. During diastole, the IABP is inflated, increasing diastolic pressure, thus augmenting flow not only into the coronary arteries but also the great vessels and the renal arteries (a). Just prior to systole, the IABP is deflated, creating a void where the inflated balloon was, thus increasing forward flow into the aorta and to the periphery (b).

Table 21.3 Hemodynamic effects of IABP therapy.

Decreased left ventricular afterload

Decreased aortic SBP

Decreased pulmonary capillary wedge pressure

Decreased LV volume

Decreased LV end-diastolic pressure

Increased coronary blood flow

Increased cardiac output

impedance (Figure 21.1). The primary hemodynamic benefits of IABP treatment are diastolic pressure augmentation and afterload reduction (Table 21.3). Diastolic augmentation can increase coronary perfusion pressure, mean arterial blood pressure, and systemic perfusion, although these effects have not been consistently found in all studies. As shown in Figure 21.2, diastolic pressure augmentation by aortic counterpulsation can be a major support of mean arterial blood pressure in patients with cardiogenic shock. Afterload reduction can decrease left ventricular filling pressures and decrease myocardial oxygen demand. The decrease in

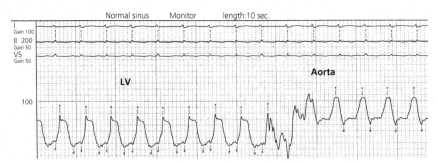

Figure 21.2 Aortic counterpulsation in a patient with cardiogenic shock, left ventricle to aortic pullback. The patient was a 48-year-old male who presented with an extensive anterior–lateral myocardial infarction. An IABP was placed via the left femoral artery. An end-hole catheter was inserted into the left ventricle and pressures were recorded as the catheter was withdrawn into the aorta. Note the decreased left ventricular systolic pressure and increased left ventricular end-diastolic pressure. IABP diastolic augmentation is a major contributor to aortic pressure.

afterload generally results in a decrease in left ventricular end-diastolic pressure (LVEDP) during counterpulsation, with preservation or increase of the left ventricular stroke volume and ejection fraction. Left ventricular work is decreased by a reduction in afterload, which results in lower myocardial oxygen demand. The decrease in systolic pressure is generally less than the increase in diastolic pressure, resulting in an increase in mean arterial blood pressure.

Because an IABP works via diastolic pressure augmentation and afterload reduction, the beneficial effects are dependent on heart rate, cardiac output, and blood pressure. Diastolic augmentation is limited in patients with poor cardiac output independent of how well the IABP is functioning. This is in contradistinction from extracorporeal membrane oxygenation (ECMO) or an LVAD, in which hemodynamic support is generally independent of intrinsic cardiac activity.

Counterpulsation has many metabolic effects on both ischemic and non-ischemic myocardium. In general, aortic counterpulsation results in decreased myocardial metabolic demands. Increased end-organ perfusion is probably an important contributor to the overall improvement in patient status associated with aortic counterpulsation among those with hemodynamic compromise, such as in cardiogenic shock.

There is a surprisingly limited amount of data on the hemodynamic effects of IABP. In a study of 41 patients with cardiogenic shock with acute myocardial infarction randomized to IABP vs. LVAD, the IABP group (n = 20) showed an increase in cardiac power index, from 0.22 (IQR 0.18–0.30) to 0.28 W/m^2 (IQR 0.24–0.36), cardiac output, from 3.0 (2.5–4.0) to 3.3 (2.9–4.3) L/min; and mean arterial pressure, from 64 (57–74) to 67 (62–84) mm Hg; and a decrease in pulmonary capillary wedge pressure, from 27.0 (20.0–30.0) to 21.5 (17.0–26.0) mm Hg. This study found that a percutaneous LVAD (Tandem Heart™,

Cardiac Assist, Pittsburgh, PA, USA) provided more hemodynamic support but resulted in more complications [1].

The IABP Cardiogenic Shock Trial was a prospective, randomized, single-center trial looking at the effects of IABP vs. inotropic therapy (i.e., dobutamine and/or norepinephrine) in 40 patients with acute myocardial infarction complicated by cardiogenic shock, treated by PCI within 12 hours of onset of hemodynamic instability. There was significant improvement in both groups in cardiac output, systemic vascular resistance, and cardiac power output, and no significant differences between the IABP group and the medical-alone group in cardiac output or systemic vascular resistance after 24, 48, 72, or 96 hours [2].

Intra-aortic balloon pump timing

To achieve optimal effects of counterpulsation, inflation and deflation need to be correctly timed to the patient's cardiac cycle. This can be accomplished by using the patient's ECG signal, the patient's arterial waveform, or an intrinsic pump rate. The most common method of triggering the IABP is from the R wave of the patient's ECG signal (Figure 21.3). On identification of the R wave the balloon deflates. Balloon inflation is generally set to start automatically in the middle of the T wave. Tachyarrhythmias, cardiac pacemakers, and poor ECG signals may cause difficulties in obtaining synchronization when the ECG mode is used. In such cases the arterial waveform may be useful for triggering.

For optimal efficacy, the IABP should inflate during early diastole (after the aortic valve closes, which is identified by the dicrotic notch) and deflate just prior to systole (just before the aortic valve opens). IABP inflation and deflation timing, as well as ratio of counterpulsations to cardiac cycles, can be adjusted to optimize performance (Figures 21.4 and 21.5). In general, optimal assistance from the IABP occurs when each cardiac cycle is augmented in a 1:1 ratio. In patients with tachycardia (e.g., rapid atrial fibrillation), a lower assist ratio (1:2 or 1:3) can be used to allow gas delivery to and removal from the balloon.

The most common cause of inadequate balloon counterpulsation is the inaccurate timing of inflation and deflation. Some errors associated with IABP timing will simply result in poor hemodynamic response to IABP, but others are more dangerous for patients with already tenuous cardiovascular situations. Understanding IABP pressure waveforms is critical to use this device properly. The timing errors can be divided into two groups: systolic errors (early and late inflation) and diastolic errors (early and late deflation).

Early inflation
Inflation of the IABP prior to aortic valve closure will increase afterload, since the heart must eject blood against an inflated balloon. This increases myocardial wall stress and LVEDP, thereby increasing LV work, reducing cardiac output, and potentially precipitating early closure of the aortic valve. On the

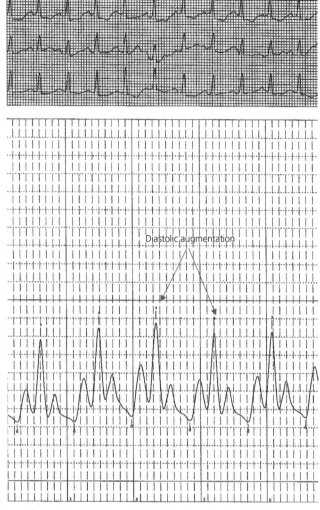

Figure 21.3 IABP set on a 1:2 ratio in a 60-year-old male with cardiogenic shock in the setting of acute myocardial infarction (200 mm Hg scale).

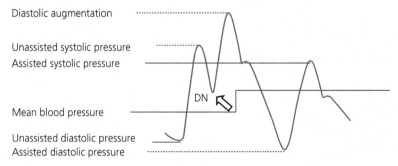

Figure 21.4 Correct IABP timing and hemodynamic effects. Normal timing of the IABP (arrow) with inflation at the dicrotic notch (DN) and good diastolic augmentation, which increases coronary blood flow and increases mean blood pressure. Assisted systolic and end-diastolic pressures are lower than unassisted systolic and end-diastolic pressures.

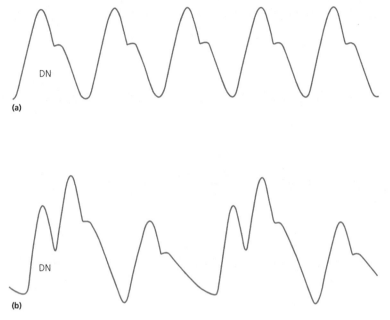

Figure 21.5 Aortic pressure with and without IABP. Aortic pressure waveforms prior to (a) and after initiation of IABP at 1:2 ratio (b). [DN=dicrotic notch]

hemodynamic tracing, a sharp or rapid rise in the augmented pressure will be seen prior to the dicrotic notch (Figure 21.6).

Late inflation

Although probably the least dangerous error, late IABP inflation can preclude the patient from obtaining optimal hemodynamic support. Here, the IABP inflates too long after the aortic valve closes. This delay does not allow for adequate diastolic augmentation. There is a blunting or complete lack of the diastolic augmentation waveform (Figure 21.7). Associated with this is a lack of end-diastolic pressure decrease (afterload reduction) and no increase in diastolic perfusion pressure.

Early deflation

Early deflation, similar to late inflation, is not a particularly dangerous situation, although the patient will not receive optimal balloon counterpulsation. The hemodynamic tracing reveals a normal diastolic augmentation, but then a long-drawn-out U-shaped wave prior to the assisted systolic waveform (Figure 21.8). Notice that there is inadequate preload reduction and therefore no change in assisted and unassisted systolic pressure. Simply prolonging the balloon inflation will quickly improve the hemodynamic support that the balloon pump can provide.

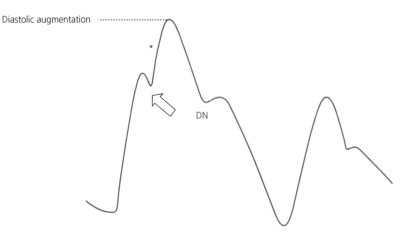

Figure 21.6 Incorrect IABP timing—early inflation. Aortic pressure waveform demonstrating early inflation of the IABP (arrow) prior to the dicrotic notch (DN) and prior to the closure of the aortic valve. There is a rapid rise in augmented diastolic pressure (*) with the aortic valve still open, which causes a dramatic increase in afterload and reduces cardiac output.

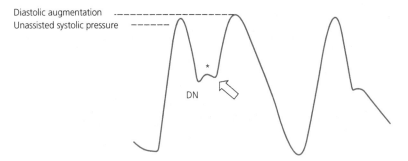

Figure 21.7 Incorrect IABP timing—late inflation. Aortic pressure waveform demonstrating late inflation of the IABP. The notable hemodynamic changes are the clearly visible dicrotic notch (DN) with the IABP inflation following (arrow). There is a prolonged dip or U wave (*), then a blunted or decreased diastolic augmentation.

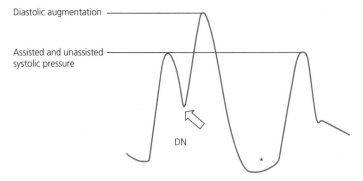

Figure 21.8 Incorrect IABP timing—early deflation. Aortic pressure waveform demonstrating early deflation of the IABP. Early deflation of the IABP in diastole does not affect the diastolic augmentation, but does prevent optimal end-diastolic pressure decrease. This is evident by a prolonged dip and U wave (*) post augmentation. There is no reduction in assisted systolic pressure, which is equal to the unassisted systolic pressure, representing a lack of afterload reduction. Large arrow denotes beginning of IABP inflation.

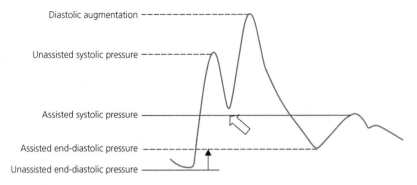

Figure 21.9 Incorrect IABP timing—late deflation. Aortic pressure waveform demonstrating late deflation of the IABP. Late deflation of the IABP in diastole causes a dramatic increase in afterload, since systole begins with higher intra-aortic pressure. This causes late opening of the aortic valve and severely reduces the cardiac output. The pressure waveform reveals an assisted end-diastolic pressure that is higher than the unassisted end-diastolic pressure and a drastically reduced assisted systolic pressure. Large arrow denotes beginning of IABP inflation.

Late deflation

Late IABP deflation is potentially the most critical timing error. If the balloon remains inflated when the left ventricle enters systole, the left ventricle is forced to contract against the inflated balloon. The result can be acute hypotension and cardiac arrest. The hemodynamic tracing reveals a long inflation time with an elevated end-diastolic pressure and a severely reduced assisted systolic pressure (Figure 21.9).

Conclusion

The IABP is a widely used device in the management of patients suffering from the ill effects of acute and chronic cardiovascular disease. Understanding the characteristic hemodynamic tracings of balloon counterpulsation is critical for proper functioning and ensuring the maximal therapeutic benefit. In turn, recognizing the possible complications and pitfalls of IABP timing is crucial to minimizing potential adverse effects.

Since IABP is widely used, it is surprising that there are so few data demonstrating clinical efficacy. Studies in high-risk PCI, acute MI complicated by cardiogenic shock, and acute MI without cardiogenic shock have shown no benefit to IABP use [3,4].

Review of IABP tracings

Match the tracing with the diagnosis. All tracings are taken with the IABP on a 1:2 ratio.
a Accurate timing
b Early balloon inflation
c Early balloon deflation
d Late balloon inflation
e Late balloon deflation

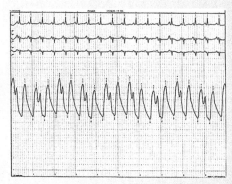

Tracing 1

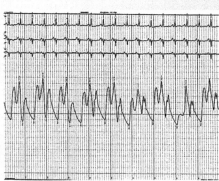

Tracing 2

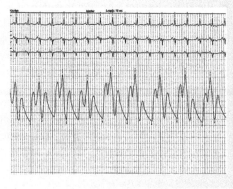

Tracing 3

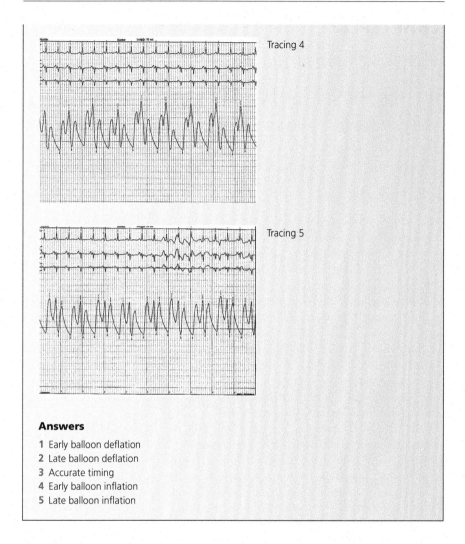

Tracing 4

Tracing 5

Answers

1 Early balloon deflation
2 Late balloon deflation
3 Accurate timing
4 Early balloon inflation
5 Late balloon inflation

References

1 Thiele H, Sick P, Boudriot E. *et al.* Randomized comparison of intra-aortic balloon support with a percutaneous left ventricular assist device in patients with revascularized acute myocardial infarction complicated by cardiogenic shock. *Eur Heart J* 2005;**26**(13):1276–1283.
2 Prondzinsky R, Unverzagt S, Russ M, *et al.* Hemodynamic effects of intra-aortic balloon counterpulsation in patients with acute myocardial infarction complicated by cardiogenic shock: the prospective, randomized IABP shock trial. *Shock* 2012;**37**(4):378–384.
3 Perera D, Lumley M, Pijls N, Patel MR. Intra-aortic balloon pump trials questions, answers, and unresolved issues. *Circ Cardiovasc Interv* 2013;**6**(3):317–321.
4 Ahmad Y, Sen S, Shun-Shin MJ, *et al.* Intra-aortic balloon pump therapy for acute myocardial infarction: a meta-analysis. *JAMA Intern Med* 2015;**175**(6):931–939.

CHAPTER 22

Hemodynamics of left ventricular assist device implantation

Brett C. Sheridan and Jason N. Katz

The modern history of left ventricular assist devices (LVAD) dates back to the late 1970s and early 1980s with the development of the Jarvik artificial heart. In 1982, surgeons at the University of Utah implanted the Jarvik 7 prototype (Figure 22.1) in a patient named Barney Clark, who ultimately survived 112 days on mechanical support [1]. At the same time, Dr. Norman Shumway and his group at Stanford University were improving the surgical technique for cardiac transplantation, and found durable success thanks in large part to the pharmacologic discovery of inducible immune tolerance. Research and development resources were concentrated on improving on the early promise of heart transplantation as the primary strategy for treating end-stage heart failure, given its biologic symmetry compared to the Frankensteinian mechanical support alternatives. This slowed the evolution of mechanical support technologies throughout the 1980s and into the 1990s.

The conventional wisdom at the time was that heart replacement therapy would require two pumps to support both the left and right ventricular chambers, and this concept created additional barriers to the maturation of mechanical circulatory support (MCS) as a field. A turning point came in 2001 with the publication of the Randomized Evaluation of Mechanical Assistance for the Treatment of Congestive Heart Failure (REMATCH) trial [2]. This pivotal study was the first to demonstrate a durable advantage of LVAD therapy for transplant-ineligible patients with advanced heart failure. With a pneumatically driven pulsatile left ventricular support system (Figure 22.1; HeartMate XVE, Thoratec Corp., Pleasanton, CA, USA), investigators showed a nearly 50% reduction in all-cause mortality compared to optimal medical management alone. These results validated two critical concepts: (a) that univentricular (i.e., left-sided) support could work in advanced, biventricular heart failure; and (b) that MCS could improve outcomes versus medical therapy for individuals with extremely advanced heart failure.

Cardiovascular Hemodynamics for the Clinician, Second Edition. Edited by George A. Stouffer.
© 2017 John Wiley & Sons Ltd. Published 2017 by John Wiley & Sons Ltd.

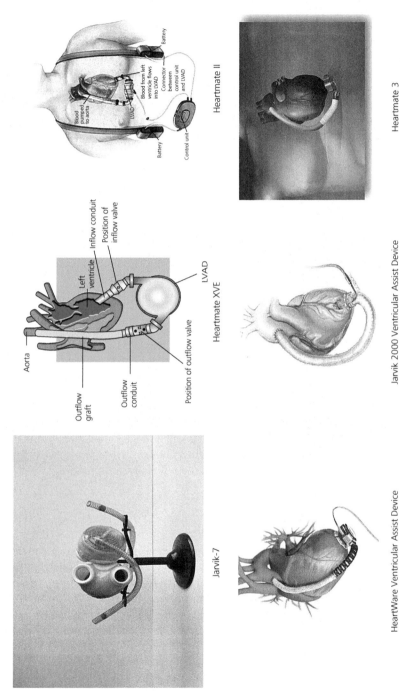

Jarvik-7

Heartmate XVE

Heartmate II

Heartmate 3

HeartWare Ventricular Assist Device

Jarvik 2000 Ventricular Assist Device

Figure 22.1 Different types of mechanical cardiac support devices.

Although the utilization of LVAD therapy slowly increased following REMATCH, it became apparent that the early pulsatile devices (e.g., HeartMate XVE; Novacor, World Heart Corp., CA, USA) were imperfect solutions to the heart failure epidemic. Limitations of these first-generation LVAD included their large size and limited durability. Many of these barriers were addressed with the creation of second-generation, axial-flow pumps (Figure 22.1; HeartMate II, Thoratec Corp., CA, USA). Results from a multicenter trial of 133 nonrandomized patients receiving the HeartMate II device as a bridge to transplantation, published in 2007 [3], demonstrated that patients could be successfully stabilized until cardiac transplantation with the use of a continuous-flow LVAD. In addition, the HeartMate II device was found to be easier to implant, more durable, and had fewer complications that its pulsatile predecessors. The HeartMate II was also tested as an alternative to the first-generation HeartMate XVE in a transplant-ineligible heart failure population. Although both devices improved quality of life, the axial-flow HeartMate II device allowed for greater survival free from stroke, with less risk of device failure [4].

With validation of LVAD therapy as both a bridge to transplantation and a destination-therapy option, other industry participants began to enter the MCS space. Currently, the HeartWare ventricular assist device (HVAD) and Jarvik 2000 ventricular assist device are being studied in a variety of heart failure groups, while the St. Jude Corporation has embarked on a randomized controlled trial of its third-generation, magnetically levitated, centrifugal-flow HeartMate 3 device (Figure 22.1).

Predictably, the utilization of LVAD has increased at a remarkable rate since about 2008, and continues to accelerate thanks in large part to rapidly evolving technology, increasing operator experience (with improved outcomes), decreasing donor organ availability, and a burgeoning population of aging heart failure patients. To better understand patient eligibility, appropriate timing of implantation, and the management of LVAD-supported individuals in both the acute and chronic post-operative settings, it is critical to understand their hemodynamic profiles.

Initial evaluation

There are multiple factors that should be considered when assessing a patient's eligibility for LVAD. It is critical to evaluate not only their expected tolerability of the initial operative insult, but also the likelihood that the patient will reap durable benefits from mechanical support. Those individuals most likely to thrive with univentricular support include those with pre-operative hemodynamics most suggestive of pure left-sided cardiac dysfunction. On the other hand, individuals with isolated right-sided heart failure, or those with biventricular failure in whom right ventricular dysfunction is not modifiable, are poor candidates for LVAD therapy and should not undergo device implantation. The following are some hemodynamic examples to guide operative assessment.

Left-sided heart failure

The ideal LVAD patient has predominantly advanced left ventricular dysfunction. These individuals will have elevated left-sided cardiac filling pressures, and often secondarily increased right-sided filling pressures (Table 22.1). As stroke volume diminishes, mean systemic perfusion (mean arterial pressure, MAP) will decrease as well. In addition, mixed venous oxygen saturation (SVO_2) will be low. If, on the other hand, left-sided filling pressures are not found to be elevated, it can be surmised that the LVAD will be unlikely to provide incremental left ventricular unloading, and hence device implantation would result in little benefit at the expense of increased complication.

Right-sided heart failure

While right ventricular function does not have to be normal for LVAD support, the right ventricle does have to be strong enough to deliver blood across the usually low-pressure, low-resistance pulmonary arterial circulation to the left heart. For those with either pure right-sided heart failure (with no left ventricular failure) or biventricular failure and unmodifiable right ventricular dysfunction, suboptimal

Table 22.1 Hemodynamic parameters of ventricular failure and VAD complications.

Condition	RA	PAP	PCWP	MAP	SVO_2
LV failure	↑	↑	↑	↓	↓
RV failure	↑ or ↓	↑ or ↓	↓	↓	↓
Hypovolemia	↓	↓	↓	↓	↓
Hypertension	↔	↑	↑	↑	↔
Tamponade	↑	↑	↑	↓	↓
Device failure	↑	↑	↑	↓	↓
LVAD thrombosis	↑	↑	↑	↓	↓
Aortic insufficiency	↔	↑	↑	↓	↓

left-sided preload will lead to device complications if LVAD implantation is pursued (Table 22.1). While it can be challenging to define the severity of right ventricular failure, those most likely to fail left-sided, univentricular support include those with markedly elevated central venous pressures (e.g., CVP ≥20 mm Hg) and those with narrow gradients between the CVP and the PCWP (e.g., PCWP – CVP <5 mm Hg or CVP/PCWP ≥0.8). In addition, the Right Ventricular Stroke Work Index [RVSWI = (meanPAP – meanRAP) × HR/CI] is often calculated in the pre-LVAD setting. For those with an RVSWI less than approximately 300 mm Hg, the risk of complications after LVAD implantation goes up considerably [5].

Early post-implantation period

After LVAD implantation, the time course of hemodynamic stabilization and homeostasis of end-organ perfusion is usually longer than the typical cardiac surgical case. A myriad of confounding variables contribute to this observation, but one factor that always generates discussion is the alteration in the arterial wave form post implant. Patients supported with continuous-flow (CF) ventricular support pumps persistently demonstrate pulsatility even with complete closure of the aortic valve (Figure 22.2). This pulsatility is explained by the physics of wave generation. The right ventricle and even the unloaded left ventricle continue to beat, creating a wave that varies in height depending on preload conditions and the intrinsic contractility of the left ventricle. Once created, this wave is continuously transmitted through the column of fluid present within the pump and to the systemic aortic circulation, albeit in a muted fashion.

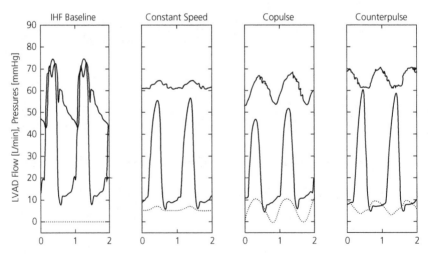

Figure 22.2 LV pressure, aortic pressure, and cardiac output in advanced systolic heart failure and with various types of mechanical support.

The majority of patients are weaned from cardiopulmonary bypass with the simultaneous support of parenteral vasoactive agents. These medications are then slowly withdrawn with invasive hemodynamic guidance in the intensive care setting. Several potential complications must be identified quickly and immediately rectified in order to avoid additional patient or device complications. Of note is that echocardiographic evaluation of the heart and LVAD, either by transthoracic or transesophageal modalities, proves complementary to invasive monitoring of hemodynamics in a perturbed state. The most frequently encountered of these clinical situations are hypovolemia, right ventricular failure, hypertension, tamponade, and device failure.

Hypovolemia

Volume loss is common during the perioperative period, and occurs secondary to hemodilution (as seen with cardiopulmonary bypass), bleeding, and third-spacing. When identified, rapid volume resuscitation and/or transfusion of blood products are mandatory. In addition, the cause of volume loss should be identified and corrected where appropriate. From an LVAD perspective, hypovolemia will often result in diminished pump flows and reduced power consumption, along with decreased blood pulsatility within the device (Figure 22.3a).

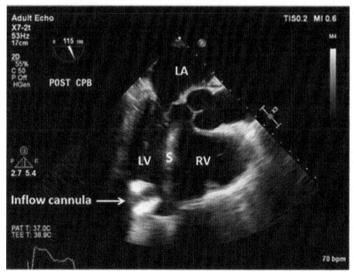

Hypovolemia and a suction event

(a)

Figure 22.3 TEE findings in patients with hemodynamic changes after VAD implantation. (a) Hypovolemia and suction event. 2D TEE mid-esophageal long-axis view showing a suction event due to high pump speed relative to volume. The inflow cannula turned and faced the interventricular septum.

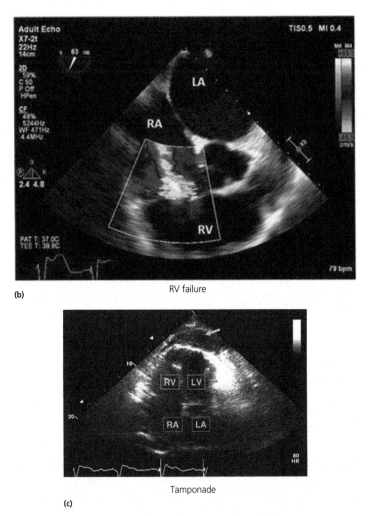

(b)   RV failure

(c)   Tamponade

Figure 22.3 (Continued) (b) RV failure. 2D mid-esophageal RV inflow–outflow view with color flow Doppler demonstrating moderate to severe tricuspid regurgitation (TR). (c) A localized apical thrombus resulting in tamponade. Post left ventricular assist device implantation there was hemodynamic compromise. An apical thrombus (arrow) compressing the left ventricular (LV) cavity resulted in cardiac tamponade. Surgical removal of the thrombus resulted in restoration of normal hemodynamics. [LA = left atrium; LV = left ventricle; RA = right atrium; RV = right ventricle; S = interventricular septum; TEE = transesophageal echocardiography.]

Right ventricular failure

It is critical to monitor for right ventricular failure, whether induced by elevated pulmonary vascular resistance, volume overload, or inadequate inotropic support. The short- and longer-term mortality of patients after durable LVAD implantation increase considerably if mechanical right ventricular support (i.e., RVAD placement) is necessary [6]. In addition to the hemodynamic changes outlined in Table 22.1, there will often be declining LVAD flows, reduced power consumption, and decreasing device pulsatility in the setting of progressive RV failure (Figure 22.3b).

Hypertension

The majority of contemporary LVAD pumps are highly sensitive to increasing afterload. As a result, marked systemic hypertension can result in decreased device flow and hence less robust left ventricular unloading. If LVAD flows diminish due to acute hypertension, pharmacologic vasodilator therapy is often needed as right ventricular inotropic support is weaned.

Cardiac tamponade

When present, cardiac tamponade can result hemodynamically in a rise and equalization of diastolic pressures. If not treated rapidly, hypotension and end-organ dysfunction often ensue. One of the earliest signs of tamponade in an LVAD patient is the near abrupt cessation of urination due to impaired renal perfusion and cardiorenal perturbations. In addition to the classic invasive hemo-dynamic changes, LVAD flows will decrease in the setting of cardiac tamponade (Figure 22.3c and Table 22.1).

Pump failure

The hemodynamic picture of a patient with LVAD failure will look similar to that of a patient with cardiogenic shock and left ventricular dysfunction. The failing LVAD will be unable to unload the congested left heart adequately. Depending on the cause of device malfunction, LVAD interrogation may show elevated or normal power consumption, elevated or low estimated device flows, and diminished pulsatility.

The chronic LVAD patient

After an LVAD patient leaves the hospital following their implant, careful outpatient follow-up is still necessary. These individuals remain susceptible to complications secondary to both patient factors and to abnormal patient–device interactions. The following are examples of conditions that may arise during chronic LVAD support.

Hypovolemia

Like in the early postoperative period, LVAD patients are at risk for hypovolemia during the chronic phase of their care. This is particularly true when robust LVAD unloading leads to enhanced renal perfusion and frequent urination. It is also a common complication of excessive diuretic therapy. As already discussed, hypovolemia can result in decreased LVAD flows, diminished pulsatility, and an associated decrease in power consumption. If the left ventricular preload is low enough, suction events—in which the LVAD inflow cannula directly contacts the opposing interventricular septum—may occur.

Late right ventricular failure

Even if LVAD patients tolerate device implantation without requiring right ventricular mechanical support, they can occasionally develop late right ventricular dysfunction. These individuals will often present with right heart failure symptoms, including hepatic congestion, ascites, peripheral edema, fatigue, and end-organ dysfunction. Progressive right heart failure can also lead to impaired left ventricular filling, diminished LVAD flows, suction events, and electrical instability (in the form of ventricular arrhythmias).

LVAD thrombosis

Increasing attention has recently focused on the risk of device thrombosis [7]. This can lead to LVAD failure, hemolysis and its downstream sequelae, cerebro-vascular events, and even death. If a clot forms directly on the pump rotor, power consumption will increase and calculated flows will often rise (then ultimately decline with subsequent pump failure). As device malfunction ensues, invasive hemodynamics will reflect cardiac decompensation and a state of volume overload (Table 22.1).

Aortic valve insufficiency

In some patients, destruction and invagination of the aortic valve leaflets can result from chronic LVAD unloading. This aortic valvopathy may lead to progressive aortic regurgitation. The presence of progressive aortic insufficiency may be suggested by an LVAD interrogation that reveals escalating power, rising flows, and diminishing device pulsatility (Table 22.1).

Conclusion

Hemodynamic assessment will continue to be a pivotal tool for guiding appropriate patient selection, assisting with patient management, and monitoring for potential sequelae of LVAD therapy. Combining invasive hemodynamic data with LVAD interrogation and selected imaging studies can help to ensure that patients continue to derive the greatest benefit possible from durable mechanical support.

References

1 DeVries WC, Anderson JL, Joyce LD, *et al.* Clinical use of the total artificial heart. *N Engl J Med* 1984;**310**:273–278.
2 Rose EA, Gelijns AC, Moskowitz AJ, *et al.* Long-term use of a left ventricular assist device for end-stage heart failure. *N Engl J Med* 2001;**345**:1435–1443.

3 Miller LW, Pagani FD, Russell SD, *et al.* Use of a continuous-flow device in patients awaiting heart transplantation. *N Engl J Med* 2007;**357**:885–896.

4 Slaughter MS, Rogers JG, Milano CA, *et al.* Advanced heart failure treated with continuous-flow left ventricular assist device. *N Engl J Med* 2009;**361**:2241–2251.

5 Ochiai Y, McCarthy PM, Smedira NG, *et al.* Predictors of severe right ventricular failure after implantable left ventricular assist device insertion: analysis of 245 patients. *Circulation* 2002;**106**(suppl I):I198–I202.

6 Lazar JF, Swartz MF, Schiralli MP, *et al.* Survival after left ventricular assist device with and without temporary right ventricular support. *Ann Thorac Surg* 2013;**96**:2155–2159.

7 Starling RC, Moazami N, Silvestry SC, *et al.* Unexpected abrupt increase in left ventricular assist device thrombosis. *N Engl J Med* 2014;**370**:33–40.

PART VI
Coronary hemodynamics

CHAPTER 23

Coronary hemodynamics

David P. McLaughlin, Samuel S. Wu and George A. Stouffer

Basic principles of coronary blood flow

The coronary arteries are the first vessels to branch off the aorta and through them the heart receives about 5% of the cardiac output when the body is at rest, or 250 mL/min.

The heart has the highest oxygen (O_2) consumption per tissue mass of all human organs. Under basal conditions, myocardium extracts approximately 75% of delivered oxygen (the myocardium has a basal metabolic requirement that is approximately 15–20 times that of resting skeletal muscle and approximately equal to that of skeletal muscle under severe acidotic conditions). The heart has the highest arterial–venous difference in O_2 concentration of any major organ (10–13 mL/100 mL) and the oxygen saturation in the coronary sinus is one of the lowest in the body (Figure 23.1).

Determinants of myocardial oxygen demands include preload, afterload, heart rate, contractility, and basal metabolic rate. Other than basal metabolic rate, these are factors that influence stroke volume. Systolic wall tension uses approximately 30% of myocardial oxygen demand. Wall tension itself is affected by intraventricular pressure, afterload, end-diastolic volume, and myocardial wall thickness.

Because there is little room for increased oxygen extraction and the heart has minimal capacity for anaerobic metabolism, increased metabolic demands of the heart are met primarily via increases in coronary blood flow (i.e., flow is tightly coupled to oxygen demand). In the absence of obstructive epicardial coronary artery disease, coronary blood flow is primarily controlled by changes in resistance in the small arteries and arterioles. Resistance within the microvessels plays an important role in myocardial perfusion in general and in regional and transmural distribution.

Cardiovascular Hemodynamics for the Clinician, Second Edition. Edited by George A. Stouffer.
© 2017 John Wiley & Sons Ltd. Published 2017 by John Wiley & Sons Ltd.

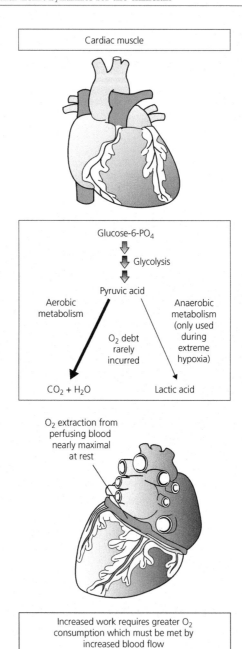

Figure 23.1 Oxygen extraction in cardiac muscle.

Camici and Crea describe a three-compartment system in the coronary circulation [1]. The proximal compartment includes the large epicardial coronary arteries, which offer little resistance to coronary blood flow in the absence of obstructive disease. The intermediate compartment includes prearterioles, which offer some resistance to flow and there is a measureable pressure drop along their length. The specific function of the prearterioles is to maintain pressure at the origin of arterioles within a narrow range despite changes in perfusion pressure or flow (important in autoregulation). The more distal compartment includes intramural arterioles and there is a considerable drop in pressure. The function of the distal compartment is to match myocardial blood supply and oxygen consumption.

For the purpose of understanding clinical applications of physiologic testing of coronary blood flow, the intermediate and distal compartments can be lumped together (labeled the microvasculature), creating a two-component model. Normal epicardial coronary arteries provide little if any resistance to myocardial blood flow even at maximal flow, and are commonly referred to as conductance vessels. In contrast, the microcirculation provides the majority of resistance to flow under normal resting conditions. This chapter will not discuss microvascular dysfunction, but it is important to keep in mind that microvasculature dysfunction has been reported in patients with prior myocardial infarction and coronary artery disease risk factors [2].

Five important principles of coronary physiology

1 Myocardial cell contraction and relaxation are aerobic, O_2-requiring processes.
2 Oxygen extraction in the coronary bed is near maximal in the baseline state (80% versus 30–40% in skeletal muscle); therefore to increase O_2 delivery, flow must increase.
3 In the normal heart, the major resistance to coronary flow occurs in the microvasculature (small, distal arterioles). There is little resistance to flow in the visible epicardial arteries.
4 The primary mechanism to increase coronary flow is via a decrease in microvascular resistance (regulated by metabolic demands).
5 The presence of hemodynamically significant epicardial disease reduces microvasculature resistance at baseline so that coronary blood flow is maintained. This limits the ability of the myocardium to increase flow in response to increased demand.

Regulation of coronary blood flow

Coronary blood flow can increase two- to fivefold in the normal heart. In one study of adult patients with angiographically normal vessels and coronary artery disease risk factors, coronary blood flow increased by 2.7 ± 0.6 times with maximal coronary vasodilation [3]. The ratio of maximal coronary flow to resting coronary blood flow is labeled coronary flow reserve (CFR). Maximal coronary blood flow can be achieved experimentally using any one of three different mechanisms. Reactive hyperemic flow is that flow that occurs following a transient period of flow cessation. Metabolites of ischemia accumulate during interruption of flow and vasodilate the microcirculation. When flow is reestablished, the resistance of the microcirculation is markedly diminished and coronary blood flow increases. Maximal coronary blood flow can also be achieved using exercise or another physiologic stimulus to increase flow. Lastly, maximal coronary flow can be achieved by intracoronary administration of potent microcirculation vasodilators such as adenosine.

Coronary blood flow is primarily controlled by release of local metabolites such as adenosine or nitric oxide. Hypoxia is a more potent coronary vasodilator than either hypercapnea or acidosis. Neural influences on coronary blood flow are relatively minor. Sympathetic activation to the heart results in transient vasoconstriction, followed by coronary vasodilation due to increased metabolic activity. Parasympathetic stimulation of the heart directly stimulates coronary vasodilation, but this effect is modest.

Coronary blood flow is unique in that it primarily occurs during diastole because of systolic compression of myocardial arteriolars and capillaries by the contracting myocardium. Systolic compressional forces are much greater in the subendocardial layers than in the epicardial arteries. Flow in the left coronary artery has a greater diastolic predominance than the right coronary artery because the compressive forces of the right ventricle (underlying a portion of the right coronary artery) are less than those of the left ventricle. At least 85% of coronary flow in the left anterior descending occurs in diastole, whereas the right coronary artery blood flow is more or less equal in systole and diastole. The predominance of flow during diastole exacerbates myocardial ischemia during tachycardia. With increased heart rates, oxygen supply is reduced (because diastole is shortened) while demand increases.

The heart has the ability to maintain coronary blood flow in the presence of varying perfusion pressures (termed autoregulation). Autoregulation maintains consistent coronary flow over a range of perfusion pressures from 60 to 150 mm Hg (Figure 23.2), although there is evidence that autoregulation is exhausted at a higher pressure (approximately 70 mm Hg) in patients with left ventricular hypertrophy [4]. In the setting of maximum vasodilation of coronary resistance vessels, coronary blood flow is no longer autoregulated and varies linearly with perfusion pressure. One example of an autoregulatory mechanism is the Bayliss phenomenon in which increased perfusion pressure causes reflex vasoconstriction. The ability of autoregulation to maintain flow when perfusion pressures are decreased is especially important in the presence of epicardial coronary stenoses.

The garden hose analogy

One way to understand coronary blood flow is to think of the coronary circulation as a garden hose with a nozzle on the end. Under regular conditions, the nozzle is used to adjust flow through the hose, being opened further when more flow is needed and partially closed when less flow is needed. If someone is stepping on the hose, the nozzle has to be opened further to maintain basal flow and it is difficult to increase flow further since the nozzle is already wide open. The more resistance to flow from the person stepping on the hose, the less control you have at the nozzle. The impact of someone stepping on a garden hose is similar to the presence of a stenosis in a coronary artery.

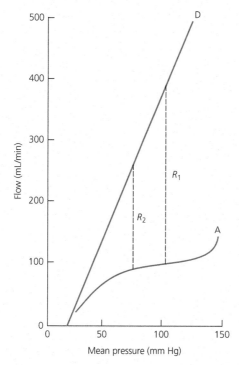

Figure 23.2 Coronary autoregulation. Source: Polese 1991 [4]. Reproduced with permission of Wolters Kluwer.

Clinical measurement of coronary hemodynamics in the cardiac catheterization laboratory: Doppler and pressure wires

There are several ways to measure coronary blood flow directly, but these are generally difficult, time consuming, and unable to measure rapid changes in coronary flow. More commonly, angioplasty wires with Doppler probes or pressure transducers are used to make clinical decisions and to study coronary physiology. The Doppler wire (an angioplasty wire with a Doppler transducer placed near the tip) is used to measure coronary flow velocity at rest and then under conditions of maximal flow. If coronary artery diameter at the location of the probe is assumed to be constant, then the ratio of velocities is the same as CFR. This technique has largely been supplanted in clinical medicine by use of the pressure wire (an angioplasty wire with a pressure transducer near the tip), which measures blood pressure distal to a stenosis. By comparing distal perfusion pressure with aortic pressure under conditions of maximal flow, fractional flow reserve (FFR) can be calculated (more detail on the derivation of FFR is included in Chapter 24).

Measurement of coronary blood flow

1 *Clearance methods.* These techniques involve introducing an inert gas (usually nitrous oxide) into the circulation via the lungs and following the progressive saturation of cardiac tissue. The increases in the systemic arterial and coronary sinus concentrations of indicator are measured over the time until arteriovenous difference reaches zero. The reciprocal of this time reflects the blood flow in milliliters per minute per 100 grams of tissue.

2 *Thermodilution.* As originally implemented in the coronary circulation, this technique requires placement of a catheter into the coronary sinus and then a continuous infusion of cold saline through a lumen near the tip at a constant rate. The temperature of the blood at a site several centimeters back from the tip of the catheter is measured with a thermistor. The method uses the form of the Fick equation dealing with continuous (rather than bolus) infusion of indicator.

3 *Flowmeter techniques.* Electromagnetic and Doppler flowmeters have been used at surgery, where they are best suited for measurement of the flow in vein grafts. The native coronary vessels are never dissected for the sole purpose of placing a flowmeter.

4 *Doppler wire.* See text for further description.

5 *Fractional flow reserve wire.* Pressures proximal and distal to a stenosis are measured as a surrogate for flow.

Doppler wire and coronary flow reserve

The physiologic principle underlying the use of CFR is that clinically significant atherosclerosis will impair coronary blood flow responses during hyperemic stresses. Coronary blood flow under resting conditions is generally 15–20% of maximal blood flow in patients with normal coronary arteries and is not altered by gender or age. As atherosclerosis progresses, maximal coronary blood flow is initially reduced, followed in the severe stages by a reduction in resting coronary blood flow. CFR, the ratio of maximal blood flow to basal blood flow, will decrease with progressive obstruction of the lumen of an epicardial coronary artery by atherosclerosis.

In humans, CFR was originally measured with probes and then subsequently with a pulsed Doppler catheter placed during cardiac surgery. There were problems with widespread use of both these techniques, as epicardial coronary artery probes were limited to patients undergoing surgery and the size of the Doppler catheter prevented placement distal to coronary stenoses. Both of these problems were overcome with the development of an 0.014 inch guidewire with a 12 MHz piezoelectric transducer mounted on its tip. To determine CFR, these wires are placed in the coronary artery of interest distal to the lesion and phasic

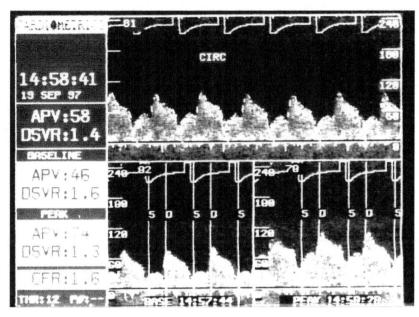

Figure 23.3 Measurement of CFR in the left circumflex with a Doppler FloWire following the administration of adenosine. The top window represents a real-time measurement of coronary velocity. The bottom left window is a "baseline" measurement and the bottom right window is velocity as measured after administration of adenosine. [APV = time-averaged distal peak velocity; CFR = coronary flow reserve; D = diastole; DSVR = diastolic/systolic flow–velocity ratio; S = systole.]

spectral blood flow velocity is measured (Figure 23.3). It is assumed that there are minimal changes in coronary diameter, thus enabling velocity to be used in place of flow (flow = velocity × area). Measurements of blood velocity under basal conditions are taken and then the patient is given a hyperemic stimulus, velocity is remeasured, and CFR is calculated. Adenosine is commonly used to induce hyperemia, since it causes less hemodynamic and ECG changes than papaverine [5].

Although the Doppler wire has great theoretical advantages, it is not widely used because of several important limitations. First, conditions other than atherosclerosis can affect CFR. These include factors that raise basal coronary blood flow (e.g., fever, hypoxia, tachycardia, anemia, or ventricular hypertrophy) and factors that impair vasodilatory responses of the microvasculature (e.g., ventricular hypertrophy or diabetes mellitus). Second, accurate measurements are dependent on correct positioning of the Doppler flow wire. The transducer should be pointing away from the vessel wall and into the flow stream to avoid vessel wall artifacts. Gray scale signal amplitude and peak velocity can be used as indicators of proper positioning. Third, there is a lack of consensus on what value of CFR is consistent with a hemodynamically significant lesion. In various clinical studies, CFR cutoff values between 1.6 and 2.5 were used to determine ischemia-causing lesions.

Since CFR cannot discriminate between epicardial lesions and microvascular dysfunction, the concept of "relative CFR" (rCFR) was developed. This approach requires that CFR be measured in a coronary artery without epicardial disease in order to interpret the value of CFR in an artery with epicardial disease. If CFR is abnormal in the artery without disease, this result implies an impaired microvasculature. The use of rCFR has several caveats, including the requirement for a vessel without significant epicardial disease and the assumption that microvasculature function is consistent across different vascular beds (an obvious problem in the case of prior myocardial infarction).

Pressure wire and fractional flow reserve

The development of a pressure transducer mounted on an angioplasty guidewire allows measurement of the pressure distal to a coronary stenosis. The concept of using pressure gradient as a technique to assess stenosis severity has existed since the early days of endovascular intervention. It is of historical interest that the original description of percutaneous transluminal coronary angioplasty (PTCA) reported a decrease in translesional pressure gradients from 58 to 19 mm Hg in the 32 patients in whom PTCA was successful [6]. Early attempts to measure pressures distal to a stenosis were hampered by the use of fluid-filled tubes, which, because of their size, increased the translesional gradient. The advent of a pressure transducer mounted on a 0.014 inch angioplasty wire overcame these difficulties and enabled the introduction of the concept of pressure-derived FFR [7,8].

The concept of pressure as a surrogate for flow requires review of Ohm's law:

Flow = pressure / resistance

FFR is defined as maximum myocardial blood flow in the presence of a stenosis divided by the theoretical maximum flow in a normal vessel (i.e., the absence of any stenosis). Under maximum arteriolar vasodilatation, the resistance imposed by the normal myocardial bed is minimal and blood flow is proportional to driving pressure. Thus, FFR represents that fraction of normal maximum flow that is achievable in the presence of epicardial coronary stenosis. Since myocardial ischemia occurs in a patient when maximum blood flow is insufficient to meet myocardial demands, FFR aims to measure perfusion pressure during maximum coronary flow to establish the physiologic significance of a stenosis. FFR is independent of changes in systemic blood pressure, heart rate, or myocardial contractility.

A full description of the theoretical basis of FFR and its clinical utility is included in Chapter 24.

> **Definitions of coronary hemodynamic measurements used clinically**
> - *Coronary flow reserve* (CFR)—Ratio of maximal coronary flow to basal coronary flow.
> - *Relative coronary flow reserve* (rCFR)—Used to minimize the influence of microvasculature on assessment of the hemodynamic severity of an epicardial stenosis. It is the ratio of CFR in the diseased vessel to CFR in a "normal" vessel (rCVR = $CVR_{target}/CVR_{reference}$).
> - *Fractional flow reserve* (FFR)—Maximum myocardial blood flow in the presence of a stenosis divided by the theoretical maximum flow in the absence of the stenosis.

References

1 Lanza GA, Crea F. Primary coronary microvascular dysfunction clinical presentation, pathophysiology, and management. *Circulation* 2010;**121**:2317–2325.

2 Camici PG, Crea F. Coronary microvascular dysfunction. *New Engl J Med* 2007;**356**:830–840.

3 Kern MJ, Bach RG, Mechem CJ, *et al.* Variations in normal coronary vasodilatory reserve stratified by artery, gender, heart transplantation and coronary artery disease. *J Am Coll Cardiol* 1996;**28**:1154–1160.

4 Polese A, De Cesare N, Montorsi P, *et al.* Upward shift of the lower range of coronary flow autoregulation in hypertensive patients with hypertrophy of the left ventricle. *Circulation* 1991;**83**:845–853.

5 Sonoda S, Takeuchi M, Nakashima Y, Kuroiwa A. Safety and optimal dose of intracoronary adenosine 5'-triphosphate for the measurement of coronary flow reserve. *Am Heart J* 1998;**135**:621–627.

6 Gruentzig AR, Senning A, Siegenthaler WE. Non-operative dilation of coronary artery stenosis. *N Engl J Med* 1979;**301**:61–68.

7 Pijls NH, de Bruyne B, Peels K, *et al.* Measurement of fractional flow reserve to assess the functional severity of coronary-artery stenoses. *N Engl J Med* 1996;**334**:1703–1708.

8 Pijls NH, Van Gelder B, Van der Voort P, *et al.* Fractional flow reserve. A useful index to evaluate the influence of an epicardial coronary stenosis on myocardial blood flow. *Circulation* 1995;**92**:3183–3193.

CHAPTER 24

Fractional flow reserve

Paul M. Johnson, Shriti Mehta, Prashant Kaul and George A. Stouffer

Concept of fractional flow reserve

The ability accurately to assess the physiologic significance of a coronary stenosis in clinical practice is critical. For clinicians in the cardiac catheterization laboratory, it is difficult to determine by angiography alone if an intermediate coronary lesion is responsible for ischemic symptoms. Lesions that are responsible for inducible ischemia are associated with worse outcomes, and those patients may benefit from revascularization, either by percutaneous intervention (PCI) or coronary artery bypass grafting (CABG). On the other hand, lesions that do not produce inducible ischemia are associated with a favorable prognosis and medical treatment alone is reasonable.

Due to the practical limitations of the Doppler wire and other methods to calculate coronary flow reserve (CFR; Figure 24.1), the use of a pressure transducer to measure pressure-derived fractional flow reserve (FFR) has gained wide acceptance as a clinically useful tool to assess the hemodynamic significance of coronary stenosis. Early efforts to measure pressure gradients across a stenosis with small fluid-filled catheters were limited because the catheters were large enough to increase artifactually the translesional gradient in diseased arteries. The development of a pressure transducer mounted on a 0.014 inch coronary guidewire overcame this limitation and made measurement of the pressure gradient across a coronary lesion efficient and safe.

The basic principle of FFR is that when resistance is constant, changes in pressure are proportional to changes in flow. Since pressure is easier to measure than flow, FFR has replaced CFR for clinical use. Ohm's Law, which describes the relationship between pressure, flow, and resistance, forms the hemodynamic basis for FFR:

Ohm's Law: Flow = pressure/resistance

Cardiovascular Hemodynamics for the Clinician, Second Edition. Edited by George A. Stouffer.
© 2017 John Wiley & Sons Ltd. Published 2017 by John Wiley & Sons Ltd.

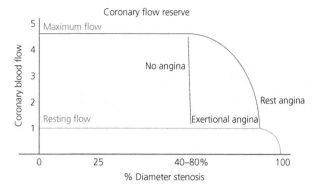

Figure 24.1 Simplified graph of coronary flow reserve. The ability to increase coronary flow is essential to meet metabolic demands during physiologic stress. Resistance to flow from a stenosis in an epicardial artery can compromise the ability of coronary flow to increase.

As described in Chapter 23, the heart has the ability to maintain adequate coronary blood flow across a range of perfusion pressures because of the autoregulatory system. The resistance of the myocardial microcirculation is regulated to vary coronary blood flow based on the oxygen demand of the myocardium. FFR is measured when microvasculature resistance is at a minimum and coronary flow is at a maximum, which enables determination of maximal pressure loss across a stenosis in an epicardial coronary artery (Figure 24.2). FFR is defined as the maximum myocardial blood flow in the presence of a stenosis divided by the theoretical maximum myocardial blood flow in a normal coronary vessel (i.e., in the absence of a stenosis). Thus, it represents the fraction of normal coronary blood flow that is achievable in the presence of an epicardial coronary stenosis. This index is independent of heart rate, systemic blood pressure, or myocardial contractility.

FFR can be represented in the following equation. The perfusion pressure across the myocardium is equal to the mean aortic pressure, P_a, minus the central venous pressure, P_v. When a coronary stenosis is present, this gradient is equal to the pressure distal to a stenosis, Pd, minus the central venous pressure, P_v.

$$FFR = \frac{(P_d - P_v)/R_{min}}{(P_a - P_v)/R_{min}}$$

At maximal hyperemia, resistance of the myocardium is minimized, R_{min}, and can thus be removed from the equation:

$$FFR = \frac{(P_d - P_v)}{(P_a - P_v)}$$

Furthermore, the venous pressure is minimal compared to the arterial pressure and can be removed from the equation:

$$FFR = \frac{P_d}{P_a}$$

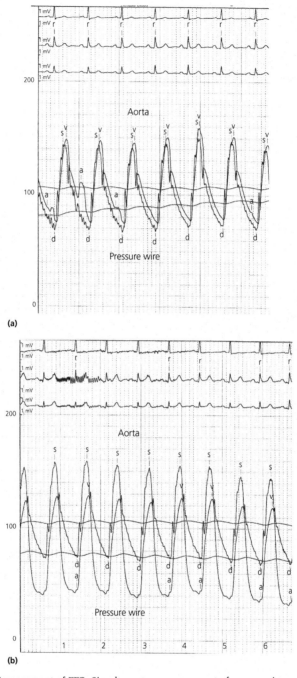

Figure 24.2 Measurement of FFR. Simultaneous measurement of pressure in aorta and distal LAD (labeled pressure wire) at rest (a) and following intracoronary administration of adenosine (b) in a 63-year-old male with chest pain and an intermediate lesion on angiography. Under basal conditions, there is a 7 mm Hg difference in mean pressures between the distal left anterior descending coronary artery (measured with the pressure wire) and the aorta (measured with the guide catheter) and the FFR was 0.94. Following administration of 60 μg of adenosine, distal perfusion pressure decreased, the difference in mean pressures increased, and the FFR decreased to 0.58.

Thus in practical terms, FFR is obtained by simultaneously measuring the mean aortic pressure (from the distal tip of a coronary catheter) and coronary pressure distal to a stenosis (from the pressure transducer of the guidewire distal to a lesion) at maximal hyperemia. It is important to remember that several assumptions have to be made to enable the use of pressure data as a surrogate for coronary flow.

Various vasodilators can be used to induce maximal hyperemia, including adenosine, nitroglycerin, or paparavine. Adenosine, which is safe and effective at producing maximal hyperemia, is the most frequently used vasodilator in clinical practice. It can be administered either by intracoronary bolus or intravenously, with clinical studies requiring the IV route to ensure that a steady state of hyperemia is achieved.

A description of some clinical scenarios (see also Figure 24.3) illustrates the relationship between FFR and coronary flow:

• A 70% stenosis in a large artery is more likely to be hemodynamically significant than a 90% stenosis in a small artery.
• Given the same degree of stenosis, flow will be decreased and FFR will be increased in an area of the heart following myocardial infarction (MI).
• The presence of collaterals supplied by a stenosed artery will result in a decrease in FFR because of increased flow.

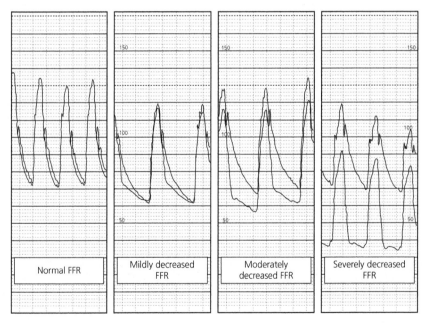

Figure 24.3 Examples of FFR measurements in four patients with coronary disease of different hemodynamic severity. Simultaneous pressure recordings, following intracoronary administration of adenosine, from the aorta and distal coronary artery in four different patients showing normal FFR and mildly, moderately, and severely decreased FFR.

Key clinical studies of FFR

Initial studies done to determine the appropriate threshold of FFR for identifying patients who would benefit from revascularization compared FFR to noninvasive stress testing. Pijls *et al* performed bicycle stress testing, thallium scintigraphy, and stress echocardiography in 45 consecutive patients with chest pain and moderate coronary stenosis. In the 21 patients with FFR <0.75, all had at least one stress test with a positive result. Using a cutoff of 0.75 for FFR produced a sensitivity of 88%, specificity of 100%, and accuracy of 93% in this population. Furthermore, after revascularization of patients with FFR <0.75, all of the positive FFR results reverted to normal [1]. Subsequent studies (most noticeably the FAME studies) modified the FFR threshold to 0.80, which is used in clinical practice today.

There are many clinical scenarios in which measurement of FFR has been shown to be clinically useful. Some of the most important studies are summarized here:

1 *Use of FFR to guide PCI in patients with multivessel coronary artery disease (CAD).* Use of FFR, compared to angiography, to determine lesions needing revascularization in patients with multivessel CAD reduced major adverse cardiovascular events in the FAME I trial. In this study, 1005 patients with multivessel coronary artery disease were randomized to undergo PCI guided by angiography or by FFR. Patients in the angiography group received drug-eluting stents to all significant lesions, whereas those in the FFR group received stents only if FFR was ≤0.80. The event rate at one year for the combined primary end-point of death, nonfatal myocardial infarction, and repeat revascularization was 18.3% in the angiography group versus 13.2% in the FFR-guided group (p = 0.02). There was also a significant reduction in the number of stents placed in the FFR group [2].

2 *Rationale for revascularization in patients with stable ischemic heart disease and intermediate angiographic stenosis with FFR ≤0.80.* In FAME 2, PCI significantly reduced major adverse cardiovascular events when compared to optimal medical therapy alone. The results of the COURAGE trial, published in 2007, found similar outcomes with and without PCI in very low-risk patients with stable ischemic heart disease treated with optimal medical therapy [3]. In the FAME 2 trial, published five years later, patients with stable ischemic heart disease referred for PCI with at least one lesion with FFR ≤0.8 were randomized to PCI plus optimal medical therapy versus optimal medical therapy alone. The primary outcome of death, MI, or urgent revascularization occurred in 12.7% of patients in the medical therapy group, and only 4.3% of the PCI plus medical therapy group at one year; HR 0.32 (0.19–0.53 for 95% CI). It should be noted that the event rate was largely driven by the need for urgent revascularization [4].

FFR is now standard of care for evaluation of intermediate angiographic lesions in stable ischemic disease. In a recent study, the supervising cardiologist was asked to determine a management strategy (PCI, medical therapy, CABG) after diagnostic angiography in 200 patients with stable chest pain [5]. Then FFR was performed on all vessels >2.25 mm and the supervising cardiologist was asked to determine a second management strategy, based on angiography and the results of FFR testing. The addition of FFR to angiography changed the management plan in 26% of the patients, and the number and location of lesions changed in 32%.

3 *Safe deferral of PCI in patients with intermediate lesions and non-significant FFR*. In the DEFER trial, Bech *et al.* measured FFR in 325 patients with moderate coronary stenosis referred for coronary intervention [6]. PCI was performed in all patients with FFR <0.75, but patients with FFR >0.75 were randomized to receive either PCI or medical management (deferral of PCI). The rate of adverse cardiovascular events in those with FFR >0.75 was lower in the medical management group compared to the performance of the PCI group. Furthermore, in long-term follow-up, those with FFR >0.75 who received medical management had a very low event rate [7].

4 *Left main lesions*. The DEFER and FAME trials excluded patients with left main disease, but subsequent prospective cohort studies demonstrated that revascularization can be safely deferred in patients with angiographically significant left main disease but non-significant FFR. A meta-analysis of 525 patients showed that patients who did not undergo revascularization based on FFR >0.75 (one study with FFR >0.80) had similar rates of all-cause mortality and nonfatal myocardial infarction, but higher rates of subsequent revascularization compared to patients who had FFR <0.75 and underwent revascularization [8].

To measure FFR of a left main lesion, intravenous adenosine should be used to induce maximal hyperemia. The guide should be disengaged to avoid ostial narrowing causing obstruction of blood flow with pressure damping in the aortic tracing and false elevation of the FFR value. The pressure sensor should be placed distal to the lesion. It has been suggested that FFR is not useful to assess left main lesions in the presence of severe disease in the left anterior descending or circumflex arteries [9], although other studies have simulated how downstream disease has a small but not clinically significant difference on the FFR value of the left main lesion, and thus FFR is still valid in that scenario [10].

5 *Acute coronary syndromes*. In ACS, microvascular dysfunction from myocardial injury can persist up to six months and can impair maximal hyperemia in infarct-related and non-infarct-related myocardium. Theoretically, microvasculature dysfunction reduces coronary flow under hyperemic conditions when contrasted with intact microvascular function. A reduction in coronary flow would lead to a smaller gradient and a higher FFR value for a given stenosis. Observational studies and post hoc analyses, including that of the FAME trial, have suggested that FFR is reliable and that deferral of revascularization based on FFR is safe in ACS. A recent expert consensus statement concluded that FFR is a valid measure in ACS, including nonculprit lesions in

the setting of ST-elevation MI (STEMI). However, the statement acknowledged the effect of microvascular dysfunction on FFR in ACS, and the potential for error in certain clinical situations [11]. A recent retrospective study demonstrated that FFR values between 0.81 and 0.85 in patients with lesions deferred for revascularization in the setting of ACS were associated with a significantly higher rate of adverse cardiac events [12].

6 *Determining the success of PCI.* The prognostic value of FFR after PCI has not been investigated extensively, but studies suggest that post-PCI FFR <0.90 predicts an increased risk of restenosis [13]. Indeed, a multicenter registry found that event rates at six months were 4.9%, 6.2%, 20.3%, and 29.5% in patients with FFR >0.95, 0.90–0.95, <0.90, or <0.80, respectively [1]. Lower FFR values can be caused by inadequate dilation of the treated segment and/or disease within the rest of the artery.

7 *Tandem lesions.* Theoretically, in the presence of serial lesions the flow through each lesion is affected by other lesions and thus overestimates the FFR value. However, a gradual pullback of the distal pressure sensor toward the guide under maximal hyperemia identifies the area of maximum pressure drop. FFR can be measured again in the vessel after PCI of the primary lesion to determine if PCI of other lesions needs to be performed [13]. It has been shown that the technique of measuring FFR during wire pullback to guide revascularization is safe and effective [14].

8 *Bifurcation lesions.* Use of FFR to guide side branch revascularization has been shown to reduce the need for intervention of short ostial side branch lesions after main branch stenting, with comparable clinical outcomes to an angiograph-guided strategy [15]. FFR of the side branch lesion before intervention can also be performed, but its value is decreased by a proximal main branch lesion. Thus, a pullback pressure recording should be performed along the length of the side branch to determine if there is a significant pressure step-up [16].

Limitations of FFR measurement

There are several limitations that must be kept in mind when using FFR. There is the need for adenosine, which increases the time, cost, and risk of side effects. Moreover, technical aspects such as removing the introducer, clearing the guide of contrast, disengaging the guide for an ostial lesion, and ensuring absence of drift are important to ensure an accurate FFR value [17].

From a theoretical standpoint, several assumptions have to be made to simplify the equation from $FFR = \dfrac{(P_d - P_v)/R_{min}}{(P_a - P_v)/R_{min}}$ to $FFR = \dfrac{P_d}{P_a}$ as detailed earlier, including that venous pressure and resistance are negligible. However, if either central venous pressure or resistance is elevated, the FFR value may be overestimated.

Lastly, recent studies suggest that FFR has a continuous and independent relationship with clinical outcomes rather than a defined threshold value [18]. The role of FFR in ischemic risk stratification continues to evolve.

Instantaneous wave-free ratio

Instantaneous wave-free ratio (iFR) is a recently developed measurement of the hemodynamic significance of a coronary artery stenosis that relies on comparison of pressures during diastole in the absence of hyperemia. It is measured during the wave-free period of mid to late diastole, when flow during the cardiac cycle is the highest and the microcirculatory resistance is the lowest. During this period, pressure and flow velocity are linearly related, allowing pressure ratios to be used to determine the limitation to flow of a lesion. Unlike in FFR assessment, hyperemia (and thus adenosine) is not required.

Using an FFR threshold of 0.80 as the gold standard, an iFR threshold of <0.90 has been proposed for revascularization based on the RESOLVE study [19]. The ADVISE studies took a different approach and proposed a hybrid iFR–FFR approach, which involves performing revascularization for iFR <0.86, deferral for iFR >0.93, and using FFR to guide revascularization if iFR is between 0.86 and 0.93. This approach allowed a 95% classification agreement between the hybrid strategy and FFR while sparing 60% of patients from adenosine [20]. Further outcome studies, including DEFINE-FLAIR and iFR-SWEDEHEART, are being performed to determine the safety of using iFR to guide revascularization.

Case study

A 61-year-old female with diabetes and hypertension reported the recent onset of exertional angina. An exercise treadmill test was performed, during which she developed chest pain and 2 mm of ST depression 2 minutes into the Bruce protocol. At angiography, her coronary arteries were unremarkable except for a 60% lesion involving the ostium of the left anterior descending coronary artery (Figure 24.4a). Because of the intermediate nature of the lesion, FFR analysis was performed using the pressure wire. FFR was 0.94 at baseline and 0.73 following intracoronary administration of 60 μg of adenosine (Figure 24.4b). QCA of the proximal LAD revealed a size of 3.3 mm and therefore a 3.0 mm Cypher drug-eluting stent was placed at 12 atmospheres. Angiography revealed a satisfactory result (Figure 24.4c); however, FFR was 0.82 following intracoronary administration of 60 μg of adenosine. Intravascular ultrasound showed that the vessel diameter was much larger than it appeared on angiography and that the stent was underdeployed (Figure 24.4d). The Cypher stent was dilated to 3.8 mm and angiography repeated (Figure 24.4e). Pressure wire analysis showed that the FFR was now 0.98 at baseline and 0.95 following intracoronary administration of 60 μg of adenosine.

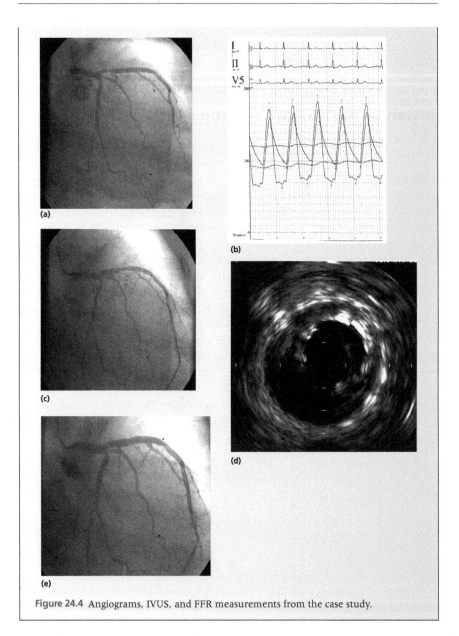

Figure 24.4 Angiograms, IVUS, and FFR measurements from the case study.

References

1 Pijls NH, De Bruyne B, Peels K, *et al*. Measurement of fractional flow reserve to assess the functional severity of coronary-artery stenoses. *N Engl J Med* 1996; **334**:1703–1708.
2 Tonino PA, De Bruyne B, Pijls NH, *et al*. Fractional flow reserve versus angiography for guiding percutaneous coronary intervention. *N Engl J Med* 2009; **360**:213–224.

3 Boden WE, O'Rourke RA, Teo KK, *et al.* Optimal medical therapy with or without PCI for stable coronary disease. *N Engl J Med* 2007;**356**:1503–1516.

4 De Bruyne B, Pijls NH, Kalesan B, *et al.* Fractional flow reserve-guided PCI versus medical therapy in stable coronary disease. *N Engl J Med* 2012;**367**:991–1001.

5 Curzen N, Rana O, Nicholas Z, *et al.* Does routine pressure wire assessment influence management strategy at coronary angiography for diagnosis of chest pain? The RIPCORD study. *Circ Cardiovasc Interv* 2014;**7**:248–255.

6 Bech GJ, De Bruyne B, Pijls NH, *et al.* Fractional flow reserve to determine the appropriateness of angioplasty in moderate coronary stenosis: a randomized trial. *Circulation* 2001; **103**:2928–2934.

7 Pijls NH, van Schaardenburgh P, Manoharan G, *et al.* Percutaneous coronary intervention of functionally nonsignificant stenosis: 5-year follow-up of the DEFER Study. *J Am Coll Cardiol* 2007;**49**:2105–2111.

8 Mallidi J, Atreya AR, Cook J, *et al.* Long-term outcomes following fractional flow reserve-guided treatment of angiographically ambiguous left main coronary artery disease: a meta-analysis of prospective cohort studies. *Cathet Cardiovasc Interv* 2015;**86**:12–18.

9 Ragosta M. Left main coronary artery disease: importance, diagnosis, assessment, and management. *Curr Probl Cardiol* 2015;**40**:93–126.

10 Fearon WF, Yong AS, Lenders G, *et al.* The impact of downstream coronary stenosis on fractional flow reserve assessment of intermediate left main coronary artery disease: human validation. *JACC Cardiovasc Interv* 2015;**8**:398–403.

11 Lotfi A, Jeremias A, Fearon WF, *et al.* Expert consensus statement on the use of fractional flow reserve, intravascular ultrasound, and optical coherence tomography: a consensus statement of the Society of Cardiovascular Angiography and Interventions. *Cathet Cardiovasc Interv* 2014;**83**:509–518.

12 Mehta SM, Depta JP, Novak E, *et al.* Association of lower fractional flow reserve values with higher risk of adverse cardiac events for lesions deferred revascularization among patients with acute coronary syndrome. *J Am Heart Assoc* 2015;**4**(8):e002172. doi:10.1161/JAHA.115.002172

13 Kakouros N, Rade JJ. Role of fractional-flow reserve in guiding percutaneous revascularization in stable coronary artery disease. *Curr Atheroscler Rep* 2015;**17**:530.

14 Kim HL, Koo BK, Nam CW, *et al.* Clinical and physiological outcomes of fractional flow reserve-guided percutaneous coronary intervention in patients with serial stenoses within one coronary artery. *JACC Cardiovasc Interv* 2012;**5**:1013–1018.

15 Koo BK. Fractional flow reserve for coronary bifurcation lesions: can fractional flow reserve-guided side branch intervention strategy improve clinical outcomes compared with angiography-guided strategy? *JACC Cardiovasc Interv* 2015;**8**:547–549.

16 Park SH, Koo BK. Clinical applications of fractional flow reserve in bifurcation lesions. *J Geriatr Cardiol* 2012;**9**:278–284.

17 Jeremias A, Stone GW. Fractional flow reserve for the evaluation of coronary stenoses: limitations and alternatives. *Cath Cardiovasc Interv* 2015;**85**:602–603.

18 Johnson NP, Toth GG, Lai D, *et al.* Prognostic value of fractional flow reserve: linking physiologic severity to clinical outcomes. *J Am Coll Cardiol* 2014;**64**:1641–1654.

19 Nijjer SS, Sen S, Petraco R, Davies JE. Advances in coronary physiology. *Circulation* 2015;**79**:1172–1184.

20 Escaned J, Echavarria-Pinto M, Garcia-Garcia HM, *et al.* Prospective assessment of the diagnostic accuracy of instantaneous wave-free ratio to assess coronary stenosis relevance: results of ADVISE II international, multicenter study (ADenosine Vasodilator Independent Stenosis Evaluation II). *JACC Cardiovasc Interv* 2015;**8**:824–833.

PART VII
Miscellaneous

CHAPTER 25

Right ventricular myocardial infarction

Robert V. Kelly, Mauricio G. Cohen and George A. Stouffer

Right ventricular (RV) dysfunction occurs to some degree in approximately 30–50% of inferior wall and 10% of anterior wall infarcts. Severe RV dysfunction leading to the classic hemodynamic changes occurs in approximately 10% of inferior myocardial infarctions and is associated with higher rates of mortality, cardiogenic shock, sustained ventricular arrhythmias, and advanced atrioventricular (AV) block. Patients in cardiogenic shock with RV involvement have significantly higher in-hospital mortality compared to patients without RV involvement. While RV dysfunction during acute arterial occlusion has classically been labeled RV infarction, profound RV ischemia may be more accurate, since patients with RV infarctions who survive their initial hospitalization tend to do well in the long term and RV function generally recovers.

The effects of ischemia on the right ventricle

The RV is pyramidal shaped with a triangular base and a thin crescentic free wall. It is designed as a volume pump ejecting into the low-resistance pulmonary circulation. The RV is less susceptible to ischemia than the left ventricle (LV) for two reasons: oxygen demand is less and the blood supply is more redundant. Oxygen demand is lower due to the smaller muscle mass of the RV (approximately 15% of muscle mass of LV), lower preload, and lower afterload. Less oxygen extraction at rest means that the RV has greater extraction reserve during stress.

The RV receives its blood supply from several sources. The septum is perfused by the left anterior descending (LAD) artery and posterior descending artery, the lateral wall by marginal branches of the right coronary artery (RCA), and the anterior wall by the conus branch of the RCA and the moderator branch artery of the LAD. The RV is also thought to receive oxygen directly from the ventricular cavity by diffusion.

Cardiovascular Hemodynamics for the Clinician, Second Edition. Edited by George A. Stouffer.

Coronary perfusion to the RV occurs approximately equally during systole and diastole, both under normal conditions and with collateral perfusion during RCA occlusion. RV perfusion during systole is greater than LV perfusion because of lower systolic intramyocardial pressure and less diastolic intracavitary pressure.

The vast majority of RV infarcts occur with occlusion of the RCA, although the LAD and circumflex can also cause RV infarcts. There is a large interindividual variation in the number and origin of RV branches from the RCA (Figure 25.1), but a direct correlation exists between more proximal occlusion of the RCA occlusion and a larger extent of RV infarction.

Clinical presentation, ECG changes, and echocardiographic findings in RV infarction

The diagnosis of RV myocardial infarction is made using the clinical presentation in combination with echocardiogram (ECG), echocardiographic, and/or hemodynamic criteria. The classic clinical triad described with RV infarction is hypotension, clear lung fields, and elevated jugular venous pressure in the setting of an inferior wall myocardial infarction.

The ECG with right-sided leads is very useful in the diagnosis of RV myocardial infarction. The sensitivity of ST elevation in V4R, V3R, and V1 is 93%, 69%, and 28%, respectively, while the specificity is 95%, 97%, and 92%.

Echocardiographic findings that support the diagnosis of RV infarction include RV dilation, RV wall motion abnormalities, paradoxical motion of the interventricular septum, tricuspid regurgitation, decreased descent of the RV base, and plethora of the inferior vena cave (IVC).

Hemodynamics of RV infarction

In proximal RCA occlusion there is compromised perfusion to the RV free wall, with RV dyskinesis and depressed RV function, which is reflected in the RV waveform as a sluggish upstroke, depressed broadened systolic peak, delayed relaxation phase, and diminished RV stroke work (Figure 25.2). RV systolic dysfunction reduces transpulmonary delivery of LV preload, leading to decreased cardiac output despite intact LV contractility. RV dysfunction is compensated for by augmented RA contraction and by left ventricular septal contraction, which bulges in piston-like fashion into the RV during systole and generates force against a stiff RV free wall.

In acute RV ischemia, diastolic biventricular function is key. Depressed RV contractility results in RV dilation and ischemia impairs RV relaxation. The RV becomes stiff and dilated in early diastole, resulting in increased impedance to initial RV inflow. As filling progresses during diastole, the noncompliant RV ascends a steep pressure–volume curve, leading to the pattern of rapid diastolic pressure elevation (Figure 25.2). Acute RV dilation and elevated RV diastolic pressure cause the

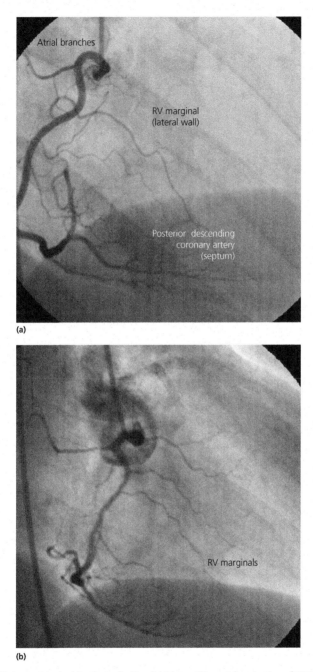

Atrial branches

RV marginal
(lateral wall)

Posterior descending
coronary artery
(septum)

(a)

RV marginals

(b)

Figure 25.1 Right ventricular blood supply. Panel (a) is an AP cranial projection of RCA demonstrating RA branches, a large RV marginal branch, and the posterior descending coronary artery.
Panel (b) is an RAO projection of RCA from a different patient and demonstrates several RV
marginal branches originating from the mid-portion of the RCA. From this angiogram, it is easy to
see that the more proximal the occlusion in the RCA, the greater the extent of RV ischemia.

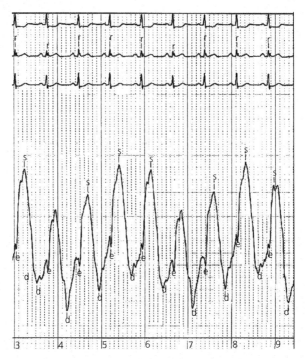

Figure 25.2 RV pressure tracing in a patient with RV ischemia.

interventricular septum to bulge into the LV during diastole, leading to impaired LV compliance and potentially limiting LV filling.

Abrupt RV dilatation within a noncompliant pericardium leads to elevated intrapericardial pressure. As both ventricles fill during diastole and compete for space within the pericardium, the effects of pericardial constraint cause a pattern of equalized diastolic pressures and the RV "dip and plateau" pattern suggestive of constrictive pericarditis. Right atrial (RA) waveforms in RV infarction are characterized by diastolic impedance imposed by a stiff dilated RV. Reduced inflow velocity across the tricuspid valve gives rise to a blunted Y descent (more prominent in expiration) rather than a rapid Y descent, as seen in constrictive pericarditis. In the RA, the blunted Y descent signifies pandiastolic RV dysfunction (Figure 25.3).

The ischemic RV causes preload and afterload of the right atrium to increase, resulting in enhanced RA contractility, reflected in a "W" pattern in the RA waveform characterized by a rapid upstroke and increased peak A wave amplitude, sharp X descent reflecting atrial relaxation, and blunted Y descent of pandiastolic RV dysfunction. Early studies reported that a prominent Y descent was frequently found in RV infarction; however, later studies that timed RA events to RV events (rather than to the ECG) showed that the X descent was predominant [1]. Patients with intact RA function demonstrate prominent A waves and X descents and

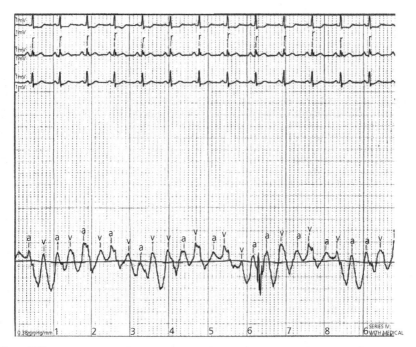

Figure 25.3 RA pressure tracing in a patient with RV ischemia. Note the "W" configuration.

diminished Y descents. An exception will be patients with tricuspid regurgitation, in whom V waves and Y descent will be prominent.

More proximal RCA occlusions compromising atrial blood supply result in atrial as well as ventricular ischemia. Atrial dysfunction results in further elevation in mean RA pressure, an "M" waveform pattern in RA tracing characterized by depressed A wave and X descent, and blunted Y descent. In proximal occlusion of the RCA resulting in acute ischemia involving both the RA and RV, there are RA dysfunction and decreased RV filling, with resultant decrements in LV preload and cardiac output.

Findings at cardiac catheterization

RV infarction is characterized by increased RA and RV diastolic pressures, low cardiac output, and systolic hypotension (Table 25.1). LV dysfunction (e.g., inferior myocardial infarction) increases RV afterload, which can further reduce cardiac output.

1 RA waveform:
  - Pressure is elevated
  - Y descent is impaired

Table 25.1 Hemodynamic principles of RV infarction.

RV systolic and diastole function are impaired.

In the setting of a large area of RV ischemia, the RV becomes merely a conduit (and a stiff one at that) from the systemic veins to the pulmonary circulation.

In the setting of a large area of RV ischemia, the difference between RA and LA pressure becomes the driving force between the systemic veins and the LV. RA transport is important in maintaining LV preload and cardiac output.

RA pressure increases and PA pulse pressure decreases.

Dilation of RV can impair LV function.

Abrupt dilation of RV can give rise to a "pseudo" constrictive pericarditis appearance to hemodynamics, including a "dip and plateau" configuration in RV tracing and a positive Kussmaul's sign.

Cardiac output is reduced.

Systemic hypotension and reduced pulse pressure are common.

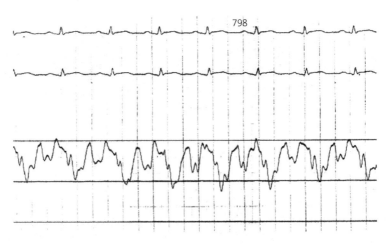

Figure 25.4 RA pressure tracing in a patient with RA and RV ischemia. Note the "M" configuration.

- Failure of RA pressure to decrease with inspiration (Kussmaul's sign) has been shown in small studies to be sensitive and specific for RV infarction.
- Comparison of X and Y descents approximates degree of RA impairment:
  (a) RV infarction with intact RA function—RA pressure tracing demonstrates increased A wave, steep X descent, and impaired Y descent ("W" pattern; Figure 25.3).
  (b) Combined RA and RV infarction—RA pressure tracing demonstrates decreased A wave and impaired X and Y descents ("M" pattern; Figure 25.4).
2 RV waveform:
  - Elevated diastolic pressures
  - Rapid rise in diastolic pressures
  - Slow upstroke in systole

- Diminished peak pressure
- Delayed relaxation
- In severe, abrupt RV dilation, RV and LV diastolic pressures are elevated and equalized and demonstrate a "dip and plateau" configuration (similar to constrictive pericarditis). The Y descent is blunted, unlike the accentuated Y descent seen in constrictive pericarditis

3 Pulmonary artery (PA) waveform:
  - Decreased PA systolic pressure
  - Pulse pressure is reduced

4 Aortic pressure
  - Relative hypotension (Figure 25.5)
  - Pulse pressure is reduced
  - Pulsus paradoxus may be present

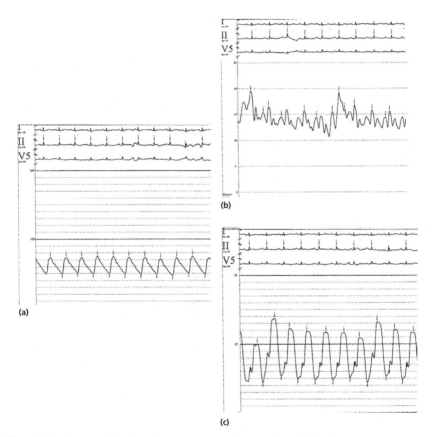

Figure 25.5 Aortic (a), RA (b) and RV (c) pressure tracings in a 64-year-old female with RV ischemia in the setting of an inferior myocardial infarction. Note the relative hypotension, increased RA pressure, and increased RV end-diastolic pressure.

Diagnosis of RV infarction with hemodynamics

Various criteria have been advanced to aid in the diagnosis of RV infarction

1 Both mean RA pressure of ≥10 mm Hg and an RA/pulmonary capillary wedge pressure (PCWP) ratio of 0.8 or more are findings that may be unmasked by volume loading. An abnormal RV radionuclide angiogram was observed in 12 of 13 patients with these hemodynamic measurements in a study of 53 patients with acute inferior myocardial infarction [2].

2 RA pressure greater than 10 mm Hg and within 1–5 mm Hg of PCWP had a sensitivity of 73% and a specificity of 100% in identifying RV infarction in 60 patients with acute myocardial infarction (22 with RV involvement) [3].

3 A severe noncompliant pattern, defined as a Y descent deeper than the X descent in RA pressure tracing, was present in 55% of patients with, and 3% of patients without, RV infarction (sensitivity of 54.5% and specificity of 97.4%) in 60 patients with acute myocardial infarction [3].

4 RA > PCWP. The sensitivity and specificity of these criteria were 45% and 100%, respectively, in a study of 60 patients with acute myocardial infarction [3].

5 Ratio of PA pulse pressure to RA pressure. In a study of 20 patients with RV dysfunction during inferior myocardial infarction compared to 50 patients with nonobstructive coronary artery disease and 14 patients presenting with acute coronary syndrome involving the left coronary artery, patients with RV dysfunction had a significantly lower ratio of PA pulse pressure to RA pressure (1.1 ± 0.6 vs. 4.3 ± 3.0 vs. 5.5 ± 4.4, respectively, p <0.01) and a higher RA:PCWP ratio (0.8 ± 0.3 vs. 0.5 ± 0.2 vs. 0.5 ± 0.3, respectively, p <0.05) [4].

Management

Management of RV infarction can be summarized as follows: early recognition + reperfusion + volume expansion ± dobutamine. The cornerstone of treatment of myocardial infarction is reperfusion, either via primary percutaneous coronary intervention or thrombolytic therapy. In this section we will concentrate on the hemodynamic management of patients with RV infarction. Aggressive fluid resuscitation is vital to restore preload and raise RV filling pressure in order to maximize cardiac output. This can require several liters of saline. Once PCWP increases above 15 mm Hg, further fluid expansion is unlikely to improve hemodynamics, since further dilation of the RV compromises LV filling.

Once RV preload is optimized, dobutamine may improve RV function and cardiac output. In one small study of patients with RV infarction, volume loading increased RA and PCWP pressure, but did not improve cardiac index. Addition of dobutamine, but not nitroprusside, increased cardiac index (by an average of 35%) and RV ejection fraction [5]. Other therapeutic options to support blood pressure include intra-aortic balloon pumping and cardiac pacing to maintain AV synchrony in the setting of advanced AV block.

References

1 Goldstein JA, Barzilai B, Rosamond TL, Eisenberg PR, Jaffe AS. Determinants of hemo-dynamic compromise with severe right ventricular infarction. *Circulation* 1990;**82**:359–368.

2 Dell'Italia LJ, Starling MR, Crawford MH, Boros BL, Chaudhuri TK, O'Rourke RA. Right ventricular infarction: identification by hemodynamic measurements before and after volume loading and correlation with noninvasive techniques. *J Am Coll Cardiol* 1984;**4**:931–939.

3 Lopez-Sendon J, Coma-Canella I, Gamallo C. Sensitivity and specificity of hemodynamic criteria in the diagnosis of acute right ventricular infarction. *Circulation* 1981;**64**:515–525.

4 Korabathina R, Heffernan KS, Paruchuri V, *et al*. The pulmonary artery pulsatility index identifies severe right ventricular dysfunction in acute inferior myocardial infarction. *Cathet Cardiovasc Interv* 2012;**80**(4):593–600.

5 Dell'Italia LJ, Starling MR, Blumhardt R, Lasher JC, O'Rourke RA. Comparative effects of volume loading, dobutamine, and nitroprusside in patients with predominant right ventricular infarction. *Circulation* 1985;**72**:1327–1335.

CHAPTER 26

Pulmonary hypertension

Lisa J. Rose-Jones, Daniel Fox, David P. McLaughlin and George A. Stouffer

The normal pulmonary circulation consists of the pulmonary arteries, which receive deoxygenated blood from the thinly walled, compliant right ventricle. The pulmonary arteries deliver this blood to the capillary beds of the respiratory parenchyma, where carbon dioxide is exchanged for oxygen. Oxygen-rich blood is then delivered to the left atrium via the pulmonary veins (Figure 26.1). This circulation is characterized by high blood flow, low pressure, and low resistance. The normal adult pulmonary vascular bed is highly distensible and capable of accommodating large increases in blood flow with minimal elevations of pressure. Normal peak systolic pressures in the pulmonary arteries range from 18–25 mm Hg and end-diastolic pressures in the pulmonary arteries range from 6–10 mm Hg, with a normal mean pressure of less than 20 mm Hg.

Pulmonary hypertension is quite simply elevated pressure in the pulmonary arteries and is defined as a mean pulmonary artery pressure (MPAP) ≥25 mm Hg. Right heart catheterization plays a crucial role in diagnosing this disease. It not only helps to determine its presence, but also aids in distinguishing the type and severity. Pulmonary hypertension may be the consequence of increased pulmonary blood flow (e.g., anemia, pregnancy, thyrotoxicosis), increased pulmonary vascular resistance, or elevated left heart pressures.

Hemodynamic profiles help to group patients into the World Health Organization (WHO) classification scheme [1]. This allows for patients to be categorized based on similar pathologic findings and guides the clinician as to what therapeutic strategies should be pursued. WHO Group 1 pulmonary arterial hypertension (PAH) is a panvasculopathy of the distal pulmonary arteries that is characterized by medial hypertrophy, intimal proliferation, and fibrosis, with ultimate plexiform lesion formation. There are numerous systemic conditions and heritable genetic mutations that are associated with the development of PAH (Table 26.1). WHO Group 2 pulmonary hypertension due to left heart disease is far and away the most prevalent. Cardiologists will often see this on an

Cardiovascular Hemodynamics for the Clinician, Second Edition. Edited by George A. Stouffer.
© 2017 John Wiley & Sons Ltd. Published 2017 by John Wiley & Sons Ltd.

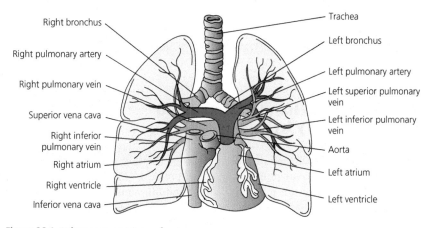

Figure 26.1 Pulmonary arteries and veins.

Table 26.1 5th World Health Organization Classification of Pulmonary Hypertension.

WHO Group 1: Pulmonary arterial hypertension (PAH)
- Idiopathic
- Heritable: BMPR2, ALK-1, ENG, SMAD9, CVA1, KCN3
- Drug/toxin: fenfluramine, aminorex
- Associated with: congenital heart disease (systemic to pulmonary shunt lesions), connective tissue disease (esp. scleroderma), portal hypertension, HIV infection, and schistosomiasis

WHO Group 2: Pulmonary hypertension owing to left heart disease
- Left ventricular systolic or diastolic dysfunction, valvular disease, and congenital/acquired left heart inflow/outflow tract obstructions

WHO Group 3: Pulmonary hypertension owing to lung diseases and/or hypoxia
- Chronic obstructive lung disease, interstitial lung disease, sleep-disordered breathing, mixed obstructive and restrictive lung diseases, alveolar hypoventilation disorders, chronic high altitude exposure, and developmental lung disease

WHO Group 4: Chronic thromboembolic pulmonary hypertension (CTEPH)

WHO Group 5: Pulmonary hypertension with unclear and multifactorial mechanisms
- Sarcoid, chronic hemolytic anemia, myeloproliferative disorders, metabolic disorders, chronic renal failure, etc.

almost daily basis. Chronic lung disease and/or hypoxia represent the causative nature in WHO Group 3 pulmonary hypertension. This is felt secondary to hypoxia-triggered vasoconstriction and vascular remodeling, as well as hyperinflation-induced compression and obliteration of alveolar vessels. Chronic thromboembolic disease makes up WHO Group 4. It is hemodynamically similar to PAH, but results in an arteriopathy as a consequence of thromboembolic material. While only about 3.8% of patients with acute pulmonary embolic events will develop this at 2 years, it is crucial to identify as it is potentially curable with surgical intervention [2]. Lastly, WHO Group 5 is composed of several different disorders that have not been as well studied. This collection of disorders has unclear and/or multifactorial mechanisms as to the causation of pulmonary hypertension (see Table 26.1).

Hemodynamic changes associated with pulmonary hypertension

The hemodynamic hallmark of pulmonary hypertension is elevated pulmonary artery pressures. A mean pulmonary artery pressure (MPAP) ≥25 mm Hg has been well accepted by the pulmonary hypertension community and is used as part of the PAH definition in all major multicenter clinical trials. While it is felt that MPAP of 21–24 mm Hg are likely not normal, much controversy exists on how to label individuals with such readings.

Pulmonary artery pressures increase in response to elevated left atrial pressure, cardiac output, or true changes in pulmonary vascular resistance from arterial remodeling. The latter, which represents PAH, has the most evidence base behind targeting management through treatment with pulmonary-specific vasodilator therapy. Thus, hemodynamics obtained through right heart catheterization are imperative to guide diagnosis and treatment options.

Hemodynamic changes in patients with elevated pulmonary pressures depend on the extent of the pulmonary hypertension. The sheer magnitude to which the pulmonary pressures are elevated is important to note; the higher the pressure, the more advanced the disease. The thin-walled, highly compliant right ventricle can accommodate acute increases in volumes at physiologic pressures (e.g., during exercise), but is not designed to overcome abrupt increases in afterload. Thus, acute RV dilation and failure can accompany sudden increases in pulmonary pressure (e.g., with acute pulmonary embolus). In chronic pulmonary hypertension, RV wall thickness increases (i.e., hypertrophy) to normalize wall stress and myocardial oxygen consumption. However, over time, as pulmonary vascular resistance increases with obliterative pulmonary artery remodeling, the right ventricle reaches a point where it can no longer overcome this afterload. It dilates and starts to fail. As right ventricular failure ensues and forward flow is impaired, the mean pulmonary artery pressure will decrease. It is important not to be fooled by these "lower" than expected MPAP. This end-stage disease progression is best detected by significant elevations in right atrial pressures (generally >20 mm Hg) associated with a low cardiac index (<2.0 L/min/m²). Both of these have been associated with worse survival [3].

In moderate cases of pulmonary hypertension, it is not uncommon to see very prominent A waves in the right atrial pressure tracings (Figure 26.2). This is a reflection of impaired RV compliance and an increase in RV end-diastolic pressure (Table 26.2). In more severe cases with significant tricuspid regurgitation, prominent V waves may be present on right atrial pressure tracings. Occasionally with

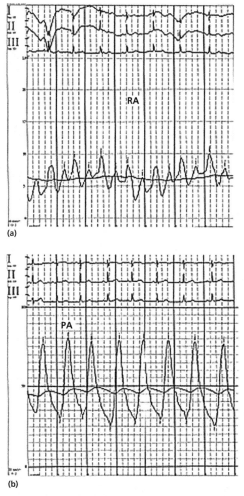

Figure 26.2 Pressure tracings in a patient with pulmonary arterial hypertension. Panel (a) shows right atrial hemodynamic tracing in a patient with portopulmonary PAH. Note the prominent A waves due to a noncompliant, hypertrophied right ventricle. Despite the extremely elevated pulmonary pressures, the patient's ability to "protect" the right atrial pressure is a good prognostic sign. Panel (b) shows a pulmonary artery pressure waveform on a 100 mm Hg scale. Note the peak systolic pressure of 80 mm Hg and mean pressures of 48–50 mm Hg.

severe cases of RV failure and tricuspid regurgitation, RA pressure tracings take on characteristics similar to ventricular pressure tracings (see Chapter 13).

In addition to MPAP ≥25 mm Hg and pulmonary capillary wedge pressure (PCWP) ≤15 mm Hg, pulmonary vascular resistance >3 Wood units is now included in the definition of PAH from the 5th World Health Symposium on

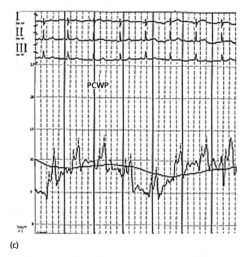

(c)

Figure 26.2 (Continued) Panel (c) shows pulmonary capillary wedge pressure (PCWP) via a balloon-tipped pulmonary artery catheter. The PCWP is crucial in excluding left heart disease as etiology of elevated pulmonary pressure. It is also necessary for calculating pulmonary vascular resistance, which is now included in the hemodynamic definition of PAH.

Table 26.2 Hemodynamic findings in pulmonary hypertension.

- ↑ Pulmonary artery pressure
- ↑ Right ventricular end-diastolic pressure
- ↑ Right atrial pressure
- Prominent A and V waves

Pulmonary Hypertension in 2013 [4]. Pulmonary vascular resistance (PVR) is calculated by dividing the transpulmonary gradient by the cardiac output:

$$PVR = (MPAP - PCWP)/CO$$

PVR is generally expressed in Wood units (1 WU = 1 mm Hg min/L = 80 dyne s/cm^5).

PVR has two components: the fixed component that resulted from vascular remodeling and cannot change acutely, as well as a dynamic component from vasoconstriction. PVR is mainly determined by the geometry of small distal resistive pulmonary arterioles and, according to Poiseuille's law, PVR is inversely related to the fourth power of arterial radius.

Assessing pulmonary vasoreactivity with pharmacologic vasodilator therapy is indicated in several instances. Patients with WHO Group 1 PAH whose etiology is felt to be idiopathic, heritable, or anorexigen induced should undergo a vasodilator challenge [5]. This test predicts response to oral calcium-channel blocker therapy and has the most evidence for treatment effect among the etiologic groups listed earlier. This is most easily accomplished with inhaled nitric oxide, although occasionally intravenous adenosine or epoprostenol is employed. A positive vaso-dilator response is defined as a reduction of the MPAP of at least 10 mm Hg to an absolute value of less than 40 mm Hg without a decline in the cardiac output [6].

Some of the highest pulmonary artery pressures will be seen in a rare condition termed Eisenmenger's syndrome. This results from longstanding, untreated large intra- and extracardiac defects that initially begin as systemic to pulmonary shunts. It is felt that high-pressure pulmonary blood flow results in vascular endothelial damage that incites the milieu to shift into the remodeling process of vasoconstriction, inflammation, and thrombosis. Eventually, resistance in the pulmonary arteries leads to elevation in right heart pressures (Figure 26.3). This leads a reversal of flow or right-to-left shunting to occur. Patients with Eisenmenger's physiology develop cyanosis, hypoxemia, and secondary erythrocytosis.

Special population: Pulmonary hypertension in patients being evaluated for cardiac transplantation

The contribution of reversible and fixed components of PVR is best illustrated in patients being evaluated for cardiac transplantation. It remains important to distinguish these components, because donor hearts are unable to pump against significant pulmonary resistance for any length of time. If there is a large component of fixed resistance, the cardiac allograft will fail, because the donor right ventricle cannot acclimate and overcome the elevated afterload. On the other hand, if the PVR is high but consists primarily of a dynamic component of vasoconstriction triggered

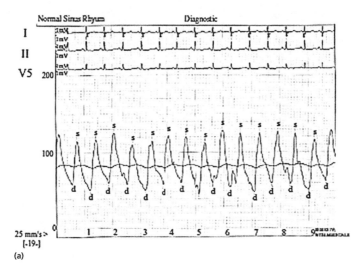

(a)

Figure 26.3 Pressure tracings from a patient with Eisenmenger's syndrome. Panel (a) shows pulmonary artery pressures on a 200 scale. Peak systolic and mean pressures of 120 mm Hg and 82 mm Hg are indicative of severe pulmonary hypertension.

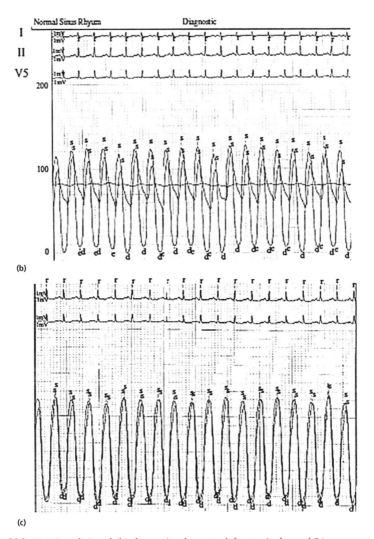

(b)

(c)

Figure 26.3 (Continued) Panel (b) shows simultaneous left ventricular and PA pressures. Panel (c) shows simultaneous measurements of right and left ventricular pressures. At this point in time, the pressures are equal in the two ventricles.

as a response to elevated left heart pressures, the patient's pulmonary resistance will drop dramatically following transplantation as left heart pressures normalize.

The International Society of Heart and Lung Transplantation (ISHLT) recommends determining the relative contributions of fixed and dynamic components. Assessment of reversibility is generally indicated when PASP >50 mm Hg, transpulmonary gradient >15 mm Hg, and/or PVR >3 Wood units [7]. Nitroprusside is the preferred agent of choice, since it induces a simultaneous decrease in both pulmonary and systemic afterload. Nitroprusside can result in a reduction in left atrial pressure, which will decrease PA pressures and theoretically reduce the possibility of pulmonary edema from selective pulmonary vasodilatation in the setting of elevated left-sided filling pressures. Inability to "reverse" pulmonary hypertension is associated with a high incidence of post-transplant mortality from right heart failure, and is thus a contraindication to heart transplantation.

Case study

The patient is a 54-year-old female with a history of end-stage ischemic cardiomyopathy and coronary artery bypass grafting 8 years prior. The left ventricular ejection fraction was severely reduced at 10–15%. She presented for work-up for cardiac transplantation as she had worsening exertional dyspnea and frequent hospitalizations for decompensated heart failure. Right heart catheterization revealed significant pulmonary hypertension that would otherwise preclude transplantation (see Table 26.3). After graduated administration of nitroprusside, the patient's pulmonary pressures were deemed "reversible" and she was cleared to proceed with transplantation.

Table 26.3 Pressures in a patient with severe systolic LV dysfunction at baseline and during nitroprusside infusion.

	Baseline	Nitroprusside infusion
Systemic BP	106/73	92/60
Mean PCWP	24	8
PA (mean)	65/34(44)	32/10 (17)
Cardiac output	2.9	4.4
PVR (Woods units)	7.0	2.0

Hemodynamic changes detected by history and physical exam

The most common symptom attributable to pulmonary hypertension is exertional dyspnea. Angina can also occur. This results from increased right ventricular myocardial oxygen demand due to high wall stress. The RV is generally perfused during both systole and diastole; however, in PH there is a drop in systolic coronary blood flow due to high RV systolic pressures in response to elevated pulmonary pressures. There can also occasionally be compression of the left main coronary by a dilated main pulmonary artery. Other common symptoms include fatigue and peripheral edema. Syncope is a sign of very advanced disease. On physical exam, increased jugular venous pressure with visually prominent A waves is typical. A left parasternal lift produced by the impulse of the hypertrophied high-pressure right ventricle is sometimes palpable. On auscultation, patients with pulmonary hypertension will have an increased pulmonic component of the second heart sound and may have a right-sided S4 heart sound and/or an early systolic ejection click due to sudden interruption of pulmonary valve opening. A mid-systolic ejection murmur caused by turbulent transvalvular pulmonary flow may also be audible.

The Graham Steell murmur of pulmonary regurgitation, an early diastolic decrescendo murmur at the left sternal border, is not uncommon in advanced cases. Other findings in patients with severe pulmonary hypertension include those associated with tricuspid regurgitation (a holosystolic murmur that augments with inspiration and prominent V waves in the jugular veins) and right ventricular failure (hepatojugular reflux, a pulsatile liver, a right ventricular S3 gallop, and peripheral edema).

Two-dimensional echocardiography in pulmonary hypertension

Assessment of the tricuspid regurgitation (TR) jet velocity by 2D echocardiography in patients with pulmonary hypertension is a useful noninvasive measure to estimate pulmonary artery systolic pressure (Figure 26.4). It is a reasonable first

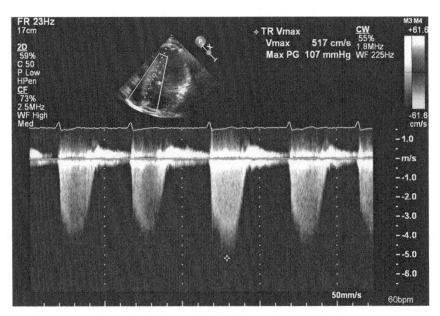

Figure 26.4 Using echocardiography to estimate pulmonary artery systolic pressure. An example of pulse-wave Doppler obtained at the level of the tricuspid valve in a patient with pulmonary hypertension.

diagnostic study when the history, symptoms, or physical exam suggest possible pulmonary hypertension. The velocity of the TR jet enables estimation of the difference between right ventricular systolic pressure and right atrial pressure via use of a modified Bernoulli equation. Pulmonary artery systolic pressure can then be estimated by adding this pressure difference to the right atrial pressure. Right atrial pressure can be either a standardized value of normal (usually 5–10 mm Hg), an estimated value based on echocardiographic characteristics of the inferior vena cava, or measured as jugular venous pulse on physical examination. These calculations assume the absence of pulmonic stenosis, which can be verified by echocardiography.

The transthoracic echocardiogram is important not only to get an assessment of the pulmonary artery systolic pressure, but also to look for signs of remodeling of the right atria and ventricle in response to increased afterload. Furthermore, it is also extremely useful to look for the most common cause of pulmonary hypertension: left-sided heart disease.

Calculation of pulmonary artery systolic pressure from echo

Pulmonary artery systolic pressure $= RAP + 4v^2$

Where:

$RAP =$ Right atrial pressure

$v =$ velocity of tricuspid regurgitation (TR "jet")

Take-home message

While a good history and physical are necessary and an echocardiogram can provide an initial assessment of pulmonary pressures, invasive hemodynamic testing is the gold standard in the diagnosis of PH. Pulmonary hypertension is a broad term that purely reflects elevated pulmonary pressures, specifically defined as MPAP ≥ 25 mm Hg. It comes in many varieties. Right heart catheterization is the next step in the diagnostic algorithm to reveal if true vascular obstruction is present and whether possible pulmonary vasodilator specific therapy is warranted.

References

1 Simonneau G, Gatzoulis M, Adatia I, *et al*. Updated clinical classification of pulmonary hypertension. *J Am Coll Cardiol* 2013;**62**(25_S). doi:10.1016/j.jacc.2013.10.029

2 Pengo V, Lensing AW, Prins MH, *et al*. Incidence of chronic thromboembolic pulmonary hypertension after pulmonary embolism. *N Engl J Med* 2004;**350**(22):2257–2264.

3 McLaughlin VV, McGoon MD. Pulmonary arterial hypertension. *Circulation* 2006; **114**:1417–1431.

4 Hoeper, MM, Bogaard HJ, Condliffe R, *et al*. Definitions and diagnosis of pulmonary hypertension. *J Am Coll Cardiol* 2013;**62**(25_S). doi:10.1016/j.jacc.2013.10.032

5 Badesch, DB, Abman SH, Ahearn GS, *et al.* American College of Chest Physicians. Medical therapy for pulmonary arterial hypertension: ACCP evidence-based clinical practice guidelines. *Chest* 2004;**126**:35s–62s.

6 McGoon M, Gutterman D, Steen V, *et al.* American College of Chest Physicians. Screening, early detection, and diagnosis of pulmonary arterial hypertension: ACCP evidence-based clinical practice guidelines. *Chest* 2004;**126**:14s–34s.

7 Mancini D, Lietz K. Contemporary reviews in cardiovascular medicine: selection of cardiac transplantation candidates in 2010. *Circulation* 2010;**122**:173–183.

CHAPTER 27

Hemodynamics of arrhythmias and pacemakers

Rodrigo Bolanos, Kimberly A. Selzman, Lukas Jantac
and George A. Stouffer

The cardiac rhythm is integral to the development of physiologic pressure wave-forms. Disturbances in electrical conduction can change atrial and ventricular filling and contraction and, hence, hemodynamic parameters. This chapter will describe changes that take place as a result of some of the most common arrhythmias encountered in the coronary intensive care unit or cardiac catheterization laboratory. Although sinus tachycardia and sinus bradycardia usually represent normal cardiac physiology, they will also be discussed in this chapter because of their important effects on pressure tracings and hemodynamic parameters. Lastly we will discuss the hemodynamic effects of pacemakers.

Premature atrial and ventricular contractions

Perhaps the most frequently encountered cardiac arrhythmia is a premature beat, either a premature atrial contraction (PAC) or a premature ventricular contraction (PVC). Although a single ectopic beat is unlikely to have a clinically significant hemodynamic effect, the pressure tracings associated with it are interesting. As a result of the earlier than normal ventricular contraction and shortened diastolic filling time, the stroke volume and arterial pulse pressure are substantially reduced. The post-ectopic beat tends to produce an increased stroke volume secondary to enhanced ventricular filling during the compensatory pause (Figure 27.1). An increase in arterial pulse pressure will also be evident.

A PVC can serve as an aid in diagnosing hypertrophic obstructive cardiomyopathy (HOCM). In HOCM, a characteristic post-extrasystolic pressure change occurs in the aorta following a PVC. This finding was first described in 1961 and is termed the Brockenbrough–Braunwald–Morrow sign (see Chapter 15 for a further description of this sign). On the sinus beat immediately following a PVC,

Cardiovascular Hemodynamics for the Clinician, Second Edition. Edited by George A. Stouffer.
© 2017 John Wiley & Sons Ltd. Published 2017 by John Wiley & Sons Ltd.

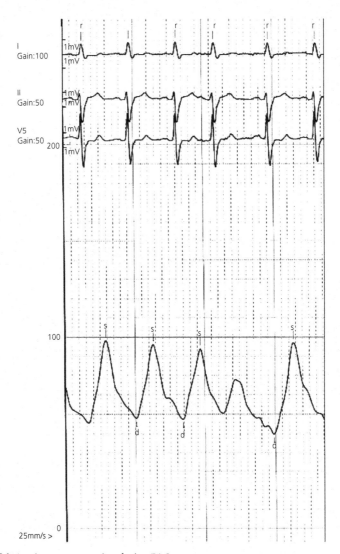

Figure 27.1 Aortic pressure tracing during PAC.

the aortic pulse pressure decreases (Figure 27.2). This finding is associated with HOCM, whereas other hemodynamic findings, including an increase in the left ventricular systolic pressure and an increase in the systolic gradient between the left ventricle and aorta, can also be seen with aortic valve stenosis. On palpation of the carotid pulse, a reduced impulse on the beat following an ectopic beat may be noted in patients with HOCM. Normally an increased impulse (i.e., increased pulse pressure) would be noted.

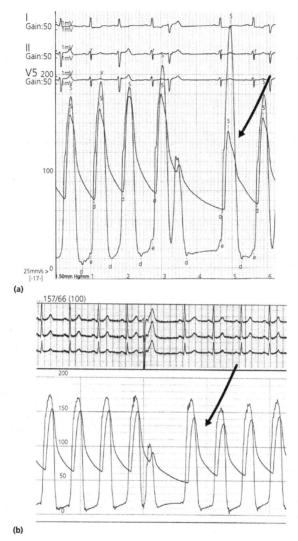

(a)

(b)

Figure 27.2 Brockenbrough–Braunwald–Morrow sign. Simultaneous recordings of LV and aortic pressures in a patient with HOCM (a) and a patient with aortic stenosis (b). Note that pulse pressure falls in the post-PVC beat in HOCM (arrow), but increases in the post-PVC beat in aortic stenosis.

Heart block

Complete heart block causes dissociation of the electrical activity of the atria and ventricles. The resulting ventricular rate is dependent on the site of pacemaker activity (i.e., junctional or ventricular) that serves as an escape rhythm. Complete heart block is generally associated with a marked slowing in rate. Systolic blood pressure may be preserved, but the long periods between ventricular contractions are associated with lower diastolic blood pressure and lower mean arterial pressure (Figure 27.3).

Cannon A waves

Large A waves on atrial pressure tracings that result from atrial contraction when the mitral or tricuspid valves are closed are termed "cannon A" waves. Cannon A waves result when ventricular contraction takes place during or just prior to atrial contraction. This increases ventricular pressure to the point where the tricuspid or mitral valve does not open during atrial contraction, which results in increased atrial pressure. Any arrhythmia that causes atrioventricular dissociation (e.g., complete heart block, pacemaker syndrome, or ventricular tachycardia) can cause random cannon A waves (Figure 27.4). More rare are arrhythmias in which the atrium is activated via retrograde conduction (e.g., AV nodal reentry or some forms of ventricular tachycardia), which can cause regular cannon A waves.

Ventricular tachycardia

Much like a PVC, ventricular tachycardia originates in the ventricles and represents an abnormal sequence of electrical as well as mechanical events. The P wave on an electrocardiogram (ECG) representing atrial activation may be visible during ventricular tachycardia. Atrial activation during this arrhythmia may take place as a result of normal antegrade activation from the sinus node or via retrograde conduction from the ventricles. Ventricular tachycardia resulting in complete atrioventricular dissociation will produce random cannon A waves. Less commonly, when atrial activation during ventricular tachycardia occurs via retrograde activation, cannon A waves will be observed in a regular fashion.

The rapid rate and loss of atrial contribution to ventricular filling that are seen in ventricular tachycardia can lead to hemodynamic deterioration (Figure 27.5). As shown in Figure 27.6, the sudden onset of ventricular tachycardia in this patient resulted in the loss of systolic pressure generation and thus a steady decay in mean blood pressure.

Junctional rhythm

During junctional rhythm, atria maybe activated via retrograde impulse originating in or around the atrioventricular node. The retrograde atrial activation is evident in leads I and II on the standard 12-lead ECG, as the P waves, if seen at all, will be inverted. Atrial systole may occur during, before, or after ventricular systole in

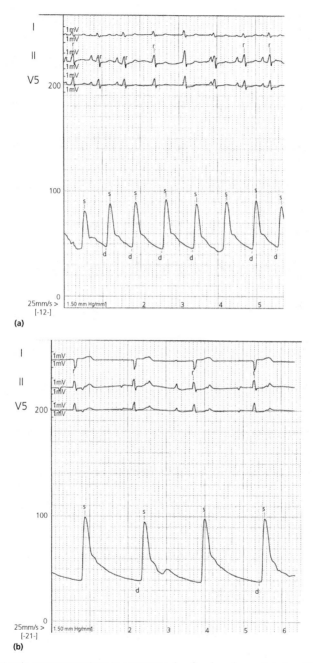

Figure 27.3 Aortic pressure tracings in a patient who developed complete heart block. Aortic pressures during a brief period (a) and sustained episode (b) of complete heart block are shown.

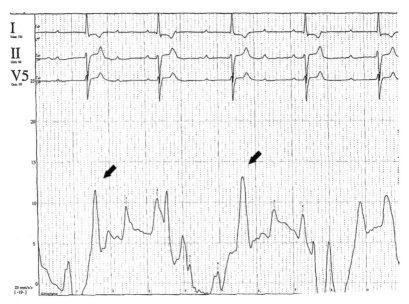

Figure 27.4 Right atrial pressure in a patient with complete heart block. Note the increase in A wave amplitude when the atrium contracts against a closed tricuspid valve (cannon A waves represented by arrows).

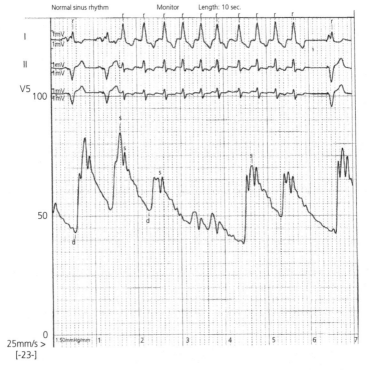

Figure 27.5 Aortic pressure in an elderly woman with a permanent pacemaker and a transient episode of ventricular tachycardia.

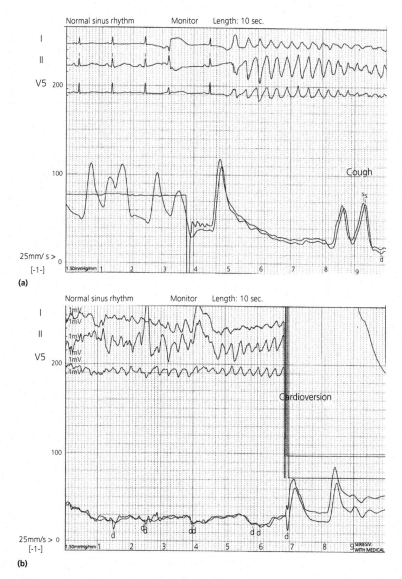

Figure 27.6 Aortic and left anterior descending (LAD) coronary artery pressure in a patient who developed ventricular tachycardia following intracoronary adenosine administration. The patient was undergoing fractional flow reserve evaluation of a lesion in the LAD when ventricular tachycardia developed (a). The increase in aortic pressure with a cough can be seen. In panel (b), the return of pulsatile blood pressure can be seen following electrical cardioversion.

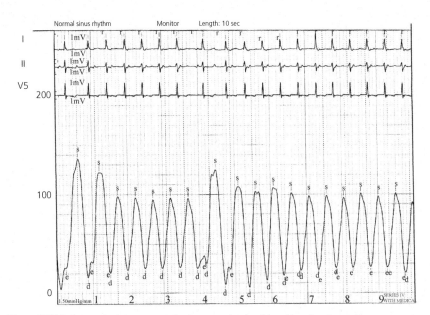

Figure 27.7 Left ventricular pressure during an episode of junctional tachycardia.

this setting. As seen with ventricular tachycardia, complete atrioventricular dissociation may also be present during a junctional rhythm. Because atria may be activated immediately following ventricular systole, cannon A waves can be observed on the right atrial (RA) hemodynamic recording. Although junctional rhythm is in general slow (40–60 bpm), accelerated junctional rhythm may compromise systolic pressure generation (Figure 27.7).

Atrial fibrillation and atrial flutter

Because atrial fibrillation implies the lack of organized atrial activity, the A wave will be absent from the pressure tracings. Depending on the size of the atrium, V waves may also be lacking if the atrium is large enough to serve as a distensible, compliant reservoir (Figure 27.8a). Occasionally, atrial activity may produce enough pressure to open and close the mitral and tricuspid valves and give rise to a C wave on the RA pressure recording. The rhythm in atrial fibrillation is irregular, with a varying length of time spent in diastole. As a result, the stroke volume and hence arterial pulse pressure may vary greatly beat to beat. In general, the longer the diastolic period, the higher the pulse pressure (Figure 27.8b).

In atrial flutter, atrial activity is more organized than in atrial fibrillation and atrial systole can occur (usually at a rate of approximately 300 bpm). The regular atrial activity is reflected on RA pressure tracings as flutter waves (Figure 27.9). Systolic pressure will vary with left ventricular filling. Almost always, atrial–ventricular block

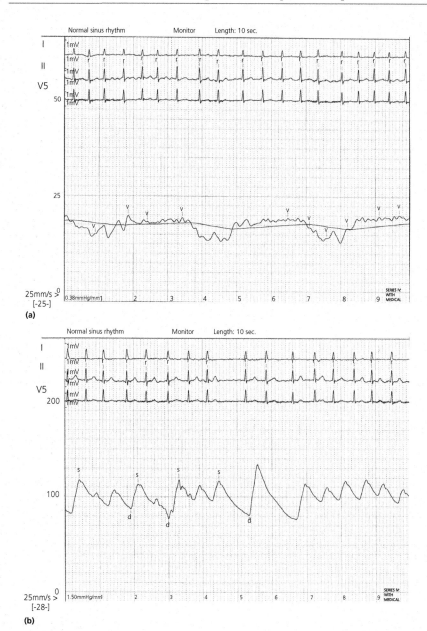

Figure 27.8 Pressure tracings in a patient with atrial fibrillation. Right atrial (a) and aortic (b) pressure tracings during atrial fibrillation. Note the increase in aortic systolic and pulse pressure when the diastolic filling period is increased.

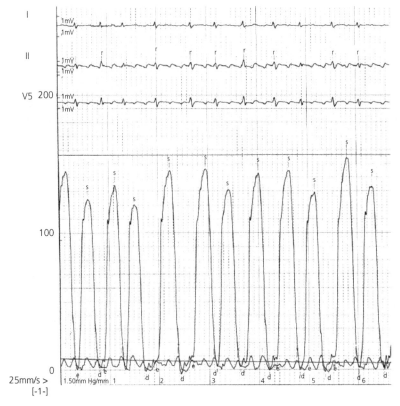

Figure 27.9 Left ventricular and right atrial pressure in a patient with atrial flutter.

exists, whereby not every atrial impulse is conducted to the ventricles. Because atrial contraction can take place against a closed mitral or tricuspid valve, an exaggerated flutter wave similar to a cannon A wave may be seen. For a detailed description of the hemodynamic importance of atrial contraction, see Chapter 5.

Sinus bradycardia or tachycardia

Sinus bradycardia or tachycardia may result in hemodynamic effects and pressure tracings that mimic other arrhythmias. During sinus tachycardia, for example, the cardiac cycle length is shortened, as evidenced by a decreased R–R interval (Figure 27.10). On the RA pressure waveform, one may not be able to distinguish separate A and V waves, because the A wave of one cycle comes progressively closer to the V wave of the preceding cycle as the heart rate increases. As a result, the tracing may resemble that of cardiac tamponade, because the Y descent will not be evident. As a result of the reduced diastolic filling time, stroke volume may be significantly reduced (although cardiac output may increase because of the increase in heart rate).

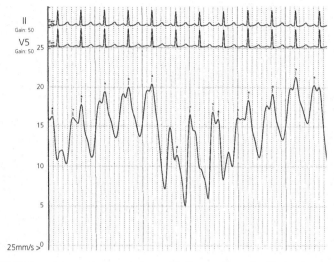

Figure 27.10 Right atrial pressure in a patient with sinus tachycardia. Notice the short time between A waves and V waves and the lack of a Y descent.

During sinus bradycardia, the R–R interval on an ECG is lengthened. As a result, a RA pressure tracing will reveal a longer diastolic period, evidenced by lengthening the interval between the V wave of one cycle and the A wave of the next cycle. On careful observation, one may be able to distinguish an additional positive deflection following the Y descent on the RA pressure waveform tracing. The etiology and significance of this waveform, termed the H wave, are unclear.

Cardiac pacing

Optimal cardiac performance is dependent on the proper timing of atrial and ventricular contraction. When the cardiac electrical conduction system becomes diseased, typically from ischemic heart disease, calcification, or a degenerative process, bradycardia or heart block may occur. These patients often require the placement of a temporary or permanent pacemaker. The first cardiac pacemaker was implanted in 1958 by Elmqvist and Senning via thoracotomy. Since that time, pacemakers have become smaller, more reliable, and more capable of mimicking natural conduction. Despite these improvements, there remain acute and chronic hemodynamic effects of pacemakers and understanding these changes in various patient populations is important in optimizing patient care and outcomes.

The most common type of pacing is a dual-chamber system in which both the RA and right ventricle (RV) are paced. Single-chamber pacemakers pace only the RA or only the RV (Figure 27.11). With biventricular pacemakers, the left ventricle (LV) is also paced, usually via a posterior lateral branch of the coronary sinus (triple-chamber pacing systems). The primary goal of pacemakers is to achieve "physiologic

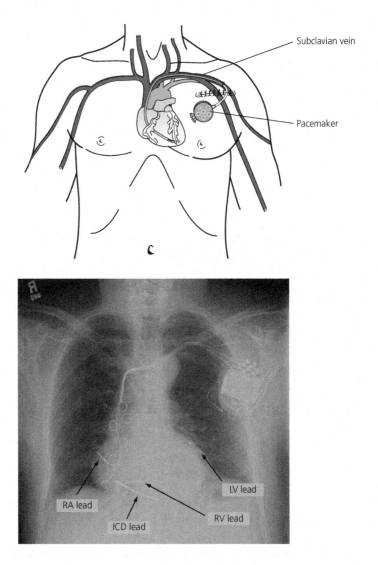

Figure 27.11 Schematic of where a permanent pacemaker lies in the chest and a chest x-ray showing four cardiac leads in a patient with an ICD and biventricular pacemaker.

pacing." The key components of physiologic pacing are optimization of atrio-ventricular (AV) synchrony, rate responsiveness, and interventricular synchrony.

AV synchrony involves the proper timing of atrial diastole and systole in relation to ventricular diastole and systole, so that ventricular preload is maximized, atrial pressures are optimal, and closure of AV valves occurs prior to ventricular systole. This is adjusted by varying the AV delay, which is programmable in all dual-chamber and biventricular pacemakers. Rate responsiveness refers to the ability of a pacemaker to increase the rate appropriately to changing physiologic demands. This is typically achieved with an accelerometer or minute ventilation sensor built into the pacemaker. Interventricular synchrony addresses the coordination of contraction between RV and LV to optimize cardiac function.

Physiology and pathophysiology of AV synchrony

Atrial contraction and AV synchrony influence cardiac output and diastolic filling pressures (Figure 27.12). Dyssynchronous or asynchronous atrial contraction results in reduced end-diastolic volume at a given end-diastolic pressure, decreased LV end-diastolic volume, reduced LV stroke volume, and reduced cardiac output.

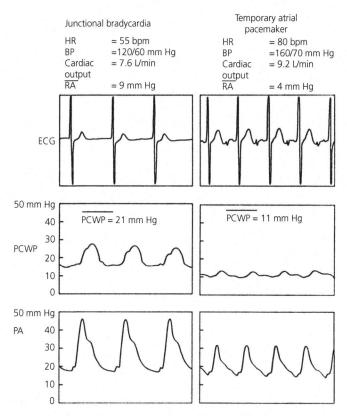

Figure 27.12 PCWP and PA pressure tracings during junctional bradycardia and atrial pacing. Source: Courtesy of WG Sanders, Jr.

Two mechanisms have been implicated in the shift in the LV pressure volume curve that is observed during impaired atrial activity: (a) the loss of atrial contraction directly influences ventricular diastolic filling; and (b) failure of the atria to empty during ventricular diastole increases volume within the pericardium and thus filling pressures [1]. In a given patient, the absence of atrial contraction and/ or loss of AV synchrony may result in altered hemodynamics, with important clinical implications.

The loss of "atrial kick," or ventricular diastolic filling from atrial contraction, may be particularly detrimental to patients with decreased ejection fractions or noncompliant ventricles. Atrial contraction may contribute up to 25–30% of diastolic filling in these individuals. This scenario may be observed in patients with bradycardia but preserved AV synchrony who are paced from the RV at a rate higher than the intrinsic rate (e.g., with a temporary pacing wire or a permanent single-chamber pacemaker). The loss of atrial contraction may be evident as a non-distinct atrial pressure waveform and as lower RV and LV end-diastolic pressures.

If atrial contraction is present but occurs after ventricular contraction has begun, then the atria will contract against closed AV valves, often resulting in prominent A waves or cannon A waves on atrial pressure tracings. This scenario can occur when atrial activity does not precede ventricular activity (sinus node dysfunction), atrial activity is asynchronous with ventricular systole (complete heart block with AV dissociation), or there is conduction retrograde from the ventricles to the atria (VA conduction), resulting in contraction of the atria against closed AV valves. This lack of AV synchrony may lead to impaired ventricular filling and thus increase the mean right atrial pressure and pulmonary capillary wedge pressure (PCWP).

Pacemaker syndrome is used to describe patients who respond adversely to the loss of AV synchrony during pacing. Symptoms of pacemaker syndrome range from pulsatile sensations in the neck to malaise, presyncope, or syncope in severe cases due to hypotension. This syndrome is most often seen in patients with a single lead pacing the right ventricular (RV) apex (VVI pacing mode) and intact sinus node function. The pacemaker will neither sense atrial activity nor time ventricular pacing based on atrial contractions. The development of dual-chamber pacemaker systems that sense and pace both the atrium and ventricle has decreased but not eliminated pacemaker syndrome. These symptoms can occur in patients with dual-chamber devices if the programmed parameters are inappropriate and allow asynchronous atrial and ventricular pacing. Similar to a single-lead system, a dual-chamber device with a nonfunctioning atrial lead will also lead to pacemaker syndrome symptoms.

Patients exhibit a wide range of clinical sensitivity to the loss of AV synchrony. Some patients are asymptomatic, while others are completely intolerant. Likewise, the expected clinical benefit of reestablishing AV synchrony in patients through placement of a pacemaker is quite variable. Although multiple invasive and noninvasive studies have shown significant improvement in cardiac output with AV sequential pacing, the expected benefits have not been consistently borne out in clinical trials.

Patient response is heterogeneous and it appears that patients with low or normal filling pressures benefit most from the "atrial kick" due to their position on the upslope of the Starling curve. Interestingly, patients with significantly increased filling volumes may be the least likely to have a correlation between "atrial kick" and increased cardiac output. These patients still appear to benefit from AV synchrony, but through other mechanisms, such as reestablishment of the optimal diastolic filling period and abolition of mitral regurgitation [2].

Numerous clinical trials have examined the benefits of "physiologic pacing"; that is, atrial-based pacing systems that promote AV synchrony versus single-lead systems (VVI). Generally accepted benefits of physiologic pacing include improved symptoms, a likely reduction in the risk of developing persistent atrial fibrillation, and possible trends toward fewer incidents of pacemaker syndrome and heart failure. At this time there is no uniform evidence across trials showing a mortality benefit or reduction in stroke with atrial-based systems.

Role of AV synchrony: Key points

- Loss of AV synchrony may result in ↑ PCWP, ↓ BP, and ↓ CO. Symptoms may include pulsatile sensations in the neck, malaise, presyncope, or syncope
- Loss of atrial contraction may be evident as nondistinct atrial pressure waveforms, ↓ LVEDP on ventricular pressure tracings, and ↓ BP on LV/aortic pressure waveforms
- Atrial contraction occurring against closed AV valves may be evident as cannon A waves, ↑ mean atrial pressure, and ↑ PCWP
- Pacemaker syndrome incidence can be decreased by using dual-chamber pacing rather than RV single-chamber pacing (VVI pacing)

Pacemakers in specific patient populations

There are specific patient populations where pacemakers often have distinctive hemodynamic effects. These include RV myocardial infarctions requiring temporary pacing, hypertrophic obstructive cardiomyopathy (HOCM), and severe congestive heart failure from dilated cardiomyopathy with left ventricular dysfunction.

Right ventricular infarction

Myocardial infarction involving the RV is complicated by bradyarrhythmias (usually in the form of sinus bradycardia or AV block) in 10–33% of cases. Complete heart block due to an RV infarction is most often transient; however, it can last several days or longer. Correction of bradycardia is occasionally necessary to maintain hemodynamic stability. Although some patients may respond to atropine or aminophylline, most patients with RV infarction and heart block require temporary pacing during the peri-infarct period. This is typically done with a temporary transvenous pacing wire, which is placed in the RV.

Some patients may experience hemodynamic deterioration with the initiation of VVI pacing, possibly due to loss of AV synchrony with loss of atrial contribution to ventricular filling, development of tricuspid regurgitation, or development of asynchronous contraction between the right and left ventricles. These patients may be better served by temporary pacing of both the atrium and ventricle with maintenance of AV synchrony. Topol *et al.* reported four patients who had low cardiac output during RV infarctions. Ventricular pacing resulted in increased heart rates, but had no effect on cardiac output. In contrast, atrial pacing increased cardiac output by 25–63% [3]. Love *et al.* subsequently reported seven patients with loss of AV synchrony during RV infarction. Restoration of AV synchrony resulted in increased systolic blood pressure, cardiac output (by an average of 50%), and stroke volume [4].

Hypertrophic obstructive cardiomyopathy

Dual-chamber pacemakers have been advocated as a therapeutic treatment option for patients with HOCM. The theory underlying the use of dual-chamber pacing with a short-programmed AV delay resulting in continuous RV pacing in these patients is that activation of the RV will cause asynchronous contraction of the septum and LV free wall, with resultant increased LV outflow tract diameter, decreased pressure gradient, and decreased systolic anterior motion of the mitral valve. Early studies reported marked decreases in LV outflow tract gradients and improvement in symptoms in most patients with dual-chamber pacing (an example of a dramatic response to pacing is shown in Figure 27.13). The initial enthusiasm was dampened by subsequent randomized crossover trials, which revealed that reductions in LVOT gradients varied significantly from patient to patient and were more modest than initially reported. A significant placebo effect emerged, with subjective symptom improvement but no difference in objective measures of exercise capacity between periods of active pacing and periods when the pacemaker was set to backup mode. Based on available data at this time, dual-chamber pacing for HOCM is not recommended as first-line therapy for relief of

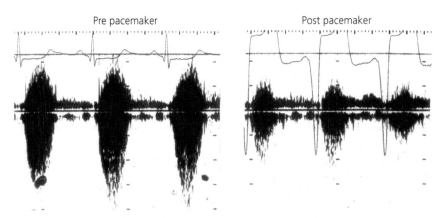

Pre pacemaker   Post pacemaker

Figure 27.13 Effect of pacing on outflow tract gradient (as determined by Doppler interrogation) in a patient with HOCM. Source: Courtesy of WG Sanders, Jr.

symptoms and outflow tract obstruction [5]. In patients with significant LVOT gradient and severe symptoms (NYHA class III or IV), surgical myectomy or alcohol septal ablation is considered prior to pacing. Pacing is generally reserved for selected patient subgroups such as those >65 years old who may not be good candidates for invasive treatment, or perhaps in patients who receive an implantable cardiac defibrillator (ICD) for prevention of sudden cardiac death.

Role of pacemakers in HOCM: Key points

- Dual-chamber pacemakers with continuous pacing of the RV apex may result in 25–40% reduction in LVOT gradient
- Reduction of LVOT and symptom relief varies widely between patients
- Use of permanent pacemakers in HOCM is reserved for patients with significant outflow gradient and severe symptoms who are not candidates for myectomy or alcohol septal ablation and/or who have another indication for permanent pacing or ICD therapy

---

Biventricular pacing in patients with heart failure and dilated cardiomyopathy

As the LV dilates in the setting of impaired systolic function, progressive adverse changes in cardiac geometry and structure can occur, resulting in increased wall stress, decreased mechanical performance, and worsening mitral regurgitation. Often accompanying the mechanical changes is the development of disordered electrical timing, resulting in a prolonged AV delay and asynchronous contraction between the ventricles of the heart. These electrical changes are manifest on the ECG as a prolonged PR interval and widened QRS duration or bundle branch block. Pacemaker therapy in dilated cardiomyopathy has thus evolved not only to correct coexisting sinus node and AV node dysfunction, but also directly to address interventricular dyssynchrony from disordered electrical timing.

Role of pacemakers in heart failure from systolic dysfunction: Key points

- Dual-chamber pacing can acutely increase CO and contractility
- Dual-chamber pacemakers with chronic, frequent (i.e., >40%) pacing of the RV may exacerbate heart failure
- Cardiac resynchronization therapy leads to ↓ PCWP, ↑ CI, and ↑ stroke work
- Patients with class III/IV experience ↑ exercise capacity, improved functional capacity, and quality of life with cardiac resynchronization therapy (CRT) with a 75–80% patient response rate
- CRT decreases hospitalizations and mortality in patients with class III/IV HF who have evidence of dyssynchrony and who are on optimal medical therapy

---

Initial pacing efforts in patients with decreased LV ejection fraction focused on reducing AV conduction delay using dual-chamber devices pacing the RA and RV

(AV synchronous pacing). Shortening the AV interval has several theoretical advantages, including lengthening the diastolic filling time, changing the diastolic filling pattern to more physiologically balanced early and late (atrial) filling components compared to primarily early filling (resulting in lower mean atrial pressures), and reducing mitral regurgitation. Initial studies of acute effects revealed improved hemodynamics, improved contractility, increased cardiac output, and, in some patients, decreased mitral regurgitation. Early enthusiasm for pacing strategies that reduced AV delay but only paced the RA and RV in patients with dilated cardiomyopathy was dampened by several large trials that failed to show improved outcomes.

In fact, there is now growing evidence that frequent RV pacing may be associated with worsening heart failure and that longer AV delays should perhaps be tolerated to promote intrinsic ventricular contraction. Sweeney *et al.* showed in a population of patients with sinus node dysfunction and narrow QRS that DDR pacing resulting in RV pacing >40% of the time was a strong predictor of heart failure hospitalization and atrial fibrillation, despite maintenance of AV synchrony [6]. In the Dual Chamber and VVI Implantable Defibrillator (DAVID) Trial, DDDR pacing at 70 bpm versus backup VVI pacing at 40 bpm resulted in a 10.6% absolute increase in risk at 1 year of the composite endpoint of mortality and hospitalization for heart failure, likely as a result of the ventricular dyssynchrony imposed by ventricular pacing even when AV synchrony is preserved [7].

The focus has now shifted to addressing directly the interventricular asynchrony that exists in patients with a dilated cardiomyopathy and a wide QRS complex. The wide QRS is felt to be an electrical marker for mechanical dyssynchrony between the two ventricles. The reestablishment of concerted LV and RV contraction via simultaneous electrical stimulation of the RV and LV is commonly known as cardiac resynchronization therapy (CRT). The concept of CRT is that pacing of the LV may correct interventricular conduction delays, leading to improved hemodynamics and contraction. The term CRT was coined by Cazeau and colleagues in 1994 when they placed four epicardial leads in a 54-year-old man with LBBB, dilated cardiomyopathy, and class IV congestive heart failure, with an immediate decrease in PCWP and increase in cardiac output [8]. Six weeks later the patient's symptoms had improved to class II, accompanied by drastic weight loss and resolution of peripheral edema.

Acute hemodynamic improvements are seen with LV pacing in patients with dilated cardiomyopathy, decreased systolic function, and left bundle branch block (LBBB; Figure 27.14). For example, Kass *et al.*, in a study of 18 patients with dilated cardiomyopathy and prolonged QRS, found that LV free-wall pacing increased dP/dt_{max} (a measurement of LV contractile performance) by $23.7 \pm 19.0\%$, pulse pressure (by $18.0 \pm 18.4\%$), and stroke work. Biventricular pacing yielded less improvement, whereas RV apical or mid-septal pacing had negligible effects [9]. AV delay had less influence on LV function than the ventricular pacing site. Nelson *et al.* found that LV pacing and biventricular pacing improved arterial pulse pressure, cardiac output, and dP/dt_{max}, while simultaneously reducing energy

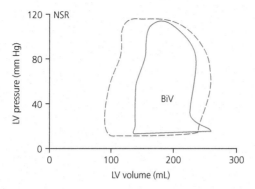

Figure 27.14 Pressure–volume loops in a patient with left bundle branch block and dilated cardiomyopathy taken during normal sinus rhythm (NSR) and during biventricular pacing (BiV). Source: Kass [9]. Reproduced with permission of Wolters Kluwer.

demands (8% reduction in myocardial oxygen consumption; MVO_2). In contrast, administration of dobutamine at a level to achieve a similar effect on dP/dt_{max} increased MVO_2 by 22% [10]. Evidence that pacing the LV at the site of greatest activation delay without concurrent RV pacing has hemodynamic benefits similar to biventricular pacing in some patients is intriguing, because LV-only pacing may improve intraventricular delay, but if anything worsens interventricular synchrony.

Large CRT trials have revealed improved functional capacity, exercise capacity, and quality of life for patients with dilated cardiomyopathy, severe symptoms (NYHA class III), and LBBB. CRT has also been demonstrated to foster beneficial remodeling, as evidenced by multiple echocardiographic parameters such as reduction in LV end-diastolic dimensions. When compiling the data of multiple CRT trials, a recent meta-analysis also showed a mortality benefit when compared to maximal medical therapy [11]. The Cardiac Resynchronization—Heart Failure (CARE-HF) study of 813 patients with severe LV dysfunction and class III or IV symptoms reported a mortality benefit with CRT as well as improvement in interventricular mechanical delay, end-systolic volume index, area of the mitral regurgitant jet, LV ejection fraction, symptoms, and quality of life [12]. The AHA/ACC pacemaker guidelines recommend implantation of a CRT device in patients with an LVEF ≤35%, NYHA class III symptoms, and a QRS duration ≥130 ms [13].

Additional patient populations that could benefit from CRT are being evaluated. For example, it has been postulated that patients with a right bundle branch block may benefit from pacing in the RV apex to preexcite the RV in comparison to the left. In addition, some patients with a narrow QRS by ECG but mechanical dyssynchrony by echocardiogram appear to benefit from CRT, with a resulting increase in cardiac index and decrease in pulmonary capillary wedge pressure. These patients likely have mechanical dyssynchrony despite the narrow QRS electrically [14].

References

1 Linderer T, Chatterjee K, Parmley WW, Sievers RE, Glantz SA, Tyberg JV. Influence of atrial systole on the Frank–Starling relation and the end-diastolic pressure-diameter relation of the left ventricle. *Circulation* 1983;**67**:1045–1053.

2 Nishimura RA, Hayes DL, Holmes DR Jr, Tajik AJ. Mechanism of hemodynamic improvement by dual-chamber pacing for severe left ventricular dysfunction: an acute Doppler and catheterization hemodynamic study. *J Am Coll Cardiol* 1995;**25**:281–288.

3 Topol EJ, Goldschlager N, Ports TA, *et al.* Hemodynamic benefit of atrial pacing in right ventricular myocardial infarction. *Ann Intern Med* 1982;**96**:594–597.

4 Love JC, Haffajee CI, Gore JM, Alpert JS. Reversibility of hypotension and shock by atrial or atrioventricular sequential pacing in patients with right ventricular infarction. *Am Heart J* 1984;**108**:5–13.

5 Maron BJ, McKenna WJ, Danielson GK, *et al.* American College of Cardiology/European Society of Cardiology clinical expert consensus document on hypertrophic cardiomyopathy. A report of the American College of Cardiology Foundation Task Force on Clinical Expert Consensus Documents and the European Society of Cardiology Committee for Practice Guidelines. *J Am Coll Cardiol* 2003;**42**:1687–1713.

6 Sweeney MO, Hellkamp AS, Ellenbogen KA, *et al.* Adverse effect of ventricular pacing on heart failure and atrial fibrillation among patients with normal baseline QRS duration in a clinical trial of pacemaker therapy for sinus node dysfunction. *Circulation* 2003;**107**: 2932–2937.

7 Wilkoff BL, Cook JR, Epstein AE, *et al.* Dual-chamber pacing or ventricular backup pacing in patients with an implantable defibrillator: the Dual Chamber and VVI Implantable Defibrillator (DAVID) Trial. *JAMA* 2002;**288**:3115–3123.

8 Cazeau S, Ritter P, Bakdach S, *et al.* Four chamber pacing in dilated cardiomyopathy. *Pacing Clin Electrophysiol* 1994;**17**:1974–1979.

9 Kass DA, Chen CH, Curry C, *et al.* Improved left ventricular mechanics from acute VDD pacing in patients with dilated cardiomyopathy and ventricular conduction delay. *Circulation* 1999;**99**:1567–1573.

10 Nelson GS, Berger RD, Fetics BJ, *et al.* Left ventricular or biventricular pacing improves cardiac function at diminished energy cost in patients with dilated cardiomyopathy and left bundle-branch block. *Circulation* 2000;**102**:3053–3059.

11 McAlister FA, Ezekowitz JA, Wiebe N, *et al.* Systematic review: cardiac resynchronization in patients with symptomatic heart failure. *Ann Intern Med* 2004;**141**:381–390.

12 Cleland JG, Daubert JC, Erdmann E, *et al.* The effect of cardiac resynchronization on morbidity and mortality in heart failure. *N Engl J Med* 2005;**352**:1539–1549.

13 Gregoratos G, Abrams J, Epstein AE, *et al.* ACC/AHA/NASPE 2002 guideline update for implantation of cardiac pacemakers and antiarrhythmia devices: summary article: a report of the American College of Cardiology/American Heart Association Task Force on Practice Guidelines (ACC/AHA/NASPE Committee to Update the 1998 Pacemaker Guidelines). *Circulation* 2002;**106**:2145–2161.

14 Achilli A, Sassara M, Ficili S, *et al.* Long-term effectiveness of cardiac resynchronization therapy in patients with refractory heart failure and "narrow" QRS. *J Am Coll Cardiol* 2003;**42**:2117–2124.

CHAPTER 28

Systematic evaluation of hemodynamic tracings

George A. Stouffer

This chapter includes hemodynamic tracings taken from 15 patients. Extract as much information as you can from these tracings and then check your answers at the end of the chapter. Remember that it is rare to arrive at a specific diagnosis based on hemodynamic tracings. Thus the goal is not to come up with a diagnosis, but rather to list the useful hemodynamic findings present in each tracing.

In assessing the hemodynamic status of a patient, it is important to use a systematic approach so that the maximal useful information is obtained. Here are 10 suggested steps to use in analyzing hemodynamic data:

1 *Make sure that the hemodynamic data are accurate.* It goes without saying that making clinical decisions based on incorrect data can have disastrous consequences (Figure 28.1). The equipment should be calibrated and leveled properly and the minimum amount of tubing and stop-cocks should be used. Other sources of errors in hemodynamic measurements are discussed in Chapter 2.

2 *Avoid artifacts.* Examine the pressure tracings to make sure that the pressures are not damped or distorted by incorrect catheter position (e.g., when a pigtail catheter has a side hole above the aortic valve during recording of left ventricular pressures). Some common artifacts are shown in Figure 28.1.

3 *Note whether intracardiac pressures are elevated.* Elevation in diastolic pressures is a sensitive indicator that pathology is present. Conversely, "normal" diastolic pressures may mask characteristic hemodynamic findings (e.g., in restrictive cardiomyopathy or constrictive pericarditis) and should elicit a fluid bolus if there is a high degree of clinical suspicion.

4 *Examine pressure waveforms from each cardiac chamber, the aorta, and the pulmonary artery.* Examine A and V waves and X and Y descents in atrial tracings and determine whether characteristic waveforms (e.g., W or M configuration) are

Cardiovascular Hemodynamics for the Clinician, Second Edition. Edited by George A. Stouffer.
© 2017 John Wiley & Sons Ltd. Published 2017 by John Wiley & Sons Ltd.

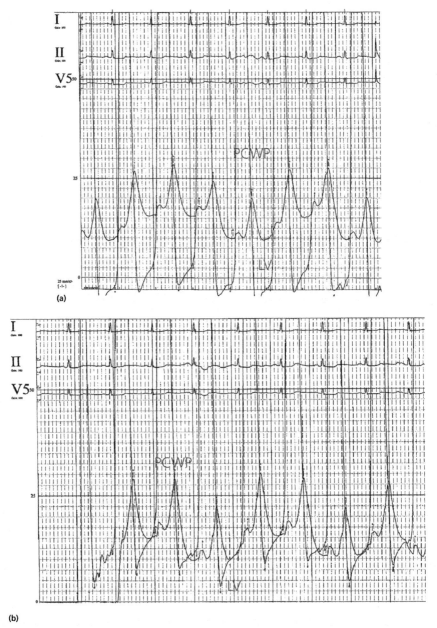

(a)

(b)

Figure 28.1 These tracings are taken from a 40-year-old female who presented with exertional dyspnea. The tracing on the left (a) is consistent with mitral stenosis, with a persistent gradient between pulmonary capillary wedge pressure and left ventricular pressure during diastole. This difference was artifactual and due to incorrect zeroing of the LV pressure transducer. Accurate tracings are shown on the right (b).

present. Similarly, in ventricular tracings, pay special attention to whether a "dip and plateau" configuration is present and to the slope of the rise in pressure during diastole. The aortic pressure tracing can provide helpful clues to many diseases, as discussed in Chapter 4.

5 *Take note of the effect of respiration.* In the normal heart, the decrease in intrathoracic pressure with inspiration is transmitted to the heart with characteristic results. If right atrial pressure does not decrease with inspiration (i.e., Kussmaul's sign), this suggests constrictive pericarditis, but can also be found in other diseases.

6 *Characterize diastolic filling.* Examination of the atrial and ventricular pressure tracings can give an indication of diastolic filling patterns. An exaggerated Y descent implies that significant ventricular filling occurs in early diastole, whereas an exaggerated X descent signifies late diastolic filling. For each patient determine whether diastolic filling occurs primarily in early diastole (e.g., constrictive pericarditis or aortic regurgitation), throughout diastole, or in late diastole (e.g., cardiac tamponade).

7 *Interpret cardiac output based on filling pressures.* Cardiac output is a function of left ventricular filling pressure. A low cardiac output in the setting of an elevated left ventricular end diastolic pressure (LVEDP) is an ominous finding, whereas low cardiac output with low LVEDP is an expected consequence of dehydration. An elevated cardiac output can be a clue to anemia, arteriovenous shunt (e.g., dialysis graft), high-output heart failure, anxiety, and so on. Note also that pulmonary artery pressure and pressure gradients across stenotic valves increase in proportion to cardiac output. For example, exercise during right heart catheterization can be a useful technique to unmask symptomatic mitral stenosis.

8 *Compare pressures measured simultaneously from two sites within the heart or major vessels.* There are numerous benefits to measuring pressures at two sites simultaneously. Comparison of pressures measured proximal and distal to a diseased valve provides information useful in determining the degree of stenosis or regurgitation. Simultaneous measurement of left ventricular and left atrial pressures (or PCWP) is useful in determining diastolic filling characteristics as well as mitral valve pathology. Also, simultaneous measurement of left ventricular/right ventricular pressures or left ventricular/right atrial pressures gives an indication of whether these chambers are independent or interdependent (e.g., in constrictive pericarditis).

9 *Perform any necessary calculations.* Calculate valve area, intracardiac shunt fraction, systemic vascular resistance, and so on as needed. Treatment decisions are often based on the severity of the condition as reflected in these calculations.

10 *Synthesize hemodynamic information with clinical presentation, ECG, past medical history, echocardiographic data, and so on* to arrive at a working diagnosis.

Unknowns

In the following images are hemodynamic data from 15 patients. See how well you do at identifying the relevant information and answering the questions.

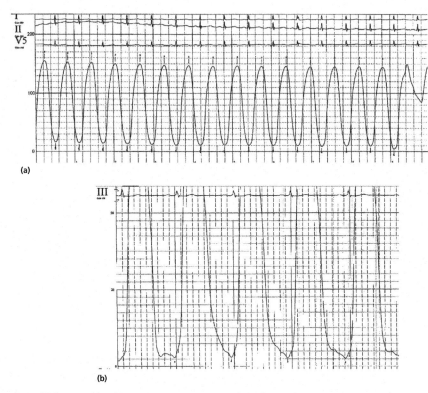

(a)

(b)

Figure 28.2 Examples of hemodynamic tracings with artifacts. The LV pressure tracing in panel (a) is a damped tracing due to an air bubble being in the line. Note the rounded appearance and lack of definition in the peak systolic and diastolic phases of the tracing. In panel (b), the LV pressure is decreasing during diastole. This is nonphysiologic and is due to a side hole of the pigtail catheter being above the aortic valve. The right atrial tracing in panel (c) has an artifact from periodically going in and out of the tricuspid valve. At first glance, it appears that RA pressures are elevated and that there is a large V wave, consistent with tricuspid regurgitation. An accurate RA tracing is shown in (d).

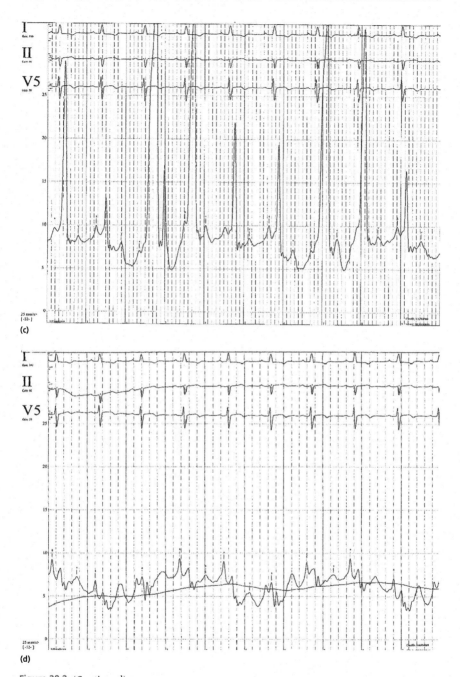

(c)

(d)

Figure 28.2 (Continued)

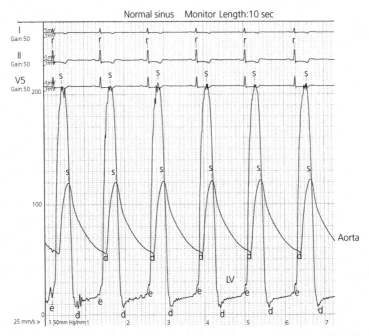

Figure 28.3 A 66-year-old male presents with exertional dyspnea and one episode of syncope. What is the diagnosis?

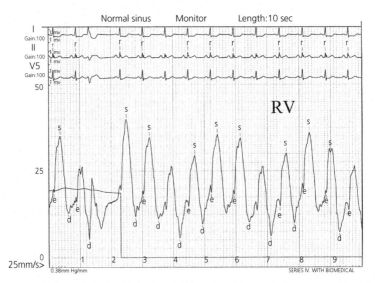

Figure 28.4 A 62-year-old female presents with acute ST elevation inferior MI. RA = 13 mm Hg and PCPW = 12 mm Hg. Does this patient have hemodynamic evidence of RV ischemia?

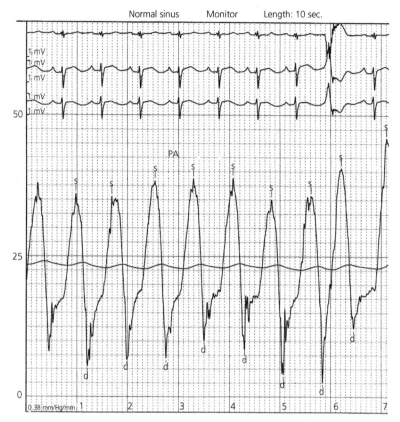

Figure 28.5 Pulmonary artery pressure in a 52-year-old female with a recent episode of endocarditis who now presents with exertional dyspnea. What is the diagnosis?

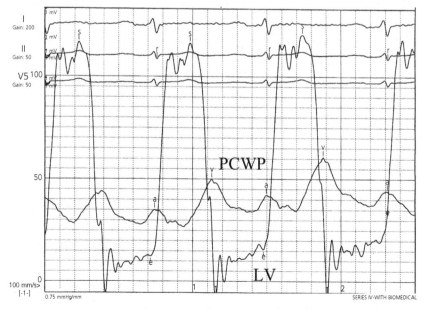

Figure 28.6 A 50-year-old male who is being evaluated after a recent hospital admission for "pneumonia." What is the diagnosis?

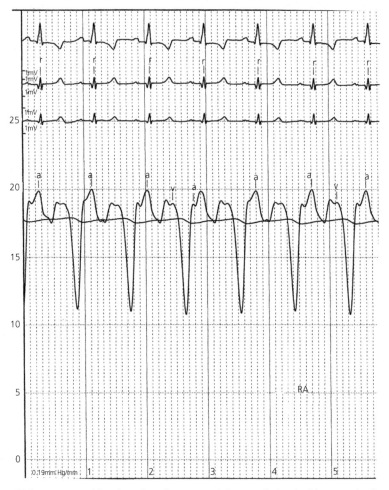

Figure 28.7 A 54-year-old male with end-stage renal disease admitted with congestive heart failure. Past medical history was remarkable for an episode of pericarditis requiring pericardiocentesis 10 years ago. What is the diagnosis?

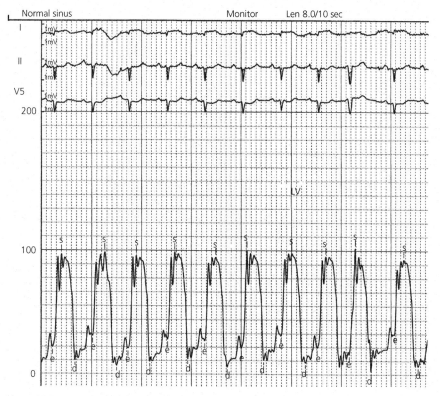

Figure 28.8 A 77-year-old female with acute anterior wall, ST elevation MI. What information is available from this pressure tracing?

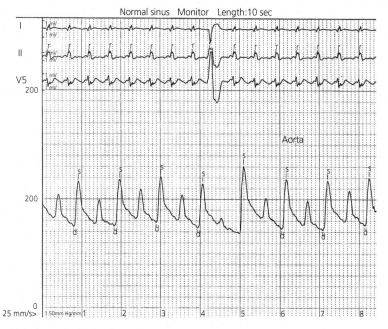

Figure 28.9 A 56-year-old male with a history of hypertension who now presents with congestive heart failure. What does the aortic pressure tracing show?

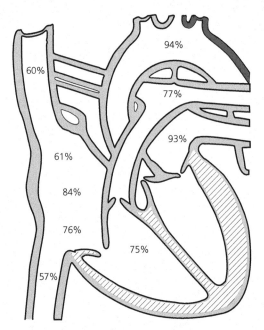

94%

60%

77%

93%

61%

84%

76%

75%

57%

Figure 28.10 A 53-year-old female with cough and shortness of breath. The oxygen saturations obtained in various chambers are listed. What is the diagnosis?

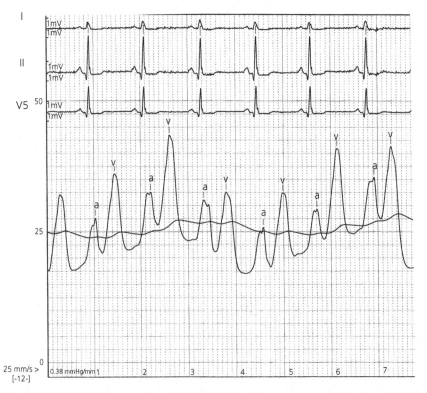

Figure 28.11 Where is this pressure tracing obtained from?

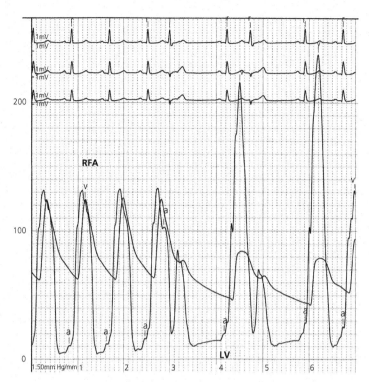

Figure 28.12 A 73-year-old white male with a history of atrial fibrillation who complains of dyspnea on exertion. What is the diagnosis?

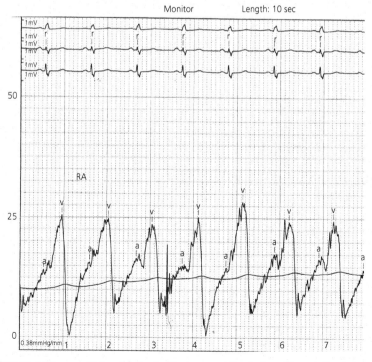

Figure 28.13 A 72-year-old female who has had recurrent episodes of "congestive heart failure." What is the diagnosis?

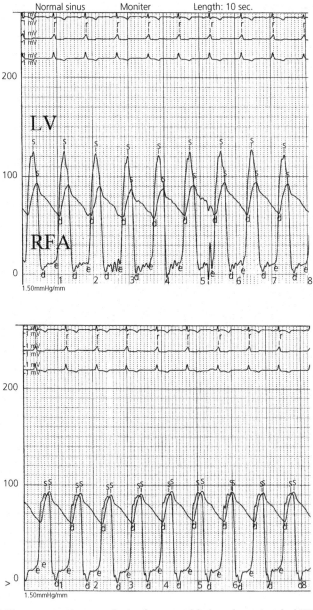

Figure 28.14 These two tracings are obtained as an end-hole catheter (marked LV) is slowly withdrawn from the LV apex to the aorta (while right femoral artery pressure is continuously recorded) in a 29-year-old female who presented with dyspnea on exertion. What is the diagnosis?

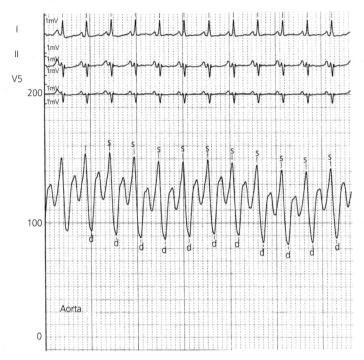

Figure 28.15 What does this aortic pressure tracing represent?

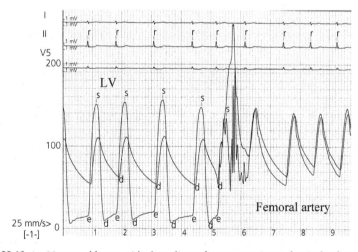

Figure 28.16 An 82-year-old man with chest discomfort on exertion. What is the diagnosis?

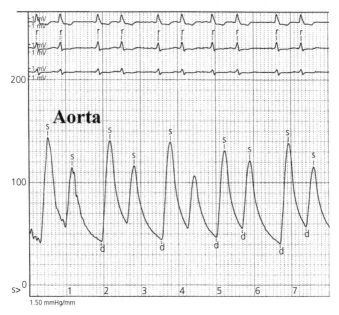

Figure 28.17 An 81-year-old female with hypertension and diabetes mellitus who presented with complaints of substernal chest pain awakening her from sleep. Cardiac enzymes are elevated. What information is available from the aortic pressure tracing?

Answers

28.3 The pressure tracings show a large gradient (approximately 90 mm Hg) between the left ventricle (LV) and the aorta. These tracings could be found in a number of conditions, including valvular aortic stenosis, hypertrophic obstructive cardiomyopathy, subvalvular aortic stenosis, or supravalvular aortic stenosis. The contour of the aortic pressure will occasionally provide some help in the diagnosis, but here there is neither bisferiens pulse (seen in hypertrophic obstructive cardiomyopathy) nor pulsus parvus et tardus (seen in aortic stenosis). Statistically, the most likely diagnosis in a 66-year-old patient is valvular aortic stenosis, which was the case here. The aortic valve area calculated to be 0.5 cm². Also note in this tracing the elevated LVEDP (approximately 25 mm Hg).

28.4 The pressure tracing shows elevated right ventricular (RV) diastolic pressure, consistent with RV ischemia. The diagnosis is confirmed by findings that RA pressure was greater than PCWP (a specificity of 100% for diagnosis of RV infarction in one study), RA pressure greater than 10 mm Hg and within 1–5 mm Hg of the PCWP (a specificity of 100% for diagnosis of RV ischemia in another study), and a mean RA pressure of 10 mm Hg or more and an RA/pulmonary capillary wedge pressure ratio of 0.8 or more (specificity of 92% in a third study).

28.5   The tracing is taken from a catheter placed in the pulmonary artery (PA). Note, however, the ventricular-like appearance, with a rise in pressure during diastole. This tracing is suggestive of severe pulmonary insufficiency (presumably from endocarditis). Also consistent with this diagnosis was the elevated RVEDP at 21 mm Hg. As the degree of pulmonic valve incompetence progresses, RV and PA pressures become similar in diastole.

28.6   The pressure tracings show a gradient between PCWP and LV that persists throughout diastole. Resistance (and thus pressure gradient) between PCWP and LV can occur either in the pulmonary venous system (e.g., veno-occlusive disease or pulmonary venous stenosis following atrial fibrillation ablation) or at the level of the mitral valve. The PCWP tracing shows distinct A and V waves (implying that the PCWP is a good surrogate for left atrial pressure) and thus the most likely diagnosis is mitral stenosis. That was the case in this patient, who had rheumatic mitral stenosis with a valve area calculated to be 0.7 cm^2.

28.7   RA pressure is elevated and the tracing shows characteristic findings of constrictive pericarditis. Note the exaggerated Y descent with a preserved X descent. Although the tracing is too short to make definitive conclusions, there also appears to be minimal variation with respiration.

28.8   This tracing shows elevated LV end-diastolic pressure (32 mm Hg) and reduced LV systolic pressure (95 mm Hg). In the setting of acute myocardial infarction, this relationship can provide important information regarding LV function. In this case, LV systolic pressure is low despite elevated filling pressures, suggesting that LV contractility is severely reduced (based on the Frank–Starling principle). The prognostic importance of LV systolic and end-diastolic pressures has been known since at least 1967, when Killip and Kimball demonstrated that mortality in the setting of acute MI was a function of LV filling pressures (in their case using physical exam findings of pulmonary edema) and aortic systolic pressure. This patient would be Killip class IV [1].

28.9   Systolic pressure alternates in a beat-to-beat fashion in this aortic pressure tracing. This is characteristic of pulsus alternans, which is found in patients with failing left ventricles. This patient had a severe nonischemic cardiomyopathy with an ejection fraction of less than 20%. Be aware of pseudo-pulsus alternans that can occur due to atrial arrhythmias and also cause beat-to-beat variation in systolic pressure.

28.10   This patient has an atrial septal defect (ASD). There is a significant "step up" in oxygen saturations between the vena cava and right ventricle. To estimate Q_p/Q_s using the short equation, first calculate mixed venous (MV) oxygen saturation. In the case of an ASD, MV oxygen saturation can be calculated using the equation of MV $O_2 = (3SVC + \{IVC)/4$. In this case, MV $O_2 = 59.25$ rounded to 59. $Q_p/Q_s = (SAO_2 - MVO_2)/(PVO_2 - PAO_2)$. If we assume $SAO_2 = PVO_2$ (a valid assumption in the absence of right-to-left shunting), $Q_p/Q_s = (94 - 59)/(94 - 77) = 2.1$.

28.11 This tracing shows left atrial pressure. Note that the mean pressure is 25 mm Hg and that there is significant respiratory variation, both consistent with atrial pressure. In the left atrium, the V wave is generally larger than the A wave; the opposite is generally true in the right atrium. These pressures were obtained from the pulmonary capillary wedge position, which explains the delay between the ECG and pressure deflections (compare the P wave on the ECG and A wave on the tracing).

28.12 This aortic pressure tracing shows findings consistent with hypertrophic obstructive cardiomyopathy. There is a minimal gradient between right femoral artery (RFA) and left ventricle (LV) at rest, but a gradient >100 mm Hg is present post PVC. Also present is a Brockenbrough–Braunwald–Morrow sign. This sign, originally described in 1961, is defined as diminished pulse pressure in a post-extrasystolic beat compared to the beat immediately preceding the premature ventricular contraction (PVC).

28.13 The RA tracings show "ventriculization," that is, the atrial pressure takes on characteristics of a ventricular pressure (an exaggerated Y descent, rapid rise in pressure during ventricular diastole, and lack of X descent). This patient had severe tricuspid regurgitation.

28.14 This patient had congenital subvalvular stenosis. The tracing on the left shows a pressure difference between the LV apex and femoral artery, with a mean gradient of 29 mm Hg. The tracing on the right was taken with an end-hole catheter just below the aortic valve. It identifies the obstruction as being subvalvular, since there is no gradient between the ventricle at this location (note the ventricular contour of the tracing) and the femoral artery.

28.15 This patient has an intra-aortic balloon pump. Note the diastolic augmentation.

28.16 At first glance this looks like aortic stenosis, since there is a pressure gradient between LV and femoral artery. Note, however, that the femoral artery pressure increases during the catheter pullback and that there is no difference between LV systolic and aortic systolic pressure. Presumably, this patient had a thrombus in the sheath that was dislodged during pullback. The cause of the chest symptoms was coronary artery disease.

28.17 At first glance this tracing looks like pulsus alternans. Note, however, that the ECG shows type 1, second-degree heart block (Wenckebach). The beat-to-beat variability in aortic systolic pressure is explained by shortened diastolic filling times in alternate beats and does not indicate severe LV failure.

Reference

1 Killip T, Kimball JT. Treatment of myocardial infarction in a coronary care unit: a two year experience of 250 patients. *Am J Cardiol* 1967;**20**:457–464.

Index

acute pericarditis 221–222
acute respiratory distress syndrome (ARDS) 18–19
adenosine 282, 285, 290–291
afterload 51, 156
AI *see* aortic insufficiency
AIx *see* augmentation index
alcohol septal ablation 196–197
ambulatory monitoring of PA pressure 209
amyl nitrate 190, 192–193, 196
amyloidosis 214
angiography
  aortic regurgitation 153
  intracardiac shunts 93
  mitral regurgitation 162
  RV myocardial infarction 303
  pulmonic valve disease 173, 175
  tricuspid valve 166, 169
aortic insufficiency (AI) – *see* aortic regurgitation
aortic pressure
  arterial pressure 58, 61–62, 66
  electrocardiography and waveform analysis 353–354
  heart failure 207–208
  normal hemodynamics 47
aortic regurgitation (AR) 143–153
  acute aortic regurgitation 147–149
  angiographic severity grading 153
  aortic pressures 144–145
  aortic stenosis 115
  case study 151–152
  chronic aortic regurgitation 143–144, 146, 148–152
  concepts and definitions 143–144
  echocardiography 147
  electrocardiography and waveform analysis 148–152

  left ventricular pressures 145
  physical examination 145–146
  severe aortic regurgitation 144, 146, 148–152
  treatment 144, 148
aortic stenosis (AS) 103–118
  adaptive and maladaptive mechanisms 103–104
  aortic regurgitation 115
  aortic valve replacement 119, 120–121
  arterial pressure 61, 63, 64
  Carrabello's sign 114, 117
  case study 116
  challenges 114–115
  common pitfalls 111–114
  concepts and definitions 103–104
  echocardiographic hemodynamics 105–110, 114–115
  electrocardiography and waveform analysis 103–104, 107–115
  etiology 103
  Gorlin formula 110–111
  invasive hemodynamics 109–117
  low flow–low-gradient aortic stenosis 120–121
  low-gradient aortic stenosis 114–115
  peripheral amplification 111–112
  physical examination 105
  presentation and prognosis 104
  pullback of pigtail catheter 113–114, 116
  severity determination 108–109
  subaortic membrane 117–118
aortic valve area (AVA) 120–121
aortic valve replacement (AVR) 119–128
  aortic insufficiency 121, 124–125
  balloon aortic valvuloplasty 122–123
  concepts and definitions 119
  effective orifice area 126–127
  expected residual gradients 125–127

Cardiovascular Hemodynamics for the Clinician, Second Edition. Edited by George A. Stouffer.
© 2017 John Wiley & Sons Ltd. Published 2017 by John Wiley & Sons Ltd.

aortic valve replacement (AVR) (*cont'd*)
  hemodynamic avoidance of common
    pitfalls 121–124
  long-term follow-up after valve
    replacement 127
  low flow–low-gradient aortic stenosis
    120–121
  patient selection 120
  rapid ventricular pacing 123
  surgical aortic valve replacement 119,
    125–127
  transcatheter aortic valve replacement
    119, 121–124
AR *see* aortic regurgitation
ARDS *see* acute respiratory distress
    syndrome
arrhythmias 321–340
  atrial fibrillation and atrial flutter 69, 85,
    138, 328–330, 351
  atrial waveform 80
  atrioventricular synchrony 332–336
  Brockenbrough–Braunwald–Morrow sign
    194-195, 197-198, 321, 323, 321, 323
  cannon A waves 324, 326, 328, 330
  cardiac resynchronization therapy 337-339
  concepts and definitions 321
  dilated cardiomyopathy 337–339
  electrocardiography and waveform
    analysis 321–331, 333, 337–339
  heart block 323–324, 325
  heart failure 337–339
  hypertrophic obstructive cardiomyopathy
    321–323, 336–337
  junctional rhythm 324, 328, 333
  pacemakers 323–324, 326, 331–339
  physiology and pathophysiology of AV
    synchrony 333–335
  premature atrial and ventricular
    contractions 321–323
  pressure–volume loops 338–339
  pulmonary artery catheter 32
  sinus bradycardia or tachycardia 321,
    330–331
  ventricular tachycardia 324, 326–327
arterial pressure 56–68
  aortic pressure 58, 61–62, 66
  augmentation index 61–62, 65
  concepts and definitions 56–58
  ejection phase 56, 61
  mean arterial pressure 58–59, 67–68

  noninvasive measurement of blood
    pressure 65–67
  oscillometric blood pressure devices 67–68
  peripheral amplification 65, 67
  pressure waveform 59–62
  pressure wave reflection 56–57
  pulse wave velocity 56–57
  respiration and aortic pressure 62, 66
  Wiggers diagram 60
AS *see* aortic stenosis
ASD *see* atrial septal defects
assumed Fick method 28–29
atherosclerosis 284
atrial fibrillation 328–330, 351
  atrial waveform 69
  cardiac output 85
  mitral stenosis 138
atrial flutter 328–330
atrial septal defects (ASD) 91–93, 97–98
atrial systole 40
atrial waveform (A wave) 69–81
  abnormalities in atrial pressures 71–77
  arrhythmias 80, 324, 326, 328,
    330–331
  cannon A waves 324, 326, 328, 330
  components of the atrial wave 69–71
  concepts and definitions 69
  conditions associated with RA pressure
    tracings 71–74
  hypertrophic cardiomyopathy 189–192
  jugular venous pulse 77, 80
  mitral stenosis 131, 133
  myocardial infarction 304–305
  normal hemodynamics 40–42, 44, 46–48
  physical examination 77–80
  prominent V waves 73–75, 76, 77
  pulmonary hypertension 312–313, 318
  systematic evaluation of hemodynamic
    tracings 341–343
  tricuspid valve 164
atrioventricular (AV) synchrony 332–336
atrioventricular (AV) valve 39–40
augmentation index (AIx) 61–62, 65
Austin Flint murmur 146
autoregulation of coronary hemodynamics
    283, 284, 289
AV *see* atrioventricular
AVA *see* aortic valve area
AVR *see* aortic valve replacement
A wave *see* atrial waveform

balloon aortic valvuloplasty 122–123
balloon pulmonary valvuloplasty (BPV)
    173, 176
Bayliss phenomenon 282
Beck's triad 243
Bernoulli equation 3–4, 12–13,
    106–107, 139
bifurcation lesions and measurement
    of FFR 294
bioimpedance systems 89
bisferiens pulse 63, 145, 190
blood flow *see* hemodynamic principles;
    normal hemodynamics
bradycardia
    arterial pressure 63
    atrial waveform 71
    junctional rhythm 333
    sinus bradycardia 321, 330–331
Brockenbrough–Braunwald–Morrow
    sign 194–195, 197–198, 321, 323

CABG *see* coronary artery bypass grafting
CAD *see* coronary artery disease
cannon A waves 324, 326
cardiac catheterization
    aortic stenosis 110
    aortic regurgitation 144
    cardiac tamponade 237
    constrictive pericarditis 227–228
    coronary hemodynamics 283–286
    effusive–constrictive pericarditis
        250–251
    heart failure 202
    hypertrophic cardiomyopathy 189
    left heart catheterization 109–117
    mitral regurgitation 158
    mitral stenosis 131
    see also pulmonary artery catheter
    pulmonic valve disease 173
    right heart catheterization 17–36
    right ventricular myocardial
        infarction 305–307
    tricuspid regurgitation 165
    tricuspid stenosis 168
cardiac index (CI) 206–207, 308
cardiac output (CO) 82–90
    aortic stenosis 115
    aortic valve replacement 122–123
    bioimpedance systems 89
    cardiac tamponade 235, 240

concepts and definitions 82–83
Doppler echocardiography 87–88
Fick method 83, 84–85, 95
heart failure 206–207
hemodynamic principles 3–5, 11–12
important formulas 83
intensive care units 88–89
intracardiac shunts 95
mitral stenosis 134
pulmonary artery catheter 17, 28–29
pulmonary hypertension 314–315
pulmonic valve disease 177
pulse contour analysis 88–89
thermodilution method 83, 85–87
cardiac resynchronization therapy (CRT)
    338–339
cardiac sarcoidosis 215–216
cardiac tamponade 234–247
    aortic valve replacement 122
    atrial waveform 79
    Beck's triad 243
    cardiac catheterization 237
    case study 244–246
    clinical progression 234, 235
    compliance of the pericardium 235
    concepts and definitions 234
    differential diagnosis 230–231,
        248–249
    echocardiography 243–245
    electrocardiography and waveform
        analysis 237–242, 246
    elevated pericardial pressure 235–236, 237
    hemodynamic findings 237–241
    hemodynamic pathophysiology
        234–237
    jugular venous distension 243
    Korotkoff sounds 241
    Kussmaul's sign 243
    left ventricular assist devices 273
    physical examination 241–243
    pulsus paradoxus 238–242
    right atrial pressure 237–241, 243–246
cardiac transplantation 315–317
cardiogenic shock 257–259
CardioMEMS 209
cardiomyopathies
    arterial pressure 63
    heart failure 200–211
    hypertrophic cardiomyopathy 185–199
    restrictive cardiomyopathy 212–217

cardiovascular magnetic resonance
(CMR) 180
Carrabello's sign 114, 117
central venous pressure (CVP)
  constrictive pericarditis 223, 226
  hemodynamic principles 5
  left ventricular assist devices 270
  normal hemodynamics 41
CF *see* continuous-flow
CFR *see* coronary flow reserve
chest X-ray 227, 250
chronic thromboembolic pulmonary
  hypertension (CTEPH) 311–312
CI *see* cardiac index
CMR *see* cardiovascular magnetic resonance
CO *see* cardiac output
computed tomography (CT) 173, 227
congestive heart failure 37, 348–349, 351
constrictive pericarditis 49, 78, 221–233
  acute pericarditis 221–222
  cardiac catheterization 227–228
  case study 231–232
  central venous pressure 223, 226
  clinical presentation and progression 221
  concepts and definitions 221–222
  differential diagnosis 213–215, 224,
    230–231
  echocardiography 229
  electrocardiography and waveform
    analysis 222, 223–225, 348
  etiology 221–222
  hemodynamics 222–226
  imaging techniques 227
  intracardial pressure 224
  physical examination 226
  pseudoconstriction 224
  respiration and blood flow 223, 226
  right atrial pressure 223, 225, 227,
    231–232
  sensitivity and specificity of hemodynamic
    findings 229
  systolic concordance and
    discordance 227–228
continuity equation 13–14, 106–108, 139
continuous-flow (CF) ventricular support
  pumps 270
continuous-wave Doppler echocardiography
  aortic regurgitation 147
  aortic stenosis 106
  hypertrophic cardiomyopathy 195–196

mitral stenosis 139–140
tricuspid valve 164
contractility
  aortic valve replacement 121
  indices of contractility 50–52
  mitral regurgitation 157
  myocardial infarction 304
coronary artery bypass grafting (CABG) 288,
  292–293
coronary artery disease (CAD) 292
coronary flow reserve (CFR) 281, 283,
  284–287, 288
coronary hemodynamics 279–287
  autoregulation 282, 283, 289
  cardiac catheterization 283–287
  clinical studies of FFR 292–294
  coronary flow reserve 281, 282, 284–287,
    288–289
  Doppler wires 283, 284–286
  electrocardiography and waveform
    analysis 289–291
  fractional flow reserve 283, 286–287,
    288–297
  garden hose analogy 283
  instantaneous wave-free ratio 295
  limitations of FFR measurement 294–295
  measurement of coronary blood flow
    284, 287
  microvascular dysfunction 281
  myocardial oxygen extraction/demand
    279, 280
  pressure wires 283, 286, 288
  principles of coronary blood flow 279–281
  regulation of coronary blood flow 281–282
  resistance 279–280, 289
coronary stenosis 289, 291–293
CRT *see* cardiac resynchronization therapy
CT *see* computed tomography
CTEPH *see* chronic thromboembolic
  pulmonary hypertension
CVP *see* central venous pressure
C wave
  arrhythmias 328
  atrial waveform 72
  normal hemodynamics 41–42
  tricuspid valve 164–166

DBP *see* diastolic blood pressure
DEFER trials 293
diabetes mellitus 354

diastole 19–20, 37–40, 43–50
diastolic augmentation 255, 257–263
diastolic blood pressure (DBP)
    aortic valve replacement 121–125
    arterial pressure 58, 68
    pulmonic valve disease 177–178
diastolic dysfunction 188
diastolic filling
    cardiac tamponade 234–235, 237–240
    constrictive pericarditis 222–223, 229
    systematic evaluation of hemodynamic
        tracings 343
diastolic murmur 139, 145–146
diastolic pressure 302–304, 306–307, 310
diastolic rumble 138–139, 146
dicrotic notch (DN) 260–262
dilated cardiomyopathy 337–339
DN *see* dicrotic notch
dobutamine 114–115, 121, 308
Doppler echocardiography
    aortic regurgitation 147
    aortic stenosis 106, 109–110
    aortic valve replacement 120
    cardiac output 87–88
    cardiac tamponade 243–245
    hypertrophic cardiomyopathy
        195–196
    left ventricular assist devices 272
    mitral stenosis 139–140
    pulmonary hypertension 318–319
    pulmonic valve disease 173
    restrictive cardiomyopathy 215
    tricuspid valve 164, 168–170
Doppler wires 283, 284–286
dynamic subvalvular stenosis 117–118

ECG *see* electrocardiography
echocardiography
    aortic regurgitation 147
    aortic stenosis 105–110, 114–115
    aortic valve replacement 120, 127
    cardiac tamponade 243–245
    constrictive pericarditis 227, 229
    effusive–constrictive pericarditis 250
    hypertrophic cardiomyopathy 194–196
    left ventricular assist devices 271–273
    mitral regurgitation 161
    mitral stenosis 139–140
    right ventricular myocardial
        infarction 302

pulmonary hypertension 318–319
pulmonic valve disease 173, 180
restrictive cardiomyopathy 215
tricuspid valve 164, 168–170
ECMO *see* extracorporeal membrane
    oxygenation
EDP *see* end-diastolic pressure
effective orifice area (EOA) 106,
    126–127
effusive–constrictive pericarditis 248–251
    cardiac catheterization 250–251
    case study 250–251
    concepts and definitions 248–249
    echocardiography 250
    electrocardiography and waveform
        analysis 249
    etiology and incidence 248
    hemodynamics 249
    imaging techniques 250
    physical examination 249–250
    presentation and differential diagnosis
        248–249
    pulsus paradoxus 249–250
Eisenmenger's syndrome 91, 98, 315
ejection fraction
    aortic regurgitation 147
    aortic stenosis 103–104, 110–111
    arterial pressure 56, 61
    heart failure 200
    intra-aortic balloon counterpulsation 258
    mitral regurgitation 156–157
    RV myocardial infarction 308
    normal hemodynamics 37
    pulmonary hypertension 318
electrocardiography (ECG) and waveform
        analysis
    answers to unknowns 354–356
    aortic regurgitation 148–152
    aortic stenosis 103–104, 107–111
    aortic valve replacement 120–121,
        125–127
    arrhythmias 321–331, 333, 337–339, 351
    arterial pressure 59–67
    atrial waveform 69–81
    cardiac tamponade 237–242, 246
    constrictive pericarditis 222, 223–225, 348
    effusive–constrictive pericarditis 249
    fractional flow reserve 289–291
    heart failure 205
    hypertrophic cardiomyopathy 189–190

electrocardiography (ECG) and waveform
analysis (*cont'd*)
  intra-aortic balloon counterpulsation
    259–264
  left ventricular assist devices 270
  mitral regurgitation 155, 158, 160
  mitral stenosis 131–132, 133, 134–136
  RV myocardial infarction 302, 304–307
  normal hemodynamics 37, 40–47, 54–55
  pulmonary artery catheter 19, 22–24, 26
  pulmonary hypertension 312–316, 318
  restrictive cardiomyopathy 214, 215–216
  systematic evaluation of hemodynamic
    tracings 341–356
  tricuspid valve 164–166
  unknowns 344–356
end-diastolic pressure (EDP)
  aortic regurgitation 144, 145, 151
  aortic valve replacement 121–122,
    124–125
  atrial waveform 75–77
  cardiac tamponade 237
  heart failure 200–201, 203–204
  hypertrophic cardiomyopathy 189–191
  intra-aortic balloon counterpulsation
    258–263
  mitral stenosis 134
  normal hemodynamics 45, 47–50
  pulmonary hypertension 312–313
  right ventricular myocardial
    infarction 307
  tricuspid valve 170
endocarditis 32, 347
end-systolic diameter (ESV) 157
EOA *see* effective orifice area
ESCAPE study 202
ESV *see* end-systolic diameter
exercise echocardiography 147
exercise hemodynamics 136
exertional dyspnea 157, 346, 352
extracorporeal membrane oxygenation
  (ECMO) 258

FAME studies 292–293
femoral artery pressure 111–112, 116
FFR *see* fractional flow reserve
Fick method
  cardiac output 83, 84–85, 95
  intracardiac shunts 95
  pulmonary artery catheter 28–29

flowmeter techniques 284
fluid resuscitation 308
fractional flow reserve (FFR) 288–297
  case study 295–296
  clinical measurement 283, 286–287
  clinical studies 292–294
  concepts and definitions 288–291
  electrocardiography and waveform
    analysis 289–291
  instantaneous wave-free radio 295
  limitations of FFR measurement
    294–295
  revascularization 288, 292–295
Frank–Starling law 9–10, 47, 202–203

Gorlin formula 110–111, 137–138
Graham Steell murmur 318

Harvey's sign 146
HCM *see* hypertrophic cardiomyopathy
heart block 323–324, 325
heart failure (HF) 200–211
  ambulatory monitoring of pulmonary
    artery pressure 209
  aortic pressure and pulsus alternans
    207–208
  arrhythmias 337–339
  cardiac output and cardiac index
    206–207
  congestive heart failure 37, 348–349, 351
  derived parameters from measured
    intracardiac pressures 206–209
  directly measured intracardiac pressures
    203–205
  electrocardiography and waveform
    analysis 348–349, 351
  etiology 200, 201
  Frank–Starling relationship 202–203
  hemodynamic findings 202, 210
  left ventricular end-diastolic pressure
    200–204
  mixed venous oxygen saturation 206
  physical examination 202
  preserved ejection fraction 200–202,
    204, 206
  pressure–volume loops 200–201, 203–204
  pulmonary artery catheter 202–203
  pulmonary artery pressure 204–205
  pulmonary capillary wedge pressures 202,
    204–205

reduced ejection fraction 200–202, 206
right atrial pressure 205
right ventricular pressure 205
right ventricular stroke work index 207
transpulmonary gradient and pulmonary
    vascular resistance 207
HeartMate 3 device 267–268
HeartWare ventricular assist device (HVAD)
    267–268
hemodynamic principles 3–16
    Bernoulli/modified Bernoulli equation
        3–4, 12–13
    cardiac output and vascular resistance
        3–5, 11–12, 14–16
    continuity equation 13–14
    cross-sectional area of blood vessel 13–14
    hydrostatic pressure 3–4
    interchangeable forms of energy in blood
        stream 3–4
    kinetic energy of blood flow 3–4
    laminar and turbulent flow: Reynold's
        number 7–9
    preload: Frank–Starling law 9–10
    pressure and fluid velocity relation 12–14
    pressure gradient and resistance 4–6
    pressure–volume relationship 11–12
    rapid increases in cardiac output 11–12
    resistance in series/parallel blood vessels
        14–16
    resistance to flow: Poiseuille's law 6–7
    wall tension: Laplace relationship 10–11
    see also normal hemodynamics
hemodynamic support
    intra-aortic balloon counterpulsation
        255–264, 308
    left ventricular assist devices 258–259,
        266–275
hemorrhage 32
HF see heart failure
HOCM see hypertrophic obstructive
    cardiomyopathy
hydrostatic pressure 3–4, 19–20
hyperemia 289, 291, 293–294
hypertension
    arterial pressure 58
    electrocardiography and waveform
        analysis 349, 354
    heart failure 204–205
    left ventricular assist devices 273
    mitral regurgitation 159

mitral stenosis 132–133
    normal hemodynamics 47
    see also pulmonary hypertension
hypertrophic cardiomyopathy (HCM)
    185–199
    anatomic variants 186
    aortic pressure 190, 192
    aortic stenosis 117–118
    Brockenbrough–Braunwald–Morrow
        sign 194–195, 197–198, 321, 323
    cardiac catheterization 189
    case study 197–198
    complications 186
    concepts and definitions 185–186
    echocardiography 194–196
    hemodynamics 188–189
    hypertrophic obstructive cardiomyopathy
        186–192, 194–195, 197–198, 321-323,
        336-337
    LV pressure 190–191
    outflow tract gradient 190–194
    physical examination 186
    presentation 185–186
    pulmonary capillary wedge pressure
        189–190
    septal reduction for refractory symptoms
        196–197
    systolic anterior motion 188–189, 195
hypertrophic obstructive cardiomyopathy
    (HOCM) 61, 186–192, 194–195,
    197–198, 321–323, 336–337
hypotension 122–123
hypovolemia
    arterial pressure 61
    cardiac tamponade 241
    left ventricular assist devices 271, 273–274
hypoxia 282, 311

IABP see intra-aortic balloon counterpulsation
ICU see intensive care units
idiopathic hypertrophic subaortic stenosis
    186–192, 194–195, 197–198
iFR see instantaneous wave-free ratio
indices of contractility 50–52
inferior vena cava (IVC) 93, 97, 229
instantaneous wave-free ratio (iFR) 295
intensive care units (ICU) 17–19, 28,
    88–89
International Society of Heart and Lung
    Transplantation (ISHLT) 316–317

intra-aortic balloon counterpulsation
255–264
cardiogenic shock 257–259
description 255–256
diastolic augmentation 255, 257–263
early deflation 261, 262
early inflation 259–261, 262
electrocardiography and waveform
analysis 259–264
hemodynamic effects 256–259
history and uses 255
indications and contraindications
255, 256
inflation and deflation of IABP 256–257,
259–263
late deflation 263
late inflation 261, 262
myocardial infarction 308
timing to cardiac cycle 259–263
intracardiac shunts 91–100
cardiac output 95
concepts and definitions 91
detection of 91–95
diagnosis at right heart catheterization 95
important formulas 96
left-to-right shunt 95–97
limitations of oximetry 94–95
mixed venous oxygen saturation 97, 98
oxygen saturation run 93–97
quantification of 93–97
right-to-left shunt 98
sample case 99
shunt management 97–98
ischemic heart disease 292–293
see also myocardial infarction
ISHLT *see* International Society of Heart and
Lung Transplantation
isovolumetric contraction 20, 37
isovolumetric ventricular relaxation 19–20, 39
IVC *see* inferior vena cava

Jarvik 2000 ventricular assist device 267–268
jugular venous distension 243
jugular venous pressure (JVP) 77, 80,
249–250
junctional rhythm 324, 328, 333
JVP *see* jugular venous pressure

Korotkoff sounds 67, 145, 241
Kussmaul's sign 223, 226, 229, 243

LAD *see* left anterior descending
laminar flow 7–9
Laplace relationship 10–11
LA pressure *see* pulmonary capillary wedge
pressure
LBBB *see* left bundle branch block
left anterior descending (LAD) coronary
artery 301, 327
left atrium (LA)
hypertrophic cardiomyopathy 189–190
mitral regurgitation 155–159, 161
mitral stenosis 129, 131–132, 134,
137–138
left bundle branch block (LBBB) 338–339
left heart catheterization 109–117
left ventricle (LV)
afterload 51
aortic regurgitation 143–145, 147–148,
151–152
aortic stenosis 103–104, 109–113
arrhythmias 328, 331–334, 338–339
arterial pressure 58–61
cardiac output 82
cardiac tamponade 241, 244
constrictive pericarditis 222–223, 227–228,
231–232
coronary hemodynamics 281
indices of contractility 50–52
intra-aortic balloon counterpulsation 255
mitral regurgitation 154–159, 161
mitral stenosis 129, 131–132, 133–138
normal hemodynamics 37, 39, 45–52
preload 47–49, 51
pressure–volume loops 50–53
pulmonary artery catheter 24
systematic evaluation of hemodynamic
tracings 342–346, 352
left ventricular assist devices (LVAD) 266–275
aortic valve insufficiency 274
cardiac tamponade 273
chronic LVAD patient 273–274
early post-implantation period 270–271
echocardiography 271–273
electrocardiography and waveform
analysis 270
hemodynamic parameters 269
history and uses 266–268
hypertension 273
hypovolemia and suction event 271,
273–274

initial evaluation 268–270
late right ventricular failure 274
left-sided heart failure 269
pump failure 273
right-sided heart failure 269–270
right ventricular failure 272–273, 274
thrombosis 274
types of device 267–268
left ventricular ejection fraction (LVEF) – *see*
ejection fraction
left ventricular end-diastolic pressure
(LVEDP)
aortic regurgitation 144, 145, 151
aortic valve replacement 121–122,
124–125
atrial waveform 75–77
cardiac tamponade 237
constrictive pericarditis 222, 227–228
heart failure 200–204
hypertrophic cardiomyopathy 189–191
intra-aortic balloon counterpulsation
258–263
mitral stenosis 134
normal hemodynamics 45, 47–50
restrictive cardiomyopathy 213–215
systematic evaluation of hemodynamic
tracings 343
left ventricular end-diastolic volume
(LVEDV) 156–157, 161, 200–202, 204
left ventricular end-systolic pressure (LVESP)
200–201
left ventricular end-systolic volume (LVESV)
157, 200–202
left ventricular hypertrophy (LVH) 185, 195
left ventricular outflow tract (LVOT) 88,
106–108, 186, 188–189, 197, 336
low flow–low-gradient (LFLG) aortic stenosis
120–121
LV *see* left ventricle
LVAD *see* left ventricular assist devices
LVEDP *see* left ventricular end-diastolic
pressure
LVEDV *see* left ventricular end-diastolic
volume
LVEF *see* ejection fraction
LVESP *see* left ventricular end-systolic
pressure
LVESV *see* left ventricular end-systolic volume
LVH *see* left ventricular hypertrophy
LVOT *see* left ventricular outflow tract

MAC *see* mitral annular calcification
magnetic resonance imaging (MRI) 173, 227
MAP *see* mean arterial pressure
MCS *see* mechanical circulatory support
mean arterial pressure (MAP) 5, 58–59,
67–68, 269
mean pulmonary artery pressure (MPAP)
310, 312–314, 319
mechanical circulatory support (MCS)
266–268
mechanical ventilation 86–87
MI *see* myocardial ischemia/infarction
mitral annular calcification (MAC) 155
mitral regurgitation (MR) 72–73, 75–78,
154–162
acute mitral regurgitation 155, 160–162
angiographic severity grading 162
aortic valve replacement 122
chronic mitral regurgitation 156–158,
160–162
compensatory mechanisms 157–158
concepts and definitions 154
echocardiography 161
hypertrophic cardiomyopathy 188–189
mitral annular calcification 155
pseudo mitral stenosis 164
pathology 154–155
physical examination 159–161
pressure–volume loops 156–158
pulmonary artery catheter 158–159
severe mitral regurgitation 160–162
mitral stenosis (MS) 129–142
atrial waveform 78
cardiac output 134
common pitfalls 137–138
concepts and definitions 129–131
echocardiography 139–140
electrocardiography and waveform
analysis 342
etiology 129
exercise hemodynamics 136
Gorlin formula 137–138
left atrium 129, 131–132, 134, 137–138
left ventricle 129, 131–132, 133–138
mitral regurgitation 162
mitral valve area, resistance, and gradient
133–135, 137–139
mitral valve surgery hemodynamics 141
percutaneous balloon mitral valvuloplasty
133, 140–141

mitral stenosis (MS) (*cont'd*)
  physical examination 138–139
  pulmonary artery 132–133
  quantification of severity of 134–136,
    137–138
  right ventricle 134
  staging 129–131
  symptoms 129
mitral valve replacement 141
modified Bernoulli equation 12–13
Morrow myectomy 196
MR *see* mitral regurgitation
MRI *see* magnetic resonance imaging
MS *see* mitral stenosis
murmur
  aortic regurgitation 145–146
  aortic stenosis 105
  mitral regurgitation 159–161
  mitral stenosis 138–139
  pulmonary hypertension 318
myocardial ischemia/infarction (MI)
  angiography 303
  aortic regurgitation 148, 149
  atrial waveform 79
  cardiac catheterization in RV
    infarction 305–307
  clinical presentation of RV infarction 302
  concepts and definitions 301
  coronary hemodynamics 281–283
  diagnosis of RV infarction with
    hemodynamics 308
  echocardiography 302
  effects of ischemia on right
    ventricle 301–302
  electrocardiography and waveform
    analysis 302, 304–307, 346, 349
  fractional flow reserve 291, 292, 294
  hemodynamics of RV infarction
    302–305, 306
  management 308
  mitral regurgitation 154
  pacemakers 335–336
  RV myocardial infarction/ischemia
    301–309
myocardial oxygen demand 279

normal hemodynamics 37–55
  afterload 51
  aorta 47
  cardiac chambers 41–46

concepts and definitions 37–40
  indices of contractility 50–52
  LA pressure/pulmonary capillary wedge
    pressure 44, 46, 52, 54
  left ventricle 37, 39, 45–52
  mechanical events of the cardiac cycle
    37–40
  normal hemodynamic values 41
  preload 47–49, 51
  pressure–volume loops 50–53
  pulmonary artery 46
  respiratory variation 52–55
  right atrium 41–43
  right ventricle 42, 43–44
  ventricular function curve 50, 53
  Wiggers diagram 37, 38

Ohm's law 5
opening snap (OS) 138–139
oscillometric blood pressure devices 67–68
outflow tract gradient 190–194
oximetry
  cardiac output 84–85
  intracardiac shunts 93–97
  pulmonary artery catheter 30–31
oxygen saturation *see* venous oxygen
  saturation

PA *see* pulmonary artery
PAC *see* premature atrial contractions
pacemakers
  arrhythmias 323–324, 326, 331–339
  atrioventricular synchrony 332–336
  cardiac pacing 331–333
  dilated cardiomyopathy 337–339
  heart block 323–324
  heart failure 337–339
  hypertrophic obstructive cardiomyopathy
    336–337
  myocardial infarction 308, 335–336
  pacemaker syndrome 334–335
  ventricular tachycardia 326
PAH *see* pulmonary arterial hypertension
pansystolic murmur 159–160
paradoxical low flow–low-gradient severe
  aortic stenosis 120
patent ductus arteriosus (PDA) 91, 93
patient–prosthetic mismatch (PPM) 126–127
PBMV *see* percutaneous balloon mitral
  valvuloplasty

PCI *see* percutaneous intervention
PCWP *see* pulmonary capillary wedge
    pressure
PDA *see* patent ductus arteriosus
peak-to-peak systolic pressure gradient in
    aortic stenosis 109–111
PEEP *see* positive end-expiratory pressure
percutaneous balloon mitral valvuloplasty
    (PBMV) 133, 140–141
percutaneous intervention (PCI) 288,
    292–293
pericardial disease
    cardiac tamponade 234–247
    constrictive pericarditis 221–233
    effusive–constrictive pericarditis 248–251
pericardiocentesis 49
peripheral amplification 65, 67, 111–112
PH *see* pulmonary hypertension
phlebostatic axis 25
physical examination
    aortic regurgitation 145–146
    aortic stenosis 105
    atrial waveform 77–80
    cardiac tamponade 241–243
    constrictive pericarditis 226
    effusive–constrictive pericarditis 249–250
    heart failure 202
    hypertrophic cardiomyopathy 186
    mitral regurgitation 159–161
    mitral stenosis 138–139
    pulmonary hypertension 317–318
    tricuspid valve 164, 168
pigtail catheter 112–114, 116
pneumonia 347
Poiseuille's law 6–7
positive end-expiratory pressure (PEEP)
    86–87
positive pressure ventilation 62, 87
pregnancy 181
preload 9–10, 47–49, 51
premature atrial contractions (PAC) 321–323
premature ventricular contractions (PVC)
    321–323
pressure waveforms *see* electrocardiography
    and waveform analysis
pressure wave reflection 56–57
pressure wires 283, 286, 288
pressure–volume loops
    arrhythmias 338–339
    heart failure 200–201, 203–204

hemodynamic principles 11–12
mitral regurgitation 156–158
normal hemodynamics 50–53
PR interval 22–24, 337–338
pseudoconstriction 224
pseudomitral stenosis 162
pseudo severe aortic stenosis 121
pulmonary arterial hypertension (PAH)
    310, 312–314
pulmonary artery (PA)
    heart failure 204–205, 209
    intracardiac shunts 93–95, 97
    mitral regurgitation 157
    mitral stenosis 132–133
    myocardial infarction 307
    normal hemodynamics 46
pulmonary artery (PA) catheter 17–37
    advantages and disadvantages of access
        sites 22
    anatomy and physiology 19–21
    aortic valve replacement 122–123
    assumed Fick method 28–29
    calculating systemic and pulmonary
        vascular resistance 29–30
    cardiac output 17, 28–29, 88
    complications 21, 32–33
    concepts and definitions 17–19
    data accuracy 24–28
    education project and case studies 33–35
    effusive–constrictive pericarditis 250–251
    electrocardiography and waveform
        analysis 19, 22–24, 26
    heart failure 202–203
    intracardiac shunts 95
    mitral regurgitation 158–160
    placement 22–24
    pulmonic valve disease 173–175,
        178–179
    thermodilution 28
    tricuspid valve 164–167, 168
    vascular access 21–22
    venous oxygen saturation monitoring
        30–31
pulmonary artery rupture 32–33
pulmonary capillary wedge pressure (PCWP)
    aortic regurgitation 150
    arrhythmias 333–335, 338
    atrial waveform 69–71, 73–75, 78
    cardiac tamponade 237, 240
    constrictive pericarditis 227–228

pulmonary capillary wedge pressure (PCWP)
(*cont'd*)
heart failure 202, 203, 204–205
hypertrophic cardiomyopathy 189–190
left ventricular assist devices 270
mitral regurgitation 155–156,
158–159, 161
mitral stenosis 131–138
myocardial infarction 308
normal hemodynamics 44, 46
pulmonary artery catheter 17, 24, 32
pulmonary hypertension 313–314
restrictive cardiomyopathy 212
systematic evaluation of hemodynamic
tracings 342–343, 347
pulmonary edema 317
pulmonary hypertension (PH) 310–320
anatomy and physiology 310, 311
cardiac transplantation 315–317
case study 317
concepts and definitions 310–312
echocardiography 318–319
Eisenmenger's syndrome 315
electrocardiography and waveform
analysis 312–316, 318
heart failure 204–205
hemodynamic changes 312–315, 317–318
history taking 317–318
mean pulmonary artery pressure 310,
312–314, 319
mitral regurgitation 159
physical examination 317–318
pulmonary capillary wedge pressure
313–314
pulmonary vascular resistance 314–316
tricuspid regurgitation 318–319
tricuspid valve 164
World Health Organization classification
scheme 310–312
pulmonary infarction 32
pulmonary regurgitation 138–139, 318
pulmonary sarcoidosis 215–216
pulmonary vascular resistance (PVR) 29–30,
207, 314–316
pulmonic valve disease 171–182
angiography 173, 175
balloon pulmonary valvuloplasty 173, 176
hemodynamic changes in chronic PR
176–178
natural history of chronic PR 180–181

non-invasive imaging 173, 180
pregnancy 181
pulmonary artery catheter 173–175,
178–179
pulmonary regurgitation 171, 176–181
pulmonary stenosis 171–172
RV function in chronic PR 178–180
severity grading 173, 176
subvalvular pulmonary stenosis 172
supravalvular pulmonary stenosis 172
treatment 173–176
valvular pulmonary stenosis 172
pulse contour analysis 88–89
pulse-wave Doppler echocardiography
mitral stenosis 139–140
pulmonary hypertension 318–319
tricuspid valve 164
pulse wave velocity (PWV) 56–57
pulsus alternans 63, 207–208
pulsus paradoxus
arterial pressure 62, 63
cardiac tamponade 238–242
constrictive pericarditis 223
effusive–constrictive pericarditis
249–250
pump failure 273
PVC *see* premature ventricular contractions
PVR *see* pulmonary vascular resistance
P wave
arrhythmias 324
atrial waveform 69–71
normal hemodynamics 40–42
PWV *see* pulse wave velocity

QRS complex
arrhythmias 337–338
normal hemodynamics 42, 43
pulmonary artery catheter 24

RA *see* right atrial; right atrium
rapid ventricular filling 19–20, 39–40, 45
rapid ventricular pacing 123
RBBB *see* right bundle branch block
RCA *see* right coronary artery
rCFR *see* relative coronary flow reserve
reduced ejection phase 61
relative coronary flow reserve (rCFR)
286–287
REMATCH trial 266–268
RESOLVE study 295

respiration 62, 66
respiratory variation 52–55
restrictive cardiomyopathy 49, 212–217
  case study 215–216
  concepts and definitions 212
  differential diagnosis 213–215, 224,
    230–231
  echocardiography 215
  hemodynamic findings 212–213
  pressure tracings for amyloidosis 214
  pressure tracings for cardiac sarcoidosis
    215–216
Reynold's number 7–9
RFA *see* right femoral artery
right atrium (RA)
  arrhythmias 328–333, 337–338
  atrial waveform 69–73
  cardiac tamponade 237–241, 243–246
  constrictive pericarditis 223, 225, 227,
    231–232
  heart failure 205
  intracardiac shunts 95
  RVmyocardial infarction 304–308
  normal hemodynamics 41–43
  pulmonary artery catheter 22–24
  pulmonic valve disease 173–175
  restrictive cardiomyopathy 212
  systematic evaluation of hemodynamic
    tracings 344–345
  tricuspid valve 163–167, 170
right bundle branch block (RBBB) during
  PA catheter insertion 32
right coronary artery (RCA) 301–303, 305
right femoral artery (RFA) pressure 352
right heart catheterization *see* pulmonary
  artery catheter
right ventricle (RV)
  arrhythmias 331–338
  cardiac tamponade 237–241, 244, 246
  constrictive pericarditis 222–223,
    227–228, 231–232
  coronary hemodynamics 281
  heart failure 205
  hypertrophic cardiomyopathy 190, 194
  intracardiac shunts 93, 95
  mitral stenosis 134
  myocardial infarction 301–309
  normal hemodynamics 42, 43–44
  pulmonic valve disease 171–181
  tricuspid valve 163–168, 170

right ventricular end-diastolic pressure (RVEDP)
  cardiac tamponade 237
  constrictive pericarditis 222, 227–228
  myocardial infarction 307
  pulmonary hypertension 312–313
  restrictive cardiomyopathy 213–215
right ventricular outflow tract (RVOT)
    172–173, 176
right ventricular (RV) failure 272–273, 274
right ventricular stroke work index
    (RVSWI) 207, 270
RV *see* right ventricle
RVEDP *see* right ventricular end-diastolic
    pressure
RVOT *see* right ventricular outflow tract
RVSWI *see* right ventricular stroke work index
RV waveform 22–24
R wave 259

SAM *see* systolic anterior motion
SBP *see* systolic blood pressure
SEP *see* systolic ejection period
septal reduction in HOCM 196–197
severe aortic regurgitation 63
sinus bradycardia 321
sinus tachycardia 321
slow filling phase 40, 45
sphygmomanometry 65–67
ST-elevation MI (STEMI) 294, 349
stroke volume (SV)
  aortic regurgitation 143
  aortic stenosis 107–108
  aortic valve replacement 120
  arrhythmias 321
  cardiac output 89
  cardiac tamponade 237, 240
  heart failure 200–201
  hemodynamic principles 11
  intra-aortic balloon counterpulsation 258
  pulmonic valve disease 176–177
subaortic membrane 117–118
subvalvular pulmonary stenosis 172
suction event 271
sudden cardiac death in HOCM 186
superior vena cava (SVC) 93, 95, 97
supravalvular pulmonary stenosis 172
surgical aortic valve replacement (SAVR)
    119, 125–127
SV *see* stroke volume
SVC *see* superior vena cava

SvO₂ *see* venous oxygen saturation
SVR *see* systemic vascular resistance
Swan–Ganz catheter *see* pulmonary artery
    catheter
systemic vascular resistance (SVR) 5–6,
    29–30, 88–89
systole 19–21, 37–40, 43–44
systolic anterior motion (SAM) 188–189, 195
systolic blood pressure (SBP)
    aortic valve replacement 122–123, 125
    arterial pressure 58, 68
    pulmonary hypertension 317–318
systolic ejection period (SEP) 110–111
systolic murmur 105, 160–161

tachycardia
    atrial waveform 71
    intra-aortic balloon counterpulsation 259
    junctional rhythm 324, 328
    mitral stenosis 134
    sinus tachycardia 321, 330–331
    ventricular tachycardia 324, 326–327
tandem lesions, interpretation of FFR 294
TAVR *see* transcatheter aortic valve
    replacement
TEE *see* transesophageal echocardiography
thermodilution
    cardiac output 83, 85–87
    coronary hemodynamics 284
    pulmonary artery catheter 28
thrombosis of LVAD 274
TPG *see* transpulmonary gradient
TR *see* tricuspid regurgitation
transcatheter aortic valve replacement
    (TAVR) 119, 121–124
transesophageal echocardiography (TEE)
    87, 127
transpulmonary gradient (TPG) 207
transthoracic echocardiogram (TTE) 127
transvalvular gradient
    aortic stenosis 110–111
    aortic valve replacement 125–127
    mitral stenosis 134–135, 138
tricuspid regurgitation (TR)
    atrial waveform 72–73, 75
    cardiac output 85–87
    left ventricular assist devices 272
    mitral stenosis 138–139
    pulmonary hypertension 318–319

tricuspid valve 163–170
    case study 169–170
    concepts and definitions 163
    echocardiography 164, 168–170
    pathophysiology 163–164
    physical examination 164, 168
    pulmonary artery catheter 164–167, 168
    treatment 167, 168
    tricuspid regurgitation 163–167
    tricuspid stenosis 167–170
TTE *see* transthoracic echocardiogram
turbulent flow 7–9
T wave
    atrial waveform 71
    intra-aortic balloon counterpulsation 259
    normal hemodynamics 42–46
    pulmonary artery catheter 22–24

Valsalva maneuver 190, 194, 196–198
valvular heart disease
    aortic regurgitation 143–153
    aortic stenosis 103–118
    aortic valve replacement 119–128
    mitral regurgitation 154–162
    mitral stenosis 129–142
    pulmonic valve disease 171–182
    tricuspid valve 163–170
valvular pulmonary stenosis 172
vascular resistance
    coronary hemodynamics 279–281, 289
    hemodynamic principles 3–4, 14–16
    pulmonary artery catheter 17, 29–30
VC *see* vena contracta
velocity time integral (VTI) 108, 110
vena contracta (VC) 106
venous oxygen saturation (SvO₂) 350
    heart failure 206
    intracardiac shunts 93–97, 98
    left ventricular assist devices 269
    pulmonary artery catheter 30–31
ventilation
    arterial pressure 62
    cardiac output 86–87
    pulmonary artery catheter 26–28
ventricular bigeminy 85
ventricular ejection 20–21
ventricular filling 223
ventricular function curve 50, 53
ventricular septal defects (VSD) 91–93, 97

ventricular tachycardia 324, 326–327
viscosity 6
VSD *see* ventricular septal defects
VTI *see* velocity time integral
V wave
  arrhythmias 330–331
  atrial waveform 70–77, 80
  heart failure 205
  hypertrophic cardiomyopathy 189–190
  mitral regurgitation 155, 158, 160
  normal hemodynamics 41–43, 46
  pulmonary hypertension 318
  systematic evaluation of hemodynamic
    tracings 341–343
  tricuspid valve 164–166

wall tension 10–11
waveform analysis *see* electrocardiography
  and waveform analysis
WHO *see* World Health Organization
Wiggers diagram 37, 38, 60
World Health Organization (WHO)
  classification scheme 310–312

X descent
  atrial waveform 69–73, 77, 80
  cardiac tamponade 237–238
  Constrictive pericarditis 223
  effusive–constrictive pericarditis 249
  myocardial infarction 304–305
  normal hemodynamics 41–42, 43
  Restrictive cardiomyopathy 213
  systematic evaluation of hemodynamic
    tracings 341–343

Y descent
  arrhythmias 330–331
  atrial waveform 70, 73, 77, 80
  cardiac tamponade 237–238
  Constrictive pericarditis 223
  effusive–constrictive pericarditis 249
  mitral stenosis 131
  myocardial infarction 304–305
  normal hemodynamics 41–42, 43
  Restrictive cardiomyopathy 213
  systematic evaluation of hemodynamic
    tracings 341–343